The Commission calls for closing the health gap in a generation

Social justice is a matter of life and death. It affects the way people live, their consequent chance of illness, and their risk of premature death. We watch in wonder as life expectancy and good health continue to increase in parts of the world and in alarm as they fail to improve in others. A girl born today can expect to live for more than 80 years if she is born in some countries – but less than 45 years if she is born in others. Within countries there are dramatic differences in health that are closely linked with degrees of social disadvantage. Differences of this magnitude, within and between countries, simply should never happen.

These inequities in health, avoidable health inequalities, arise because of the circumstances in which people grow, live, work, and age, and the systems put in place to deal with illness. The conditions in which people live and die are, in turn, shaped by political, social, and economic forces.

Social and economic policies have a determining impact on whether a child can grow and develop to its full potential and live a flourishing life, or whether its life will be blighted. Increasingly the nature of the health problems rich and poor countries have to solve are converging. The development of a society, rich or poor, can be judged by the quality of its population's health, how fairly health is distributed across the social spectrum, and the degree of protection provided from disadvantage as a result of ill-health.

In the spirit of social justice, the Commission on Social Determinants of Health was set up by the World Health Organization (WHO) in 2005 to marshal the evidence on what can be done to promote health equity, and to foster a global movement to achieve it.

As the Commission has done its work, several countries and agencies have become partners seeking to frame policies and programmes, across the whole of society, that influence the social determinants of health and improve health equity. These countries and partners are in the forefront of a global movement.

The Commission calls on the WHO and all governments to lead global action on the social determinants of health with the aim of achieving health equity. It is essential that governments, civil society, WHO, and other global organizations now come together in taking action to improve the lives of the world's citizens. Achieving health equity within a generation is achievable, it is the right thing to do, and now is the right time to do it.

Table of Contents

Acknowledgements

The work of the Commission was championed, informed, and guided by the Chair of the Commission and the Commissioners.

Report writing team: Michael Marmot, Sharon Friel, Ruth Bell, Tanja AJ Houweling, and Sebastian Taylor. The team is indebted to all those who contributed to the development of the report, including Commissioners, Knowledge Networks, country partners, civil society facilitators, and colleagues in the World Health Organization (WHO), Geneva. Special thanks are due to Ron Labonte, Don Matheson, Hernan Sandoval (Special Advisor to the Commission), and David Woodward.

The Commission secretariat (University College London) was led by Sharon Friel. Team members included Ruth Bell, Ian Forde, Tanja AJ Houweling, Felicity Porritt, Elaine Reinertsen, and Sebastian Taylor. The Commission Secretariat (WHO) was led by Jeanette Vega (2004-2007) and Nick Drager (2008). WHO staff instrumental in setting up and guiding the Commission workstreams were: Erik Blas, Chris Brown, Hilary Brown, Alec Irwin, Rene Loewenson (consultant), Richard Poe, Gabrielle Ross, Ritu Sadana, Sarah Simpson, Orielle Solar, Nicole Valentine and Eugenio Raul Villar Montesinos. Other staff contributing included: Elmira Adenova, Daniel Albrecht, Lexi Bambas-Nolan, Ahmad Reza Hosseinpoor, Theadora Koller, Lucy Mshana, Susanne Nakalembe, Giorelley Niezen, Bongiwe Peguillan, Amit Prasad, Kumanan Rasanathan, Kitt Rasmussen, Lina Reinders, Anand Sivasankara Kurup, Niko Speybroeck and Michel Thieren.

WHO has supported the Commission in many ways. In particular we thank the former Director-General JW Lee and the current Director-General Margaret Chan. The Commission thanks the Assistant Director-General Tim Evans for championing our work within the organization and the Regional Directors for continuing support: Marc Danzon, Hussein Abdel-Razzak Al Gezairy, Nata Menabde, Shigeru Omi, Samlee Plianbangchang, Mirta Roses Perialgo, and Luis Gomes Sambo. We also thank the WHO regional focal points: Anjana Bhushan, Soe Nyunt-U (WPRO); Chris Brown (EURO); Luiz Galvao,

Marco Ackerman (PAHO-AMRO); Davison Munodawafa, Than Sein (SEARO); Benjamin Nganda, Anthony Mawaya, Chris Mwikisa (AFRO); Sameen Siddiqi, Susanne Watts and Mohamed Assai (EMRO). Thanks also to the numerous other WHO colleagues who have supported the work of the Commission including the country representatives, Meena Cabral de Mello, Carlos Corvalan, Claudia Garcia-Moreno, Amine Kebe, Jacob Kumaresan, and Erio Ziglio.

We are indebted to the country partners of the Commission - the many government departments and officials who have supported our work with ideas, expert guidance, and invaluable critique, as well as financially. In particular we thank Fiona Adshead and Maggie Davies (England and United Kingdom); David Butler-Jones, Sylvie Stachenko, Jim Ball and Heather Fraser (Canada); Maria Soledad Barria, Pedro Garcia, Francisca Infante, Patricia Frenz (Chile); Paulo Buss, Alberto Pellegrini Filho (Brazil); Gholam Reza Heydari, Bijan Sadrizadeh, Alireza Olyaee Manesh (Islamic Republic of Iran); Stephen Muchiri (Kenya); Paulo Ivo Garrido, Gertrudes Machatine (Mozambique); Anna Hedin, Bernt Lundgren, Bosse Peterson (Sweden); Palitha Abeykoon, Sarah Samarage (Sri Lanka); Don Matheson, Stephen McKernan, Teresa Wall (New Zealand); and Ugrid Jindawatthana, Amphon Milintangkul (Thailand).

We thank the civil society facilitators who have both informed the work of the Commission and used its evidence base to advocate globally a social determinants approach to health and health equity: Diouf Amacodou, Francoise Barten, Amit Sen Gupta, Prem John, Mwajuma Masaiganah, Alicia Muñoz, Hani Serag, Alaa Ibrahim Shukrallah, Patrick Mubangizi Tibasiimwa, Mauricio Torres, and Walter Varillas.

We are very grateful to all members of the Knowledge Networks for their dedication to the collation and synthesis of the global evidence base on the social determinants of health and health equity. In particular, thanks to the networks' hub leaders and coordinators: Joan Benach, Josiane Bonnefoy, Jane Doherty, Sarah Escorel, Lucy Gilson, Mario Hernández, Clyde Hertzman, Lori Irwin, Heidi Johnston, Michael P Kelly, Tord Kjellstrom, Ronald Labonté, Susan Mercado, Antony Morgan, Carles Muntaner,

Piroska Östlin, Jennie Popay, Laetitia Rispel, Vilma Santana, Ted Schrecker, Gita Sen, and Arjumand Siddiqi.

Thank you also to all 25 reviewers of the Knowledge Networks' final reports and to commentators on the Commission's work, including those who attended the Vancouver meeting, in particular Pascale Allotey, Sudhir Anand, Debebar Banerji, Adrienne Germain, Godfrey Gunatilleke, and Richard Horton. We have worked closely with other academics and researchers throughout the life of the Commission. A special thanks in particular to Robert N Butler, Hideki Hashimoto, Olle Lundberg, Tony McMichael, Richard Suzman, Elizabeth Waters, and Susan Watts.

The Indigenous Health symposium held in Adelaide, Australia, the Three Cities meeting in London, United Kingdom, and the meeting in New Orleans, United States of America, provided valuable insights and evidence for the Commission. Thanks in particular to Nancy Adler, Clive Aspin, Sue Atkinson, Paula Braveman, Lucia Ellis, Daragh Fahey, Gail Findlay, Evangeline Franklin, Heather Gifford, Mick Gooda, Sandra Griffin, Shane Houston, Adam Karpati, Joyce Nottingham, Paul Plant, Ben Springgate, Carol Tannahill, Dawn Walker, and David Williams.

The Commission meetings in Brazil, Canada, Chile, China, Egypt, India, Islamic Republic of Iran, Japan, Kenya, Switzerland, and the United States would not have been possible without the support of those political leaders, government officials, WHO offices, academics, and nongovernmental organization staff who assisted us during our visits. The Commission and its various workstreams are very grateful to those agencies and countries that provided financial support including the International Development Research Centre, Open Society Institute, Public Health Agency of Canada, Purpleville Foundation, Robert Wood Johnson Foundation, Swedish National Institute of Public Health, United Kingdom Government, and WHO.

The report was copy-edited by Lucy Hyatt, designed by Ben Murray and team at BMD Graphic Design, and indexed by Liza Furnival.

Note from the chair

The Commission on Social Determinants of Health was set up by former World Health Organization Director-General JW Lee. It was tasked to collect, collate, and synthesize global evidence on the social determinants of health and their impact on health inequity, and to make recommendations for action to address that inequity.

The Commissioners, secretariat and, indeed, everyone connected to the Commission were united in three concerns: a passion for social justice, a respect for evidence, and a frustration that there appeared to be far too little action on the social determinants of health. To be sure, there were examples of countries that had made remarkable progress in health some of which, at least, could be attributed to action on social conditions. These examples encouraged us. But the spectre of health inequity haunts the global scene. A key aim of the Commission has been to foster a global movement on social determinants of health and health equity. We are encouraged by the signs.

We judge that there is enough knowledge to recommend action now while there needs to be an active research programme on the social determinants of health. The Final Report of the Commission on Social Determinants of Health sets out key areas – of daily living conditions and of the underlying structural drivers that influence them – in which action is needed. It provides analysis of social determinants of health and concrete examples of types of action that have proven effective in improving health and health equity in countries at all levels of socioeconomic development.

Part 1 sets the scene, laying out the rationale for a global movement to advance health equity through action on the social determinants of health. It illustrates the extent of the problem between and within countries, describes what the Commission believes the causes of health inequities are, and points to where solutions may lie.

Part 2 outlines the approach the Commission took to evidence, and to the indispensable value of acknowledging and using the rich diversity of different types of knowledge. It describes the rationale that was applied in selecting social determinants for investigation and suggests, by means of a conceptual framework, how these may interact with one another.

Parts 3, 4, and 5 set out in more detail the Commission's findings and recommendations. The chapters in Part 3 deal with the conditions of daily living – the more easily visible aspects of birth, growth, and education; of living and working; and of using health care. The chapters in Part 4 look at more 'structural' conditions – social and economic policies that shape growing, living, and working; the relative roles of state and market in providing for good and equitable health; and the wide international and global conditions that can help or hinder national and local action for health equity. Part 5 focuses on the critical importance of data – not simply conventional research, but living evidence of progress or deterioration in the quality of people's lives and health that can only be attained through commitment to and capacity in health equity surveillance and monitoring.

Part 6, finally, reprises the global networks – the regional connections to civil society worldwide, the growing caucus of country partners taking the social determinants of health agenda forward, the vital research agendas, and the opportunities for change at the level of global governance and global institutions – that the Commission has built and on which the future of a global movement for health equity will depend.

Our thanks are due, in particular, to the invaluable and seemingly inexhaustible commitment and contributions of the Commissioners. Their collective guidance and leadership underpins all that the Commission has achieved.

Michael Marmot, *Chair*
Commission on Social Determinants of Health

The Commissioners

Michael Marmot	William H. Foege	Pascoal Mocumbi	David Satcher
Frances Baum	Yan Guo	Ndioro Ndiaye	Anna Tibaijuka
Monique Bégin	Kiyoshi Kurokawa	Charity Kaluki Ngilu	Denny Vågerö
Giovanni Berlinguer	Ricardo Lagos Escobar	Hoda Rashad	Gail Wilensky
Mirai Chatterjee	Alireza Marandi	Amartya Sen	

A new global agenda for health equity

Our children have dramatically different life chances depending on where they were born. In Japan or Sweden they can expect to live more than 80 years; in Brazil, 72 years; India, 63 years; and in one of several African countries, fewer than 50 years. And within countries, the differences in life chances are dramatic and are seen worldwide. The poorest of the poor have high levels of illness and premature mortality. But poor health is not confined to those worst off. In countries at all levels of income, health and illness follow a social gradient: the lower the socioeconomic position, the worse the health.

It does not have to be this way and it is not right that it should be like this. Where systematic differences in health are judged to be avoidable by reasonable action they are, quite simply, unfair. It is this that we label health inequity. Putting right these inequities – the huge and remediable differences in health between and within countries – is a matter of social justice. Reducing health inequities is, for the Commission on Social Determinants of Health (hereafter, the Commission), an ethical imperative. Social injustice is killing people on a grand scale.

The social determinants of health and health equity

The Commission, created to marshal the evidence on what can be done to promote health equity and to foster a global movement to achieve it, is a global collaboration of policy-makers, researchers, and civil society led by Commissioners with a unique blend of political, academic, and advocacy experience. Importantly, the focus of attention embraces countries at all levels of income and development: the global South and North. Health equity is an issue within all our countries and is affected significantly by the global economic and political system.

The Commission takes a holistic view of social determinants of health. The poor health of the poor, the social gradient in health within countries, and the marked health inequities between countries are caused by the unequal distribution of power, income, goods, and services, globally and nationally, the consequent unfairness in the immediate, visible circumstances of peoples lives – their access to health care, schools, and education, their conditions of work and leisure, their homes, communities, towns, or cities – and their chances of leading a flourishing life. This unequal distribution of health-damaging experiences is not in any sense a 'natural' phenomenon but is the result of a toxic combination of poor social policies and programmes, unfair economic arrangements, and bad politics. Together, the structural determinants and conditions of daily life constitute the social determinants of health and are responsible for a major part of health inequities between and within countries.

The global community can put this right but it will take urgent and sustained action, globally, nationally, and locally. Deep inequities in the distribution of power and economic arrangements, globally, are of key relevance to health equity. This in no way implies ignoring other levels of action. There is a great deal that national and local governments can do; and the Commission has been impressed by the force of civil society and local movements that both provide immediate local help and push governments to change.

And of course climate change has profound implications for the global system – how it affects the way of life and health of individuals and the planet. We need to bring the two agendas of health equity and climate change together. Our core concerns with health equity must be part of the global community balancing the needs of social and economic development of the whole global population, health equity, and the urgency of dealing with climate change.

A new approach to development

The Commission's work embodies a new approach to development. Health and health equity may not be the aim of all social policies but they will be a fundamental result. Take the central policy importance given to economic growth: Economic growth is without question important, particularly for poor countries, as it gives the opportunity to provide resources to invest in improvement of the lives of their population. But growth by itself, without appropriate social policies to ensure reasonable fairness in the way its benefits are distributed, brings little benefit to health equity.

Traditionally, society has looked to the health sector to deal with its concerns about health and disease. Certainly, maldistribution of health care – not delivering care to those who most need it – is one of the social determinants of health. But the high burden of illness responsible for appalling premature loss of life arises in large part because of the conditions in which people are born, grow, live, work, and age. In their turn, poor and unequal living conditions are the consequence of poor social policies and programmes, unfair economic arrangements, and bad politics. Action on the social determinants of health must involve the whole of government, civil society and local communities, business, global fora, and international agencies. Policies and programmes must embrace all the key sectors of society not just the health sector. That said, the minister of health and the supporting ministry are critical to global change. They can champion a social determinants of health approach at the highest level of society, they can demonstrate effectiveness through good practice, and they can support other ministries in creating policies that promote health equity. The World Health Organization (WHO), as the global body for health, must do the same on the world stage.

Closing the health gap in a generation

The Commission calls for closing the health gap in a generation. It is an aspiration not a prediction. Dramatic improvements in health, globally and within countries, have occurred in the last 30 years. We are optimistic: the knowledge exists to make a huge difference to people's life chances and hence to provide marked improvements in health equity. We are realistic: action must start now. The material for developing solutions to the gross inequities between and within countries is in the Report of this Commission.

The Commission's overarching recommendations

1 Improve Daily Living Conditions

Improve the well-being of girls and women and the circumstances in which their children are born, put major emphasis on early child development and education for girls and boys, improve living and working conditions and create social protection policy supportive of all, and create conditions for a flourishing older life. Policies to achieve these goals will involve civil society, governments, and global institutions.

2 Tackle the Inequitable Distribution of Power, Money, and Resources

In order to address health inequities, and inequitable conditions of daily living, it is necessary to address inequities – such as those between men and women – in the way society is organized. This requires a strong public sector that is committed, capable, and adequately financed. To achieve that requires more than strengthened government – it requires strengthened governance: legitimacy, space, and support for civil society, for an accountable private sector, and for people across society to agree public interests and reinvest in the value of collective action. In a globalized world, the need for governance dedicated to equity applies equally from the community level to global institutions.

3 Measure and Understand the Problem and Assess the Impact of Action

Acknowledging that there is a problem, and ensuring that health inequity is measured – within countries and globally – is a vital platform for action. National governments and international organizations, supported by WHO, should set up national and global health equity surveillance systems for routine monitoring of health inequity and the social determinants of health and should evaluate the health equity impact of policy and action. Creating the organizational space and capacity to act effectively on health inequity requires investment in training of policy-makers and health practitioners and public understanding of social determinants of health. It also requires a stronger focus on social determinants in public health research.

Three principles of action

(1) Improve the conditions of daily life – the circumstances in which people are born, grow, live, work, and age.

(2) Tackle the inequitable distribution of power, money, and resources – the structural drivers of those conditions of daily life – globally, nationally, and locally.

(3) Measure the problem, evaluate action, expand the knowledge base, develop a workforce that is trained in the social determinants of health, and raise public awareness about the social determinants of health.

These three principles of action are embodied in the three overarching recommendations above. The remainder of the Executive Summary and the Commission's Final Report is structured according to these three principles.

1. Improve Daily Living Conditions

The inequities in how society is organized mean that the freedom to lead a flourishing life and to enjoy good health is unequally distributed between and within societies. This inequity is seen in the conditions of early childhood and schooling, the nature of employment and working conditions, the physical form of the built environment, and the quality of the natural environment in which people reside. Depending on the nature of these environments, different groups will have different experiences of material conditions, psychosocial support, and behavioural options, which make them more or less vulnerable to poor health. Social stratification likewise determines differential access to and utilization of health care, with consequences for the inequitable promotion of health and well-being, disease prevention, and illness recovery and survival.

EQUITY FROM THE START

Early child development (ECD) – including the physical, social/emotional, and language/cognitive domains – has a determining influence on subsequent life chances and health through skills development, education, and occupational opportunities. Through these mechanisms, and directly, early childhood influences subsequent risk of obesity, malnutrition, mental health problems, heart disease, and criminality. At least 200 million children globally are not achieving their full development potential (Grantham-McGregor et al., 2007). This has huge implications for their health and for society at large.

Evidence for action

Investment in the early years provides one of the greatest potentials to reduce health inequities within a generation (ECDKN, 2007a). Experiences in early childhood (defined as prenatal development to eight years of age), and in early and later education, lay critical foundations for the entire lifecourse (ECDKN, 2007a). The science of ECD shows that brain development is highly sensitive to external influences in early childhood, with lifelong effects. Good nutrition is crucial and begins in utero with adequately nourished mothers. Mothers and children need a continuum of care from pre-pregnancy, through pregnancy and childbirth, to the early days and years of life (WHO, 2005b). Children need safe, healthy, supporting, nurturing, caring, and responsive living environments. Preschool educational programmes and schools, as part of the wider environment that contributes to the development of children, can have a vital role in building children's capabilities. A more comprehensive approach to early life is needed, building on existing child survival programmes and extending interventions in early life to include social/emotional and language/cognitive development.

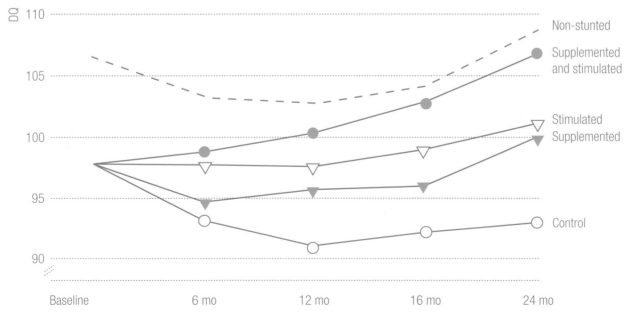

Effects of combined nutritional supplementation and psychosocial stimulation on stunted children in a 2-year intervention study in Jamaica[a].

[a] Mean development scores (DQ) of stunted groups adjusted for initial age and score compared with a non-stunted group adjusted for age only, using Griffiths Mental Development Scales modified for Jamaica. Reprinted, with permission of the publisher, from Grantham-McGregor et al. (1991).

What must be done

A comprehensive approach to the early years in life requires policy coherence, commitment, and leadership at the international and national level. It also requires a comprehensive package of ECD and education programmes and services for all children worldwide.

Commit to and implement a comprehensive approach to early life, building on existing child survival programmes and extending interventions in early life to include social/emotional and language/cognitive development.

- Set up an interagency mechanism to ensure policy coherence for early child development such that, across agencies, a comprehensive approach to early child development is acted on.

- Make sure that all children, mothers, and other caregivers are covered by a comprehensive package of quality early child development programmes and services, regardless of ability to pay.

Expand the provision and scope of education to include the principles of early child development (physical, social/emotional, and language/cognitive development).

- Provide quality compulsory primary and secondary education for all boys and girls, regardless of ability to pay. Identify and address the barriers to girls and boys enrolling and staying in school and abolish user fees for primary school.

HEALTHY PLACES HEALTHY PEOPLE

Where people live affects their health and chances of leading flourishing lives. The year 2007 saw, for the first time, the majority of human beings living in urban settings (WorldWatch Institute, 2007). Almost 1 billion live in slums.

Evidence for action

Infectious diseases and undernutrition will continue in particular regions and groups around the world. However, urbanization is reshaping population health problems, particularly among the urban poor, towards non-communicable diseases, accidental and violent injuries, and deaths and impact from ecological disaster (Campbell & Campbell, 2007; Yusuf et al., 2001).

The daily conditions in which people live have a strong influence on health equity. Access to quality housing and shelter and clean water and sanitation are human rights and basic needs for healthy living (UNESCO, 2006a; Shaw, 2004). Growing car dependence, land-use change to facilitate car use, and increased inconvenience of non-motorized modes of travel, have knock-on effects on local air quality, greenhouse gas emission, and physical inactivity (NHF, 2007). The planning and design of urban environments has a major impact on health equity through its influence on behaviour and safety.

The balance of rural and urban dwelling varies enormously across areas: from less than 10% urban in Burundi and Uganda to 100% or close to it in Belgium, Hong Kong Special Administrative Region, Kuwait, and Singapore. Policies and investment patterns patterns reflecting the urban-led growth paradigm (Vlahov et al., 2007) have seen rural communities

worldwide, including Indigenous Peoples (Indigenous Health Group, 2007), suffer from progressive underinvestment in infrastructure and amenities, with disproportionate levels of poverty and poor living conditions (Ooi & Phua, 2007; Eastwood & Lipton, 2000), contributing in part to out-migration to unfamiliar urban centres.

The current model of urbanization poses significant environmental challenges, particularly climate change – the impact of which is greater in low-income countries and among vulnerable subpopulations (McMichael et al., 2008; Stern, 2006). At present, greenhouse gas emissions are determined mainly by consumption patterns in cities of the developed world. Transport and buildings contribute 21% to CO2 emissions (IPCC, 2007), agricultural activity accounts for about one fifth. And yet crop yields depend in large part on prevailing climate conditions. The disruption and depletion of the climate system and the task of reducing global health inequities go hand in hand.

What must be done

Communities and neighbourhoods that ensure access to basic goods, that are socially cohesive, that are designed to promote good physical and psychological well-being and that are protective of the natural environment are essential for health equity.

Place health and health equity at the heart of urban governance and planning.

- Manage urban development to ensure greater availability of affordable housing; invest in urban slum upgrading including, as a priority, provision of water and sanitation, electricity, and paved streets for all households regardless of ability to pay.

- Ensure urban planning promotes healthy and safe behaviours equitably, through investment in active transport, retail planning to manage access to unhealthy foods, and through good environmental design and regulatory controls, including control of the number of alcohol outlets.

Promote health equity between rural and urban areas through sustained investment in rural development, addressing the exclusionary policies and processes that lead to rural poverty, landlessness, and displacement of people from their homes.

- Counter the inequitable consequences of urban growth through action that addresses rural land tenure and rights and ensures rural livelihoods that support healthy living, adequate investment in rural infrastructure, and policies that support rural-to-urban migrants.

Ensure that economic and social policy responses to climate change and other environmental degradation take into account health equity.

Fair Employment and Decent Work

Employment and working conditions have powerful effects on health equity. When these are good, they can provide financial security, social status, personal development, social relations and self-esteem, and protection from physical and psychosocial hazards. Action to improve employment and work must be global, national, and local.

Evidence for action

Work is the area where many of the important influences on health are played out. (Marmot & Wilkinson, 2006). This includes both employment conditions and the nature of work itself. A flexible workforce is seen as good for economic competitiveness but brings with it effects on health (Benach & Muntaner, 2007). Evidence indicates that mortality is significantly higher among temporary workers compared to permanent workers (Kivimäki et al., 2003). Poor mental health

outcomes are associated with precarious employment (e.g. non-fixed term temporary contracts, being employed with no contract, and part-time work) (Artazcoz et al., 2005; Kim et al., 2006). Workers who perceive work insecurity experience significant adverse effects on their physical and mental health (Ferrie et al., 2002).

The conditions of work also affect health and health equity. Adverse working conditions can expose individuals to a range of physical health hazards and tend to cluster in lower-status occupations. Improved working conditions in high-income countries, hard won over many years of organized action and regulation, are sorely lacking in many middle- and low-income countries. Stress at work is associated with a 50% excess risk of coronary heart disease (Marmot, 2004; Kivimäki et al., 2006), and there is consistent evidence that high job demand, low control, and effort-reward imbalance are risk factors for mental and physical health problems (Stansfeld & Candy, 2006).

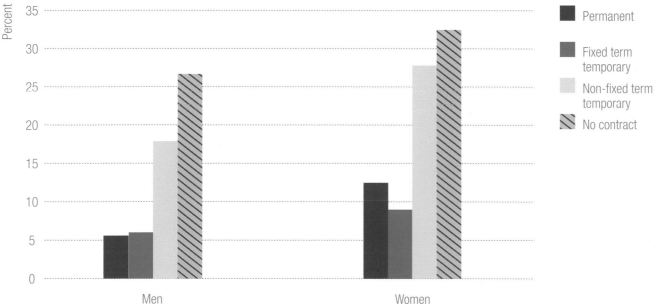

Prevalence of poor mental health among manual workers in Spain by type of contract.

Legend: Permanent; Fixed term temporary; Non-fixed term temporary; No contract

Source: Artazcoz et al., 2005

What must be done

Through the assurance of fair employment and decent working conditions, government, employers, and workers can help eradicate poverty, alleviate social inequities, reduce exposure to physical and psychosocial hazards, and enhance opportunities for health and well-being. And, of course, a healthy workforce is good for productivity.

Make full and fair employment and decent work a central goal of national and international social and economic policy-making.

- Full and fair employment and decent work should be made a shared objective of international institutions and a central part of national policy agendas and development strategies, with strengthened representation of workers in the creation of policy, legislation, and programmes relating to employment and work.

Achieving health equity requires safe, secure, and fairly paid work, year-round work opportunities, and healthy work-life balance for all.

- Provide quality work for men and women with a living wage that takes into account the real and current cost of healthy living.

- Protect all workers. International agencies should support countries to implement core labour standards for formal and informal workers; to develop policies to ensure a balanced work-home life; and to reduce the negative effects of insecurity among workers in precarious work arrangements.

Improve the working conditions for all workers to reduce their exposure to material hazards, work-related stress, and health-damaging behaviours.

Regional variation in the percentage of people in work living on US$ 2/day or less.

Legend:
- World
- Central & South East Europe
- East Asia
- South East Asia & Pacific
- South Asia
- Latin America & Caribbean
- Middle East
- North Africa
- Sub-Saharan Africa

(Chart: Percent on y-axis from 0 to 100; years 1997, 2002, 2007 on x-axis)

2007 figures are preliminary estimates.
Reprinted, with permission of the author, from ILO (2008).

SOCIAL PROTECTION ACROSS THE LIFECOURSE

All people need social protection across the lifecourse, as young children, in working life, and in old age. People also need protection in case of specific shocks, such as illness, disability, and loss of income or work.

Evidence for action

Low living standards are a powerful determinant of health inequity. They influence lifelong trajectories, among others through their effects on ECD. Child poverty and transmission of poverty from generation to generation are major obstacles to improving population health and reducing health inequity. Four out of five people worldwide lack the back-up of basic social security coverage (ILO, 2003).

Redistributive welfare systems, in combination with the extent to which people can make a healthy living on the labour market, influence poverty levels. Generous universal social protection systems are associated with better population health, including lower excess mortality among the old and lower mortality levels among socially disadvantaged groups. Budgets for social protection tend to be larger, and perhaps more sustainable, in countries with universal protection systems; poverty and income inequality tend to be smaller in these countries compared to countries with systems that target the poor.

Extending social protection to all people, within countries and globally, will be a major step towards securing health equity within a generation. This includes extending social protection to those in precarious work, including informal work, and household or care work. This is critical for poor countries in which the majority of people work in the informal sector, as well as for women, because family responsibilities often preclude them from accruing adequate benefits under contributory social protection schemes. While limited institutional infrastructure and financial capacity remains an important barrier in many countries, experience across the world shows that it is feasible to start creating social protection systems, even in low-income countries.

What must be done

Reducing the health gap in a generation requires that governments build systems that allow a healthy standard of living below which nobody should fall due to circumstances beyond his or her control. Social protection schemes can be instrumental in realizing developmental goals, rather than being dependent on achieving these goals – they can be efficient ways to reduce poverty, and local economies can benefit.

Establish and strengthen universal comprehensive social protection policies that support a level of income sufficient for healthy living for all.

- Progressively increase the generosity of social protection systems towards a level that is sufficient for healthy living.

- Ensure that social protection systems include those normally excluded: those in precarious work, including informal work and household or care work.

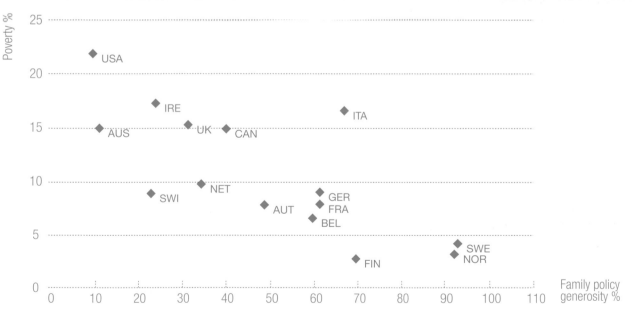

Total family policy generosity and child poverty in 20 countries, circa 2000.

Net benefit generosity of transfers as a percentage of an average net production worker's wage.
The poverty line is 50% of median equivalized disposable income.
AUS = Australia; AUT = Austria; BEL = Belgium; CAN = Canada; FIN = Finland; FRA = France;
GER = Germany; IRE = Ireland; ITA = Italy; NET = the Netherlands; NOR = Norway; SWE =
Sweden; SWI = Switzerland; UK = the United Kingdom; USA = the United States of America.
Reprinted, with permission of the publisher, from Lundberg et al. (2007).

UNIVERSAL HEALTH CARE

Access to and utilization of health care is vital to good and equitable health. The health-care system is itself a social determinant of health, influenced by and influencing the effect of other social determinants. Gender, education, occupation, income, ethnicity, and place of residence are all closely linked to people's access to, experiences of, and benefits from health care. Leaders in health care have an important stewardship role across all branches of society to ensure that policies and actions in other sectors improve health equity.

Evidence for action

Without health care, many of the opportunities for fundamental health improvement are lost. With partial health-care systems, or systems with inequitable provision, opportunities for universal health as a matter of social justice are lost. These are core issues for all countries. More pressingly, for low-income countries, accessible and appropriately designed and managed health-care systems will contribute significantly to the achievement of the Millennium Development Goals (MDGs). Without them, the chances of meeting the MDGs are greatly weakened. Yet health-care systems are appallingly weak in many countries, with massive inequity in provision, access, and use between rich and poor.

The Commission considers health care a common good, not a market commodity. Virtually all high-income countries organize their health-care systems around the principle of universal coverage (combining health financing and provision). Universal coverage requires that everyone within a country can access the same range of (good quality) services according to needs and preferences, regardless of income level, social status, or residency, and that people are empowered to use these services. It extends the same scope of benefits to the whole population. There is no sound argument that other countries, including the poorest, should not aspire to universal health-care coverage, given adequate support over the long term.

The Commission advocates financing the health-care system through general taxation and/or mandatory universal insurance. Public health-care spending has been found to be redistributive in country after country. The evidence is compellingly in favour of a publicly funded health-care system. In particular, it is vital to minimize out-of-pocket spending on health care. The policy imposition of user fees for health care in low- and middle-income countries has led to an overall reduction in utilization and worsening health outcomes. Upwards of 100 million people are pushed into poverty each year through catastrophic household health costs. This is unacceptable.

Health-care systems have better health outcomes when built on Primary Health Care (PHC) – that is, both the PHC model that emphasizes locally appropriate action across the range of social determinants, where prevention and promotion are in balance with investment in curative interventions, and an emphasis on the primary level of care with adequate referral to higher levels of care.

In all countries, but most pressingly in the poorest and those experiencing brain-drain losses, adequate numbers of appropriately skilled health workers at the local level are fundamental to extending coverage and improving the quality of care. Investment in training and retaining health-care

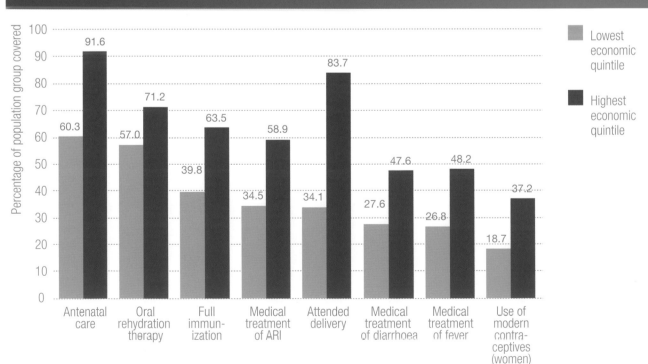

Use of basic maternal and child health services by lowest and highest economic quintiles, 50+ countries.

Reprinted, with permission of the publisher, from Gwatkin, Wagstaff & Yazbeck (2005).

workers is vital to the required growth of health-care systems. This involves global attention to the flows of health personnel as much as national and local attention to investment and skills development. Medical and health practitioners – from WHO to the local clinic – have powerful voices in society's ideas of and decisions about health. They bear witness to the ethical imperative, just as much as the efficiency value, of acting more coherently through the health-care system on the social causes of poor health.

What must be done

Build health-care systems based on principles of equity, disease prevention, and health promotion.

- Build quality health-care services with universal coverage, focusing on Primary Health Care.

- Strengthen public sector leadership in equitable health-care systems financing, ensuring universal access to care regardless of ability to pay.

Build and strengthen the health workforce, and expand capabilities to act on the social determinants of health.

- Invest in national health workforces, balancing rural and urban health-worker density.

- Act to redress the health brain drain, focusing on investment in increased health human resources and training and bilateral agreements to regulate gains and losses.

2. Tackle the Inequitable Distribution of Power, Money, and Resources

Inequity in the conditions of daily living is shaped by deeper social structures and processes. The inequity is systematic, produced by social norms, policies, and practices that tolerate or actually promote unfair distribution of and access to power, wealth, and other necessary social resources.

HEALTH EQUITY IN ALL POLICIES, SYSTEMS, AND PROGRAMMES

Every aspect of government and the economy has the potential to affect health and health equity – finance, education, housing, employment, transport, and health, just to name six. Coherent action across government, at all levels, is essential for improvement of health equity.

Evidence for action

Different government policies, depending on their nature, can either improve or worsen health and health equity (Kickbusch, 2007). Urban planning, for example, that produces sprawling neighbourhoods with little affordable housing, few local amenities, and irregular unaffordable public transport does little to promote good health for all (NHF, 2007). Good public policy can provide health benefits immediately and in the future.

Policy coherence is crucial – this means that different government departments' policies complement rather than contradict each other in relation to the production of health and health equity. For example, trade policy that actively encourages the unfettered production, trade, and consumption of foods high in fats and sugars to the detriment of fruit and vegetable production is contradictory to health policy, which recommends relatively little consumption of high-fat, high-sugar foods and increased consumption of fruit and vegetables (Elinder, 2005). Intersectoral action (ISA) for health – coordinated policy and action among health and non-health sectors – can be a key strategy to achieve this (PHAC, 2007).

Reaching beyond government to involve civil society and the voluntary and private sectors is a vital step towards action for health equity. The increased incorporation of community engagement and social participation in policy processes helps to ensure fair decision-making on health equity issues. And health is a rallying point for different sectors and actors – whether it is a local community designing a health plan for themselves (Dar es Salaam, United Republic of Tanzania's Healthy City Programme) or involving the entire community including local government in designing spaces that encourage walking and cycling (Healthy by Design, Victoria, Australia) (Mercado et al., 2007).

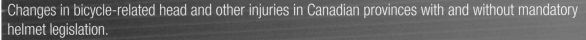

Changes in bicycle-related head and other injuries in Canadian provinces with and without mandatory helmet legislation.

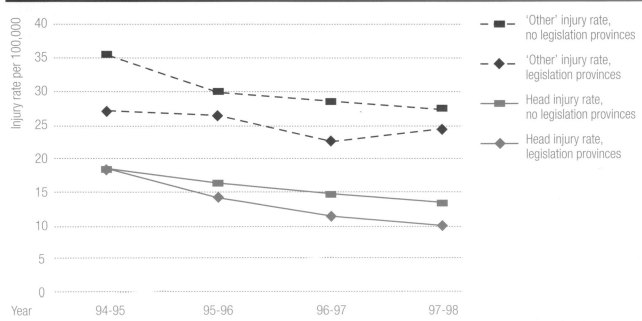

Legislation introduced across provinces between 1995 and 1997.
Reprinted, with permission of the publisher, from Macpherson et al. (2002).

Making health and health equity a shared value across sectors is a politically challenging strategy but one that is needed globally.

What must be done

Place responsibility for action on health and health equity at the highest level of government, and ensure its coherent consideration across all policies.

- Make health and health equity corporate issues for the whole of government, supported by the head of state, by establishing health equity as a marker of government performance.

- Assess the impact of all policies and programmes on health and health equity, building towards coherence in all government action.

Adopt a social determinants framework across the policy and programmatic functions of the ministry of health and strengthen its stewardship role in supporting a social determinants approach across government.

- The health sector itself is a good place to start building supports and structures that encourage action on the social determinants of health and health equity. This requires strong leadership from the minister of health, with support from WHO.

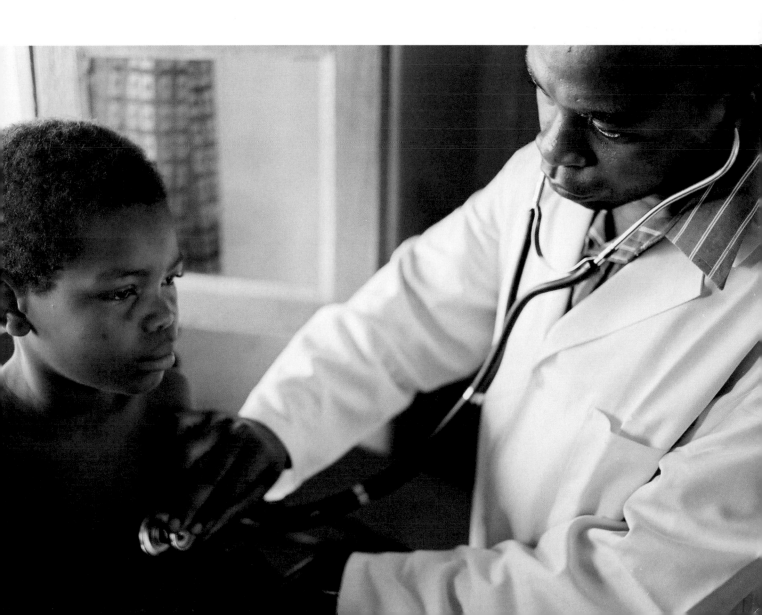

Fair Financing

Public finance to fund action across the social determinants of health is fundamental to welfare and to health equity.

Evidence for action

For countries at all levels of economic development, increasing public finance to fund action across the social determinants of health – from child development and education, through living and working conditions, to health care – is fundamental to welfare and health equity. Evidence shows that the socioeconomic development of rich countries was strongly supported by publicly financed infrastructure and progressively universal public services. The emphasis on public finance, given the marked failure of markets to supply vital goods and services equitably, implies strong public sector leadership and adequate public expenditure. This in turn implies progressive taxation – evidence shows that modest levels of redistribution have considerably greater impact on poverty reduction than economic growth alone. And, in the case of poorer countries, it implies much greater international financial assistance.

Low-income countries often have relatively weak direct tax institutions and mechanisms and a majority of the workforce operating in the informal sector. They have relied in many cases on indirect taxes such as trade tariffs for government income. Economic agreements between rich and poor countries that require tariff reduction can reduce available domestic revenue in low-income countries before alternative streams of finance have been established. Strengthened progressive tax capacity is an important source of public finance and a necessary prerequisite of any further tariff-cutting agreements. At the same time, measures to combat the use of offshore financial centres to reduce unethical avoidance of national tax regimes

could provide resources for development at least comparable to those made available through new taxes. As globalization increases interdependence among countries, the argument for global approaches to taxation becomes stronger.

Aid is important. While the evidence suggests that it can and does promote economic growth, and can contribute more directly to better health, the view of the Commission is that aid's primary value is as a mechanism for the reasonable distribution of resources in the common endeavour of social development. But the volume of aid is appallingly low. It is low in absolute terms (both generic and health specific); relative to wealth in donor countries; relative to the commitment to a level of aid approximating 0.7% of their gross domestic product (GDP) made by donors in 1969; and relative to the amounts required for sustainable impact on the MDGs. A step-shift increase is required. Independent of increased aid, the Commission urges wider and deeper debt relief.

The quality of aid must be improved too – following the Paris agreement – focusing on better coordination among donors and stronger alignment with recipient development plans. Donors should consider channelling most of their aid through a single multilateral mechanism, while poverty reduction planning at the national and local levels in recipient countries would benefit from adopting a social determinants of health framework to create coherent, cross-sectoral financing. Such a framework could help to improve the accountability of recipient countries in demonstrating how aid is allocated, and what impact it has. In particular, recipient governments should strengthen their capacity and accountability to allocate available public finance equitably across regions and among population groups.

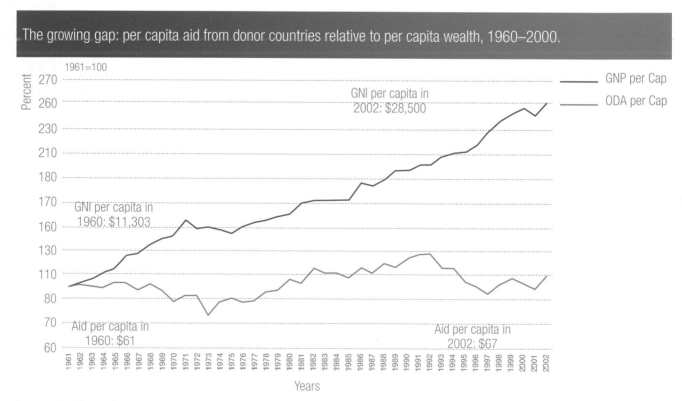

The growing gap: per capita aid from donor countries relative to per capita wealth, 1960–2000.

Reprinted, with permission of the publisher, from Randel, German & Ewing (2004).

What must be done

Strengthen public finance for action on the social determinants of health.

- Build national capacity for progressive taxation and assess potential for new national and global public finance mechanisms.

Increase international finance for health equity, and coordinate increased finance through a social determinants of health action framework.

- Honour existing commitments by increasing global aid to the 0.7% of GDP commitment, and expand the Multilateral Debt Relief Initiative; enhance action on health equity by developing a coherent social determinants of health focus in existing frameworks such as the Poverty Reduction Strategy Paper.

Fairly allocate government resources for action on the social determinants of health.

- Establish mechanisms to finance cross-government action on social determinants of health, and to allocate finance fairly between geographical regions and social groups.

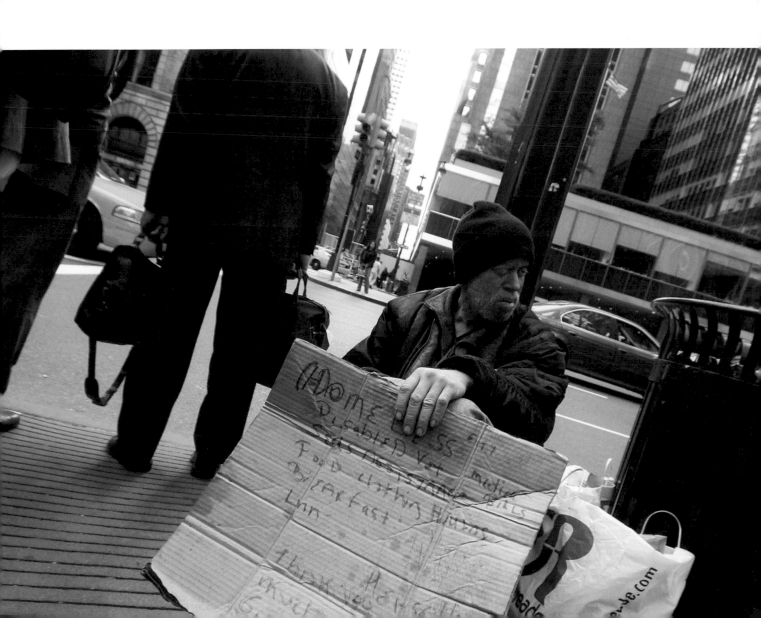

Market Responsibility

Markets bring health benefits in the form of new technologies, goods and services, and improved standard of living. But the marketplace can also generate negative conditions for health in the form of economic inequalities, resource depletion, environmental pollution, unhealthy working conditions, and the circulation of dangerous and unhealthy goods.

Evidence for action

Health is not a tradable commodity. It is a matter of rights and a public sector duty. As such, resources for health must be equitable and universal. There are three linked issues. First, experience shows that commercialization of vital social goods such as education and health care produces health inequity. Provision of such vital social goods must be governed by the public sector, rather than being left to markets. Second, there needs to be public sector leadership in effective national and international regulation of products, activities, and conditions that damage health or lead to health inequities. These together mean that, third, competent, regular health equity impact assessment of all policy-making and market regulation should be institutionalized nationally and internationally.

The Commission views certain goods and services as basic human and societal needs – access to clean water, for example, and health care. Such goods and services must be made available universally regardless of ability to pay. In such instances, therefore, it is the public sector rather than the marketplace that underwrites adequate supply and access.

With respect both to ensuring the provision of goods and services vital to health and well-being – for example, water, health care, and decent working conditions – and controlling the circulation of health-damaging commodities (for example, tobacco and alcohol), public sector leadership needs to be robust. Conditions of labour and working conditions are – in many countries, rich and poor – all too often inequitable, exploitative, unhealthy, and dangerous. The vital importance of good labour and work to a healthy population and a healthy economy demands public sector leadership in ensuring progressive fulfilment of global labour standards while also ensuring support to the growth of micro-level enterprises. Global governance mechanisms – such as the Framework Convention on Tobacco Control – are required with increasing urgency as market integration expands and accelerates circulation of and access to health-damaging commodities. Processed foods and alcohol are two prime candidates for stronger global, regional, and national regulatory controls.

In recent decades, under globalization, market integration has increased. This is manifested in new production arrangements, including significant changes in labour, employment, and working conditions, expanding areas of international and global economic agreements, and accelerating commercialization of goods and services – some of them undoubtedly beneficial for health, some of them disastrous. The Commission urges that caution be applied by participating countries in the consideration of new global, regional, and bilateral economic – trade and investment – policy commitments. Before such

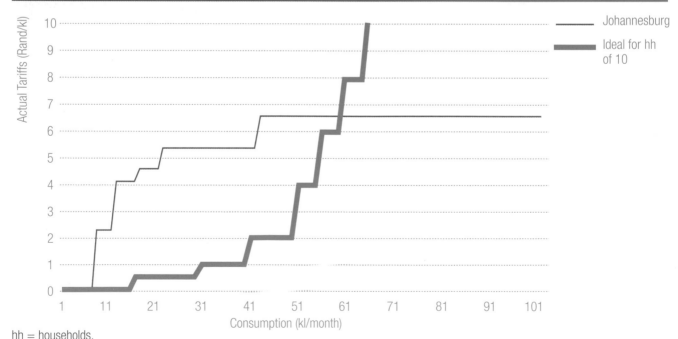

Johannesburg water pricing. The existing subsidy structure (thin line) favours richer consumers (and allows over-use), while the ideal tariff structure (thick line) favours adequate subsidized supply to poorer consumers with disincentives for higher use.

hh = households.
Reprinted, with permission of the author, from GKN (2007).

commitments are made, understanding the impact of the existing framework of agreements on health, the social determinants of health, and health equity is vital. Further, assessment of health impacts over time suggests strongly that flexibility, allowing signatory countries to modify their commitment to international agreements if there is adverse impact on health or health equity, should be established at the outset, with transparent criteria for triggering modification.

Public sector leadership does not displace the responsibilities and capacities of other actors: civil society and the private sector. Private sector actors are influential, and have the power to do much for global health equity. To date, though, initiatives such as those under corporate social responsibility have shown limited evidence of real impact. Corporate social responsibility may be a valuable way forward, but evidence is needed to demonstrate this. Corporate accountability may well be a stronger basis on which to build a responsible and collaborative relationship between the private sector and public interest.

What must be done

Institutionalize consideration of health and health equity impact in national and international economic agreements and policy-making.

- Institutionalize and strengthen technical capacities in health equity impact assessment of all international and national economic agreements.

- Strengthen representation of health actors in domestic and international economic policy negotiations.

Reinforce the primary role of the state in the provision of basic services essential to health (such as water/sanitation) and the regulation of goods and services with a major impact on health (such as tobacco, alcohol, and food).

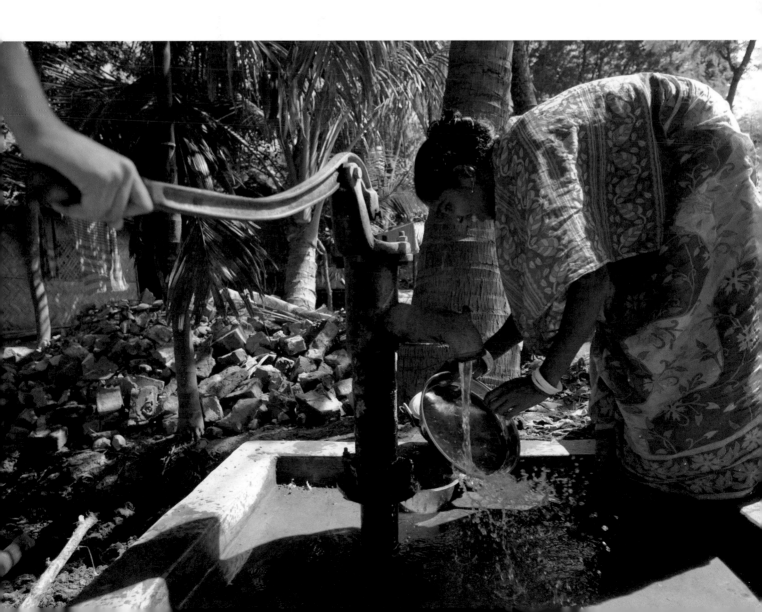

Gender Equity

Reducing the health gap in a generation is only possible if the lives of girls and women – about half of humanity – are improved and gender inequities are addressed. Empowerment of women is key to achieving fair distribution of health.

Evidence for action

Gender inequities are pervasive in all societies. Gender biases in power, resources, entitlements, norms and values, and the way in which organizations are structured and programmes are run damage the health of millions of girls and women. The position of women in society is also associated with child health and survival – of boys and girls. Gender inequities influence health through, among other routes, discriminatory feeding patterns, violence against women, lack of decision-making power, and unfair divisions of work, leisure, and possibilities of improving one's life.

Gender inequities are socially generated and therefore can be changed. While the position of women has improved dramatically over the last century in many countries, progress has been uneven and many challenges remain. Women earn less then men, even for equivalent work; girls and women lag behind in education and employment opportunities. Maternal mortality and morbidity remain high in many countries, and reproductive health services remain hugely inequitably distributed within and between countries. The intergenerational effects of gender inequity make the imperative to act even stronger. Acting now, to improve gender equity and empower women, is critical for reducing the health gap in a generation.

What must be done

Gender inequities are unfair; they are also ineffective and inefficient. By supporting gender equity, governments, donors, international organizations, and civil society can improve the lives of millions of girls and women and their families.

Address gender biases in the structures of society – in laws and their enforcement, in the way organizations are run and interventions designed, and the way in which a country's economic performance is measured.

- Create and enforce legislation that promotes gender equity and makes discrimination on the basis of sex illegal.

- Strengthen gender mainstreaming by creating and financing a gender equity unit within the central administration of governments and international institutions.

- Include the economic contribution of housework, care work, and voluntary work in national accounts.

Develop and finance policies and programmes that close gaps in education and skills, and that support female economic participation.

- Invest in formal and vocational education and training, guarantee pay-equity by law, ensure equal opportunity for employment at all levels, and set up family-friendly policies.

Increase investment in sexual and reproductive health services and programmes, building to universal coverage and rights.

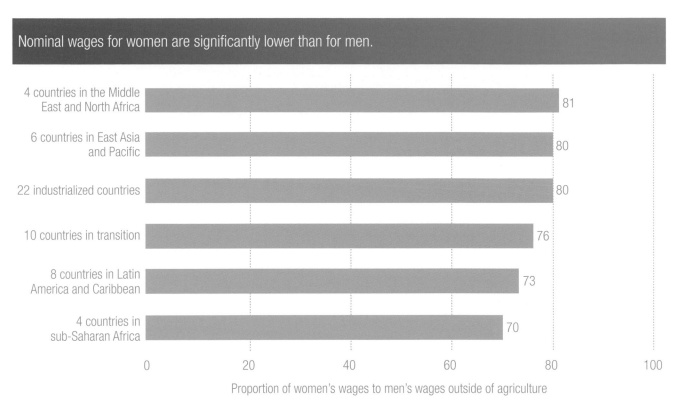

Nominal wages for women are significantly lower than for men.

4 countries in the Middle East and North Africa	81
6 countries in East Asia and Pacific	80
22 industrialized countries	80
10 countries in transition	76
8 countries in Latin America and Caribbean	73
4 countries in sub-Saharan Africa	70

Proportion of women's wages to men's wages outside of agriculture

Reprinted, with permission of the author, from UNICEF (2006).

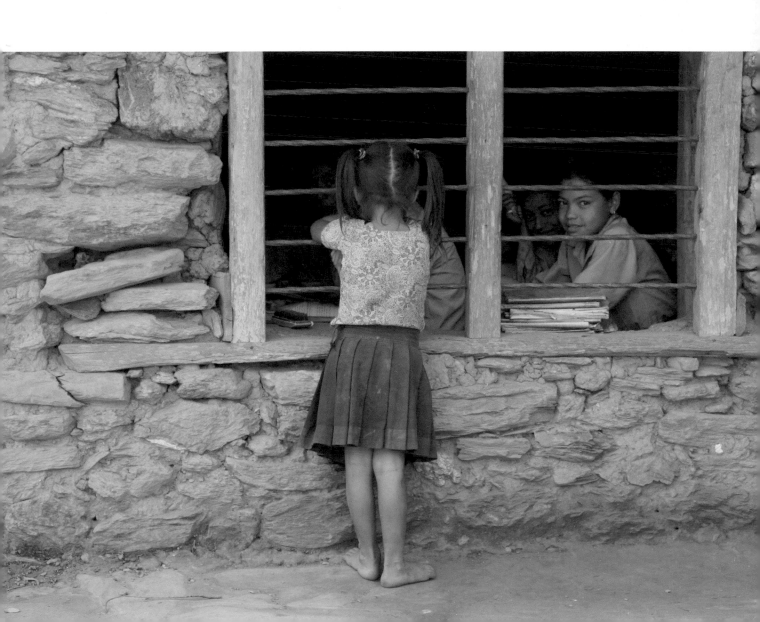

POLITICAL EMPOWERMENT – INCLUSION AND VOICE

Being included in the society in which one lives is vital to the material, psychosocial, and political empowerment that underpins social well-being and equitable health.

Evidence for action

The right to the conditions necessary to achieve the highest attainable standard of health is universal. The risk of these rights being violated is the result of entrenched structural inequities (Farmer, 1999).

Social inequity manifests across various intersecting social categories such as class, education, gender, age, ethnicity, disability, and geography. It signals not simply difference but hierarchy, and reflects deep inequities in the wealth, power, and prestige of different people and communities. People who are already disenfranchised are further disadvantaged with respect to their health – having the freedom to participate in economic, social, political, and cultural relationships has intrinsic value (Sen, 1999). Inclusion, agency, and control are each important for social development, health, and well-being. And restricted participation results in deprivation of human capabilities, setting the context for inequities in, for example, education, employment, and access to biomedical and technical advances.

Any serious effort to reduce health inequities will involve changing the distribution of power within society and global regions, empowering individuals and groups to represent strongly and effectively their needs and interests and, in so doing, to challenge and change the unfair and steeply graded distribution of social resources (the conditions for health) to which all, as citizens, have claims and rights.

Changes in power relationships can take place at various levels, from the 'micro' level of individuals, households, or communities to the 'macro' sphere of structural relations among economic, social, and political actors and institutions. While the empowerment of social groups through their representation in policy-related agenda-setting and decision-making is critical to realize a comprehensive set of rights and ensure the fair distribution of essential material and social goods among population groups, so too is empowerment for action through bottom-up, grassroots approaches. Struggles against the injustices encountered by the most disadvantaged in society, and the process of organizing these people, builds local people's leadership. It can be empowering. It gives people a greater sense of control over their lives and future.

Community or civil society action on health inequities cannot be separated from the responsibility of the state to guarantee a comprehensive set of rights and ensure the fair distribution of essential material and social goods among population groups. Top-down and bottom-up approaches are equally vital.

What must be done

Empower all groups in society through fair representation in decision-making about how society operates, particularly in relation to its effect on health equity, and create and maintain a socially inclusive framework for policy-making.

- Strengthen political and legal systems to protect human rights, assure legal identity and support the needs and claims of marginalized groups, particularly Indigenous Peoples.

- Ensure the fair representation and participation of individuals and communities in health decision-making as an integral feature of the right to health.

Enable civil society to organize and act in a manner that promotes and realizes the political and social rights affecting health equity.

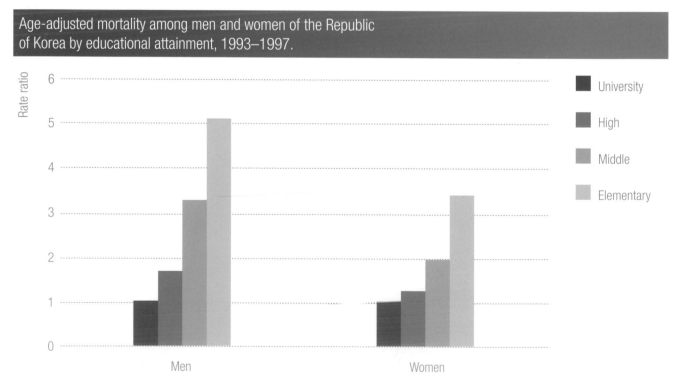

Age-adjusted mortality among men and women of the Republic of Korea by educational attainment, 1993–1997.

Source: Son et al., 2002

Good Global Governance

Dramatic differences in the health and life chances of peoples around the world reflect imbalance in the power and prosperity of nations. The undoubted benefits of globalization remain profoundly unequally distributed.

Evidence for action

The post-war period has seen massive growth. But growth in global wealth and knowledge has not translated into increased global health equity. Rather than convergence, with poorer countries catching up to the Organisation for Economic Cooperation and Development, the latter period of globalization (after 1980) has seen winners and losers among the world's countries, with particularly alarming stagnation and reversal in life expectancy at birth in sub-Saharan Africa and some of the former Soviet Union countries (GKN, 2007). Progress in global economic growth and health equity made between 1960 and 1980 has been significantly dampened in the subsequent period (1980-2005), as global economic policy influence hit hard at social sector spending and social development. Also associated with the second (post-1980) phase of globalization, the world has seen significant increase in, and regularity of, financial crises, proliferating conflicts, and forced and voluntary migration.

Through the recognition, under globalization, of common interests and interdependent futures, it is imperative that the international community re-commits to a multilateral system in which all countries, rich and poor, engage with an equitable voice. It is only through such a system of global governance, placing fairness in health at the heart of the development agenda and genuine equality of influence at the heart of its decision-making, that coherent attention to global health equity is possible.

What must be done

Make health equity a global development goal, and adopt a social determinants of health framework to strengthen multilateral action on development.

- The United Nations, through WHO and the Economic and Social Council, to adopt health equity as a core global development goal and use a social determinants of health indicators framework to monitor progress.

- The United Nations to establish multilateral working groups on thematic social determinants of health – initially early child development, gender equity, employment and working conditions, health-care systems, and participatory governance.

Strengthen WHO leadership in global action on the social determinants of health, institutionalizing social determinants of health as a guiding principle across WHO departments and country programmes.

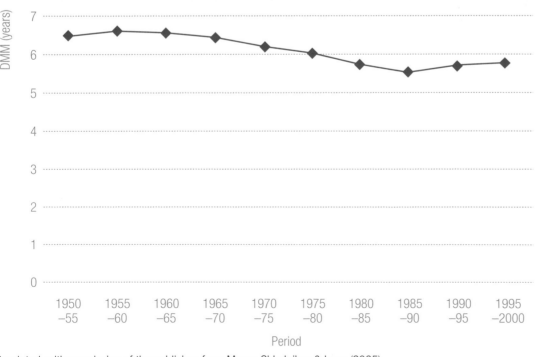

Trend in the dispersion measure of mortality (DMM) for life expectancy at birth, 1950–2000.

Reprinted, with permission of the publisher, from Moser, Shkolnikov & Leon (2005).

3. Measure and Understand the Problem and Assess the Impact of Action

The world is changing fast and often it is unclear the impact that social, economic, and political change will have on health in general and on health inequities within countries or across the globe in particular. Action on the social determinants of health will be more effective if basic data systems, including vital registration and routine monitoring of health inequity and the social determinants of health, are in place and there are mechanisms to ensure that the data can be understood and applied to develop more effective policies, systems, and programmes. Education and training in social determinants of health are vital.

The Social Determinants of Health: Monitoring, Research, and Training

No data often means no recognition of the problem. Good evidence on levels of health and its distribution, and on the social determinants of health, is essential for understanding the scale of the problem, assessing the effects of actions, and monitoring progress.

Evidence for action

Experience shows that countries without basic data on mortality and morbidity by socioeconomic indicators have difficulties moving forward on the health equity agenda. Countries with the worst health problems, including countries in conflict, have the least good data. Many countries do not even have basic systems to register all births and deaths. Failing birth registration systems have major implications for child health and developmental outcomes.

The evidence base on health inequity, the social determinants of health, and what works to improve them needs further strengthening. Unfortunately, most health research funding remains overwhelmingly biomedically focused. Also, much research remains gender biased. Traditional hierarchies of evidence (which put randomized controlled trials and laboratory experiments at the top) generally do not work for research on the social determinants of health. Rather, evidence needs to be judged on fitness for purpose – that is, does it convincingly answer the question asked.

Evidence is only one part of what swings policy decisions – political will and institutional capacity are important too. Policy actors need to understand what affects population health and how the gradient operates. Action on the social determinants of health also requires capacity building among practitioners, including the incorporation of teaching on social determinants of health into the curricula of health and medical personnel.

Unregistered births (in thousands) in 2003 by region and level of development.

Region	Births	Unregistered children, n (%)
World	133 028	48 276 (36%)
Sub-Saharan Africa	26 879	14 751 (55%)
Middle East and North Africa	9790	1543 (16%)
South Asia	37 099	23 395 (63%)
East Asia and Pacific	31 616	5901 (19%)
Latin America and Caribbean	11 567	1787 (15%)
CEE/CIS and Baltic States	5250	1218 (23%)
Industrialized countries	10 827	218 (2%)
Developing countries	119 973	48 147 (40%)
Least developed countries	27 819	19 682 (71%)

CEE = Central and Eastern Europe; CIS = Commonwealth of Independent States.

Source: UNICEF, 2005

What must be done

There is enough evidence on the social determinants of health to act now. Governments, supported by international organizations, can make action on the social determinants of health even more effective by improving local, national, and international monitoring, research, and training infrastructures.

Ensure that routine monitoring systems for health equity and the social determinants of health are in place, locally, nationally, and internationally.

• Ensure that all children are registered at birth without financial cost to the household.

• Establish national and global health equity surveillance systems with routine collection of data on social determinants and health inequity.

Invest in generating and sharing new evidence on the ways in which social determinants influence population health and health equity and on the effectiveness of measures to reduce health inequities through action on social determinants.

• Create a dedicated budget for generation and global sharing of evidence on social determinants of health and health equity.

Provide training on the social determinants of health to policy actors, stakeholders, and practitioners and invest in raising public awareness.

• Incorporate the social determinants of health into medical and health training, and improve social determinants of health literacy more widely. Train policy-makers and planners in the use of health equity impact assessment.

• Strengthen capacity within WHO to support action on the social determinants of health.

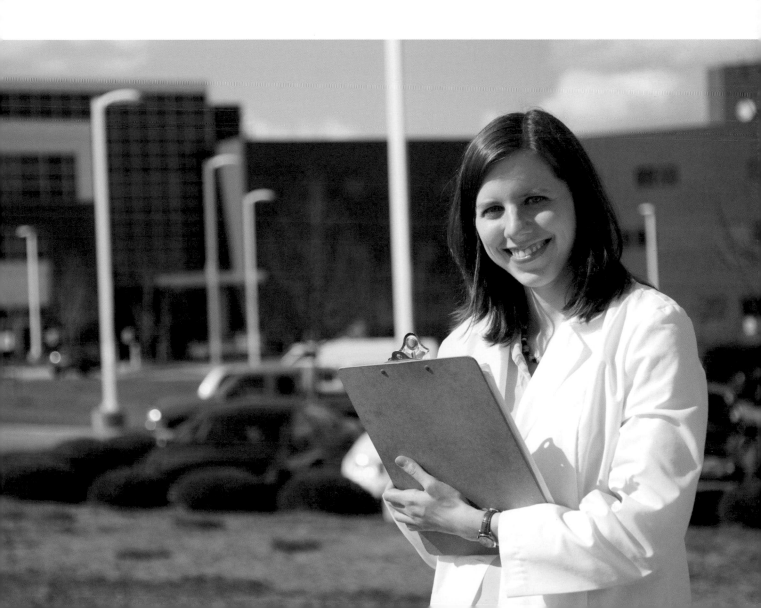

ACTORS

Above, we set out the key actions called for in the recommendations. Here, we describe those on whom effective action depends. The role of governments through public sector action is fundamental to health equity. But the role is not government's alone. Rather, it is through the democratic processes of civil society participation and public policy-making, supported at the regional and global levels, backed by the research on what works for health equity, and with the collaboration of private actors, that real action for health equity is possible.

Multilateral agencies

An overarching Commission recommendation is the need for intersectoral coherence – in policy-making and action – to enhance effective action on the social determinants of health and achieve improvements in health equity. Multilateral specialist and financing agencies can do much to strengthen their collective impact on the social determinants of health and health equity, including:

- *Coherence in global monitoring and action:* Adopt health equity as a fundamental shared goal, and use a common global framework of indicators to monitor development progress; and collaborate in multi-agency thematic working groups for coherent social determinants of health action.

- *Coherent and accountable financing:* Ensure that increases in aid and debt relief support coherent social determinants of health policy-making and action among recipient governments, using health equity and social determinants of health performance indicators as core conditions of recipient accountability.

- *Improved participation of UN Member States in global governance:* Support equitable participation of Member States and other stakeholders in global policy-making fora.

WHO

WHO is the mandated leader in global health. It is time to enhance WHO's leadership role through the agenda for action on the social determinants of health and global health equity. This involves a range of actions, including:

- *Policy coherence globally and nationally:* Adopt a stewardship role supporting social determinants of health capacity-building and policy coherence across partner agencies in the multilateral system; strengthen technical capacity globally and among Member States for representation of public health in all major multilateral fora; and support Member States in developing mechanisms for coherent policy and ISA for social determinants of health.

- *Measurement and evaluation:* Support goal-setting on health equity and monitoring progress on health equity between and within countries as a core developmental objective; support the establishment of national health equity surveillance systems in Member States, and build necessary technical capacities in countries; support Member States in development and use of health equity impact assessment tools and other health equity-related tools such as a national equity gauge; and convene a regular global meeting as part of a periodic review of the global situation.

- *Enhancing WHO capacity:* Build internal social determinants of health capacity across the WHO, from headquarters, through the Regional Offices, to Country Programmes.

National and local government

Underpinning action on the social determinants of health and health equity is an empowered public sector, based on principles of justice, participation, and intersectoral collaboration. This will require strengthening of the core functions of government and public institutions, nationally and sub-nationally, particularly in relation to policy coherence, participatory governance, planning, regulation development and enforcement, and standard-setting. It also depends on strong leadership and stewardship from the ministry of health, supported by WHO. Government actions include:

- *Policy coherence across government:* Place responsibility for action on health and health equity at the highest level of government, and ensure its coherent consideration across all ministerial and departmental policy-making. Ministers of health can help bring about global change – they will be pivotal in helping to create buy-in by the head of state and from other ministries.

- *Strengthening action for equity:* Commit to progressive building of universal health-care services; establish a central gender unit to promote gender equity across government policy-making; improve rural livelihoods, infrastructure investment, and services; upgrade slums and strengthen locally participatory health urban planning; invest in full employment and decent labour policy and programmes; invest in ECD; build towards universal provision in vital social determinants of health services and programmes regardless of ability to pay, supported by a universal programme of social protection; and establish a national framework for regulatory control over health-damaging commodities.

- *Finance:* Streamline incoming international finance (aid, debt relief) through a social determinants of health action framework, with transparent accountability; strengthen revenue through improved progressive domestic taxation; and collaborate with other Member States in the development of regional and/or global proposals for new sources of international public finance.

- *Measurement, evaluation, and training:* Build towards universal birth registration; set cross-government performance indicators for health equity through the establishment of a national health equity surveillance system; build capacity to use health equity impact assessment as a standard protocol in all major policy-making; ensure training of practitioners and policy-makers on the social determinants of health; and raise public awareness of the social determinants of health.

Civil society

Being included in the society in which one lives is vital to the material, psychosocial, and political aspects of empowerment that underpin social well-being and equitable health. As community members, grassroots advocates, service and programme providers, and performance monitors, civil society actors from the global to the local level constitute a vital bridge between policies and plans and the reality of change and improvement in the lives of all. Helping to organize and promote diverse voices across different communities, civil society can be a powerful champion of health equity. Many of the actions listed above will be, at least in part, the result of pressure and encouragement from civil society; many of the milestones towards health equity in a generation will be marked – achieved or missed – by the attentive observation of civil society actors. Civil society can play an important role in actions on the social determinants of health through:

- *Participation in policy, planning, programmes, and evaluation:* Participate in social determinants of health policy-making, planning, programme delivery, and evaluation from the global level, through national intersectoral fora, to the local level of needs assessments, service delivery, and support; and monitor service quality, equity, and impact.

- *Monitoring performance:* Monitor, and report and campaign on, specific social determinants of health, such as upgrading of and services in slums, formal and non-formal employment conditions, child labour, indigenous rights, gender equity, health and education services, corporate activities, trade agreements, and environmental protection.

Private sector

The private sector has a profound impact on health and well-being. Where the Commission reasserts the vital role of public sector leadership in acting for health equity, this does not imply a relegation of the importance of private sector activities. It does, though, imply the need for recognition of potentially adverse impacts, and the need for responsibility in regulation with regard to those impacts. Alongside controlling undesirable effects on health and health equity, the vitality of the private sector has much to offer that could enhance health and well-being. Actions include:

- *Strengthening accountability:* Recognize and respond accountably to international agreements, standards, and codes of employment practice; ensure employment and working conditions are fair for men and women; reduce and eradicate child labour, and ensure compliance with occupational health and safety standards; support educational and vocational training opportunities as part of employment conditions, with special emphasis on opportunities for women; and ensure private sector activities and services (such as production and patenting of life-saving medicines, provision of health insurance schemes) contribute to and do not undermine health equity.

- *Investing in research:* Commit to research and development in treatment for neglected diseases and diseases of poverty, and share knowledge in areas (such as pharmaceuticals patents) with life-saving potential.

Research institutions

Knowledge – of what the health situation is, globally, regionally, nationally, and locally; of what can be done about that situation; and of what works effectively to alter health inequity through the social determinants of health – is at the heart of the Commission and underpins all its recommendations. Research is needed. But more than simply academic exercises, research is needed to generate new understanding and to disseminate that understanding in practical accessible ways to all the partners listed above. Research on and knowledge of the social determinants of health and ways to act for health equity will rely on continuing commitments among academics and practitioners, but it will rely on new methodologies too – recognizing and utilizing a range of types of evidence, recognizing gender bias in research processes, and recognizing the added value of globally expanded Knowledge Networks and communities. Actions in this field of actors include:

- *Generating and disseminating social determinants of health knowledge:* Ensure research funding is allocated to social determinants of health work; support the global health observatory and multilateral, national, and local cross-sectoral working through development and testing of social determinants of health indicators and intervention impact evaluation; establish and expand virtual networks and clearing houses organized on the principles of open access, managed to enhance accessibility from sites in all high-, middle-, and low-income settings; contribute to reversal of the brain drain from low- and middle-income countries; and address and remove gender biases in research teams, proposals, designs, practices, and reports.

IS CLOSING THE HEALTH GAP IN A GENERATION FEASIBLE?

This question – is closing the health gap in a generation feasible – has two clear answers. If we continue as we are, there is no chance at all. If there is a genuine desire to change, if there is a vision to create a better and fairer world where people's life chances and their health will no longer be blighted by the accident of where they happen to be born, the colour of their skin, or the lack of opportunities afforded to their parents, then the answer is: we could go a long way towards it.

Action can be taken, as we show throughout the report. But coherent action must be fashioned across the determinants – across the fields of action set out above – rooting out structural inequity as much as ensuring more immediate well-being. To achieve this will take changes starting at the beginning of life and acting through the whole lifecourse. In calling to close the gap in a generation we do not imagine that the social gradient in health within countries, or the dramatic differences between countries, will be abolished in 30 years. But the evidence, produced in the Final Report, both on the speed with which health can improve and the means needed to achieve change, encourage us that significant closing of the gap is indeed achievable.

This is a long-term agenda, requiring investment starting now, with major changes in social policies, economic arrangements, and political action. At the centre of this action should be the empowerment of people, communities, and countries that currently do not have their fair share. The knowledge and the means to change are at hand and are brought together in this report. What is needed now is the political will to implement these eminently difficult but feasible changes. Not to act will be seen, in decades to come, as failure on a grand scale to accept the responsibility that rests on all our shoulders.

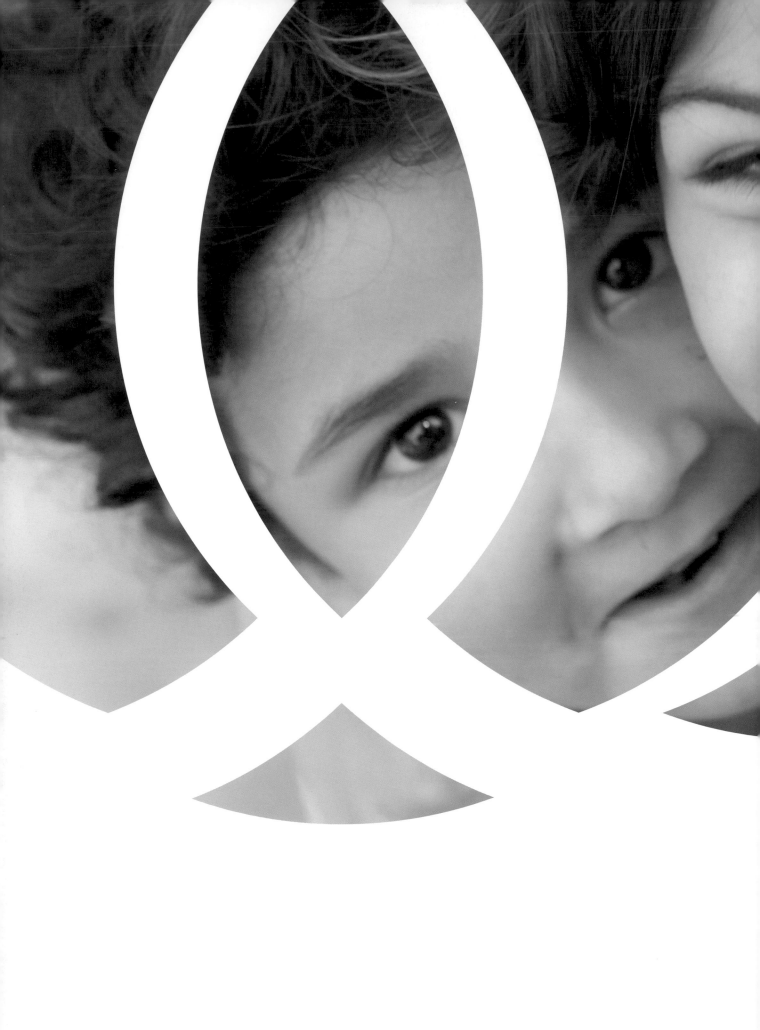

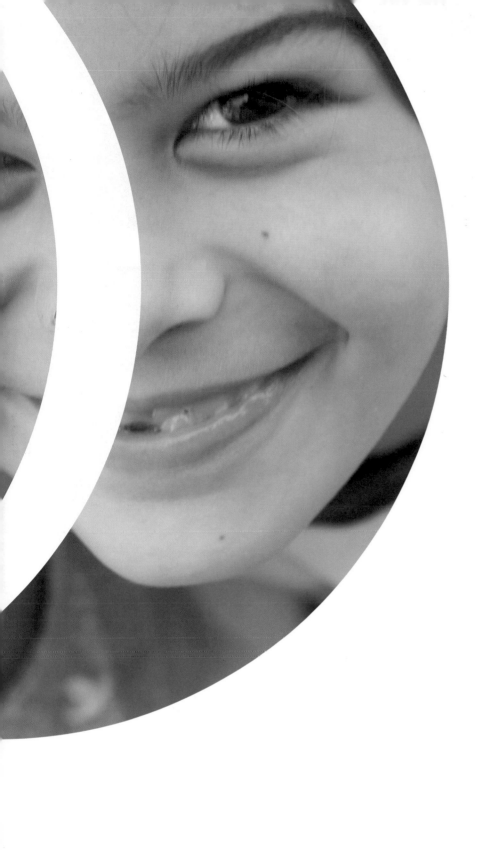

CHAPTER 1

A new global agenda – the Commission on Social Determinants of Health

Our children have dramatically different life chances depending on where they were born. In Japan or Sweden they can expect to live more than 80 years; in Brazil, 72 years; in India, 63 years; and in one of several African countries, fewer than 50 years. Within countries, the differences in life chances are dramatic and are seen in all countries – even the richest. The balance of poverty and affluence may be different in low-income countries, but it is still true that the more affluent flourish and the less affluent do not.

It does not have to be this way and it is not right that it should be like this. It is not an unfortunate cluster of random events, nor differences in individual behaviours, that consistently keep the health of some countries and population groups below others. Where systematic differences in health are judged to be avoidable by reasonable action globally and within society they are, quite simply, unjust. It is this that we label health inequity.

HEALTH EQUITY AND THE SOCIAL DETERMINANTS OF HEALTH

Traditionally, societies have looked to the health sector to deal with its concerns about health and disease. Certainly, maldistribution of health care – not delivering care to those who most need it – is one of the social determinants of health. But the high burden of illness responsible for appalling premature loss of life arises in large part because of the conditions in which people are born, grow, live, work, and age – conditions that together provide the freedom people need to live lives they value (Sen, 1999; Marmot, 2004).

Poor and unequal living conditions are, in their turn, the consequence of deeper structural conditions that together fashion the way societies are organized – poor social policies and programmes, unfair economic arrangements, and bad politics. These 'structural drivers' operate within countries under the authority of governments, but also, increasingly over the last century and a half, between countries under the effects of globalization. This toxic combination of bad policies, economics, and politics is, in large measure, responsible for the fact that a majority of people in the world do not enjoy the good health that is biologically possible. Daily living conditions, themselves the result of these structural drivers, together constitute the social determinants of health.

Putting these inequities right is a matter of social justice. Reducing health inequities is, for the Commission on Social Determinants of Health (hereafter, the Commission), an ethical imperative. The right to the highest attainable standard of health is enshrined in the Constitution of the World Health Organization (WHO) and numerous international treaties (UN, 2000a). But the degree to which these rights are met from one place to another around the world is glaringly unequal. Social injustice is killing people on a grand scale.

A NEW AGENDA FOR HEALTH, EQUITY, AND DEVELOPMENT

We start from the proposition that there is no necessary biological reason why a girl in one part of the world, say Lesotho, should have a life expectancy at birth (LEB) shorter by 42 years than a girl in another, say Japan. Similarly, there is no necessary biological reason why there should be a difference in LEB of 20 years or more between social groups in any given country. Change the social determinants of health and there will be dramatic improvements in health equity.

We call for the health gap to be closed in a generation. This reflects our judgement that action – socially, politically, and economically – would lead to dramatic narrowing of the health differences between and within countries. This is not to predict that the social gradient in health within countries, or the dramatic differences between them, will be abolished in 30 years, but it is to demand that the appalling unfairness that we see around the world be placed at the top of the agenda for global, regional, and national action. The evidence, outlined in this report, both on the speed with which health can improve and the means needed to achieve change, encourages us that significant closing of the gap is indeed achievable, but it will take action starting now.

THREE PRINCIPLES OF ACTION TO ACHIEVE HEALTH EQUITY

The Commission's analysis, following the social determinants of health as summarized above, leads to three principles of action:

1. Improve the conditions of daily life – the circumstances in which people are born, grow, live, work, and age.

2. Tackle the inequitable distribution of power, money, and resources – the structural drivers of those conditions of daily life – globally, nationally, and locally.

3. Measure the problem, evaluate action, expand the knowledge base, develop a workforce that is trained in the social determinants of health, and raise public awareness about the social determinants of health.

While the report that follows is structured around these three principles, there is not an implied order of action. Measuring the problem and taking action to resolve it must proceed at the same time. Taking action on the conditions of daily life and on the structural drivers of those conditions should proceed simultaneously. They are not alternatives.

The Commission's work embodies a new approach to development. Health and health equity may not be the aim of all social policies but they will be a fundamental result. Take the central policy importance given to economic growth: Economic growth is without question important, particularly for poor countries, as it gives the opportunity to provide resources to invest in improvement of the lives of their population. But growth for its own sake, without appropriate social policies to ensure reasonable fairness in the way its benefits are distributed, brings no benefit to health.

Health systems have an important role to play. Ministries of health also have an important stewardship responsibility. The health sector should work in concert with other sectors of society. Health and health equity are important measures of the success of social policies. But beyond the health sector, action on the social determinants of health must involve the whole of government, civil society[1] and local communities, business, global fora, and international agencies.

As processes of globalization bring us closer together as peoples and nations, we begin to see the interdependence of our aspirations – aspirations for human security, including protection against poverty and exclusion, and aspirations for human freedom (Sen, 1999), not just to grow and flourish as individuals but to grow and flourish together. We recognize the barriers to common global flourishing – particularly the entrenched interests of some social groups and countries. But we also recognize the value and necessity of collective action – nationally and globally – to correct the corrosive effects of inequality of life chances.

TWO URGENT AGENDAS – HEALTH EQUITY AND ENVIRONMENTAL CHANGE

There is, at last, widespread recognition that disruption and depletion of natural environmental systems, including climate change, is not simply a technical discussion among environmental experts but has profound implications for the way of life of people globally and for all living organisms. It was beyond the remit, and competence, of the Commission to design a new international economic order that balances the needs of social and economic development of the whole global population, health equity, and the urgency of dealing with global warming. But the sense of urgency and willingness to experiment with innovative solutions is the spirit required to deal with both issues.

THE COMMISSION AND THE WORLD HEALTH ORGANIZATION

In the spirit of social justice, the Commission was set up by the late Director-General of WHO, Dr Jong Wook Lee. He saw action on social determinants of health as the route to achieving health equity. The Commission, created to marshal the evidence on what can be done to promote health equity and to foster a global movement to achieve it, is a global collaboration of policy-makers, researchers, and civil society led by Commissioners who contribute a broad range of political, academic, and advocacy experience. Health equity is, necessarily, a truly global agenda. The current Director-General, Dr Margaret Chan, has embraced the Commission with enthusiasm. She said:

"No one should be denied access to life-saving or health-promoting interventions for unfair reasons, including those with economic or social causes. These are some of the issues being addressed by the Commission on Social Determinants of Health ... When health is concerned, equity really is a matter of life and death." (Chan, 2007)

Director-General Chan has committed WHO to action on the social determinants of health, not only because it has the power to do so, but because it has the moral authority.

FOSTERING A GLOBAL MOVEMENT FOR CHANGE

The Commission seeks to foster a global movement for change. The indications are clear: health is universally valued, and people desire fairness. Where it has been studied, there is clear evidence of concern about the unfairness of living conditions (YouGov Poll, 2007) that lead to differences in levels of health (RWJF Commission, 2008). We have already encountered a great deal of support for our core conclusions. While WHO is a central and vitally important actor in taking forward the health equity agenda, the global movement is being built by a host of stakeholders. It is clear, too, that changing the social determinants of health and health equity is a long-term agenda requiring sustained support and investment.

BEYOND 'BUSINESS AS USUAL'

A key concern of the Commission from its inception has been that implementing real change might be seen as unrealistic – that superficial changes would be more attractive to those who prefer to continue with 'business as usual'. The evidence is compelling that business as usual is increasingly unfeasible. Among the enthusiasm for the work of the Commission, we have also encountered two types of criticism aimed at the social determinants of health: "We know it all already" and "You have no evidence to support action". Between the two critiques, the Commission seeks to forge a new path to action. We know much about the social determinants of health, it is true. Yet policy-making all too often appears to happen as if there were no such knowledge available. And we *do not yet* know enough. There is a pressing need to invest in a great deal more research, bringing together different disciplines and areas of expertise, to work out how social determinants create health inequity, and how action on these determinants can produce better, fairer health.

The Commission is unusual in having inspired and supported action in the real world from its inception. Over three years, a number of countries have signed up to the Commission's vision. Brazil, Canada, Chile, Islamic Republic of Iran, Kenya, Mozambique, Sri Lanka, Sweden, and the United Kingdom each became partners of the Commission and have made progress on developing policies, across government, on tackling social determinants of health equity. More countries will follow (Argentina, Mexico, Poland, Thailand, New Zealand, and Norway have all expressed enthusiasm to join). From the rota of nations, the Commission's list of country partners is, as

---

[1] Civil society refers to the arena of uncoerced collective action around shared interests, purposes, and values. In theory, its institutional forms are distinct from those of the state, family, and market though, in practice, the boundaries between state, civil society, family, and market are complex. Civil society is often populated by organizations such as registered charities, development nongovernmental organizations, community groups, women's organizations, faith-based organizations, professional organizations, trade unions, self-help groups, social movements, business associations, coalitions, and advocacy groups.

yet, relatively small. In many places, things have not changed and will, without doubt, take much time to change. But our country partners are a powerful expression of political will and practical commitment. Is it feasible to do things differently? Yes. These countries are already doing it. As Parts 3 and 4 of this report show, partnerships with other countries, civil society, WHO, other international bodies, and opinion formers are all vital in pursuing the social determinants of health agenda.

WHY NOW?

WHO made inspiring declarations 60 years ago, at its birth, and again 30 years ago, at Alma Ata. Those declarations are consistent with the call that we are making today. Why will things be any different now?

Better knowledge

There is now a great deal more knowledge, globally circulating, on both the nature of the problem of health inequity and what can be done to address the social determinants of health.

Better development

The dominant model of development is changing. The Millennium Development Goals (MDGs) reflect an unprecedented global concern to effect real, sustainable change in the lives of people in poor countries. There is growing demand for a new approach to social development – one that moves beyond an overriding focus on economic growth to look at building well-being through the combined effects of growth and empowerment (Stern, 2004).

Stronger health leadership

Convening the Commission, WHO signalled its desire to do things differently. Its Member States, too, are increasingly calling for a new model for health – from the point of view of both social justice and increasingly unsustainable reliance on the traditional health-care model.

An unsustainable status quo

What happens in one part of the world now has an impact everywhere – financial crises, conflicts, population movement, trade and labour, food production and food security, and disease. The scale of inequity is simply unsustainable. Underpinning the call for global human justice, the inescapable evidence of climate change and environmental degradation have set clear limits to a future based on the status quo and are prompting an increasing global willingness to do things differently.

CAN THINGS CHANGE?

The question – is closing the health gap in a generation feasible – has two clear answers. If we continue as we are, there is no chance at all. If there is a genuine desire to change, if there is a vision to create a better and fairer world where people's life chances and their health will no longer be blighted by the accident of where they happen to be born, the colour of their skin, or the lack of opportunities afforded to their parents, then the answer is: we could go a long way towards it.

Achieving this vision will take major changes in social policies, in economic arrangements, and in political action. At the centre of this action should be the empowerment of people, communities, and countries that currently do not have their fair share. The knowledge and the means to change are at hand and are brought together in this Report. What is needed now is the political will to implement these difficult but feasible changes.

This is a long-term agenda, requiring investment across the lifecourse and starting now. Not to act will be seen, in decades to come, as failure on a grand scale to accept the responsibility that rests on all our shoulders.

CHAPTER 2
Global health inequity – the need for action

HEALTH INEQUITY IN ALL COUNTRIES

"There are no conditions of life to which a man cannot get accustomed, especially if he sees them accepted by everyone around him." (Tolstoy, 1877)

We have become all too accustomed to premature death and disease and to the conditions that give rise to them. But much of the global burden of disease and premature death is avoidable, and therefore unacceptable. It is inequitable. Health equity has two important strands: improving average health of countries and abolishing avoidable inequalities in health within countries. In both cases – average health of countries and distribution within countries – the aim should be to bring the health of those worse off up to the level of the best. If the infant mortality rate in Iceland (WHO, 2007c) were applied to the whole world, only two babies would die in every 1000 born alive. There would be 6.6 million fewer infant deaths in the world each year.

Yet the distribution of infant deaths is most unequal, both between countries and within them. Fig. 2.1 shows variation between countries in infant mortality from just over 20/1000 live births in Colombia to just over 120 in Mozambique. And it shows dramatic inequities within countries – an infant's chances of survival are closely related to her mother's education. In Bolivia, babies born to women with no education have infant mortality greater than 100 per 1000 live births; the infant mortality rate of babies born to mothers with at least secondary education is under 40/1000. All countries included in Fig. 2.1 show the survival disadvantage of children born to women with no education. If it is considered too unrealistic to contemplate an infant mortality rate of 2 per 1000 live births in low-income countries, we must at least acknowledge the scale of improvement in infant survival apparently offered by educating girls and women.

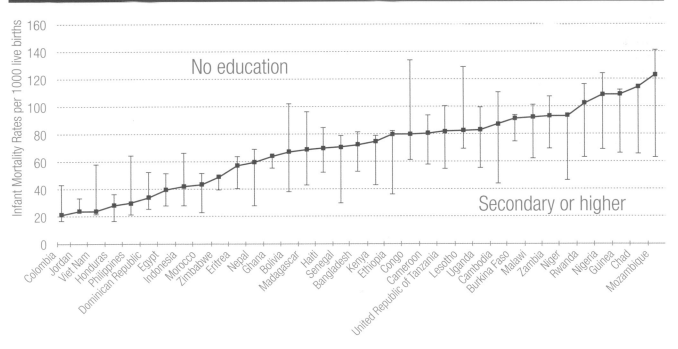

Figure 2.1: Inequity in infant mortality rates between countries and within countries by mother's education.

Data from the Demographic and Health Surveys (DHS, nd) derived from STATcompiler. The continuous dark line represents average infant mortality rates for countries; the end-points of the bars indicate the infant mortality rates for mothers with no education and for mothers with secondary or higher education.

INEQUITY IN HEALTH CONDITIONS

LEB among indigenous Australians is substantially lower (59.4 for males and 64.8 for females in the period 1996-2001) than that of all Australians (76.6 and 82.0, respectively, for the period 1998-2000) (Aboriginal and Torres Strait Islander Social Justice Commissioner, 2005).

In Europe, the excess risk of dying among middle-aged adults in the lowest socioeconomic groups ranges from 25% to 50% and even 150% (Mackenbach, 2005).

Health inequalities are observed among the oldest old. The prevalence of long-term disabilities among European men aged 80+ years is 58.8% among the lower educated versus 40.2% among the higher educated (Huisman, Kunst & Mackenbach, 2003).

In the United States of America, 886 202 deaths would have been averted between 1991 and 2000 if mortality rates between whites and African Americans were equalized. This contrasts to 176 633 lives saved by medical advances (Woolf et al., 2004).

Cardiovascular diseases (CVDs) are the number one group of conditions causing death globally. An estimated 17.5 million people died from CVDs in 2005, representing 30% of all global deaths. Over 80% of CVD deaths occur in low- and middle-income countries (WHO, nd,a).

Of people with diabetes, 80% live in low- and middle-income countries. Diabetes deaths are likely to increase by more than 50% in the next 10 years without urgent action (WHO, nd,c).

Mental health problems will become increasingly important. It is estimated that unipolar depressive disorders will be the leading cause of the burden of disease in high-income countries in 2030, and it will be number two and three in middle- and low-income countries, respectively (Mathers & Loncar, 2005).

The lifetime risk of maternal death is one in eight in Afghanistan; it is 1 in 17 400 in Sweden, (WHO et al., 2007).

Maternal mortality is three to four times higher among the poor compared to the rich in Indonesia (Graham et al., 2004).

Every day, over 13 500 people worldwide die due to tobacco. The total number of smoking deaths will increase from 5 to 8 million in the next 20 years. Soon, it will become the leading cause of death in developing countries (as it is in high-income countries) (Mathers & Loncar, 2005).

Worldwide, alcohol causes 1.8 million deaths (3.2% of the total). Unintentional injuries alone account for about one third of the 1.8 million deaths (WHO, nd,b).

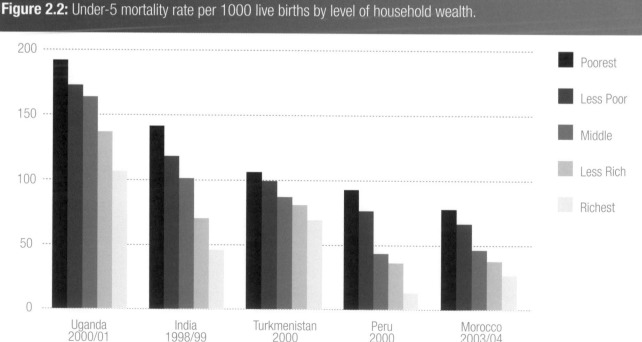

Figure 2.2: Under-5 mortality rate per 1000 live births by level of household wealth.

Source: Gwatkin et al. (2007), using DHS data.

The social gradient is not confined to poorer countries. Fig. 2.3 shows national data for some areas of the United Kingdom (England and Wales) for people classified according to levels of neighbourhood deprivation. As can be seen, the mortality rate varies in a continuous way with degrees of deprivation (Romeri, Baker & Griffiths, 2006). The range is large: the difference in mortality between the most and least deprived is more than 2.5-fold.

THE GRADIENT

The poorest of the poor, around the world, have the worst health. Those at the bottom of the distribution of global and national wealth, those marginalized and excluded within countries, and countries themselves disadvantaged by historical exploitation and persistent inequity in global institutions of power and policy-making present an urgent moral and practical focus for action. But focusing on those with the least, on the 'gap' between the poorest and the rest, is only a partial response. Fig. 2.2 shows under-5 mortality rates by levels of household wealth. The message here is clear: the relation between socioeconomic level and health is graded. People in the second highest quintile have higher mortality in their offspring than those in the highest quintile. We have labelled this the social gradient in health (Marmot, 2004).

The social gradient is not confined to poorer countries. Fig. 2.3 shows national data for some areas of the United Kingdom (England and Wales) for people classified according to levels of neighbourhood deprivation. As can be seen, the mortality rate varies in a continuous way with degrees of deprivation (Romeri, Baker & Griffiths, 2006). The range is large: the difference in mortality between the most and least deprived is more than 2.5-fold.

THE POOREST OF THE POOR AND THE SOCIAL GRADIENT IN HEALTH

The implications of Figs. 2.1, 2.2, and 2.3 are clear. We need to be concerned with both material deprivation – the poor material conditions of the 40% of the world's population that live on US$ 2/day or less – and the social gradient in health that affects people in rich and poor countries alike.

Poverty is not only lack of income. The implication, both of the social gradient in health and the poor health of the poorest of the poor, is that health inequity is caused by the unequal distribution of income, goods, and services and of the consequent chance of leading a flourishing life. This unequal distribution is not in any sense a 'natural' phenomenon but is the result of policies that prize the interests of some over those of others – all too often of a rich and powerful minority over the interests of a disempowered majority.

People at the bottom of the range in Fig. 2.3 are rich by global standards. They are all living on well above US$ 2/day. They have clean water to drink, sanitary living conditions, and infant mortality rates below 10 per 1000 live births, yet they have higher mortality rates than those in the middle of the socioeconomic range. Those in the middle certainly are not materially deprived in the sense just described, but they too have higher mortality than those above them – the greater the social disadvantage, the worse the health. The steepness of the gradient varies over time and across countries. It is likely, then, that action on the social determinants of health would reduce the social gradient in health (Marmot, 2004).

In rich countries, low socioeconomic position means poor education, lack of amenities, unemployment and job insecurity, poor working conditions, and unsafe neighbourhoods, with their consequent impact on family life. These all apply to the socially disadvantaged in low-income countries in addition to the considerable burden of material deprivation and vulnerability to natural disasters. So these dimensions of social disadvantage – that the health of the worst off in high-income countries is, in a few dramatic cases, worse than average health in some lower-income countries (Table 2.1) – are important for health.

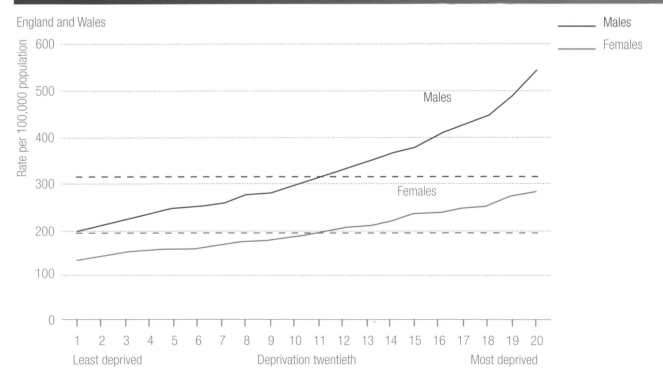

Figure 2.3: Death rates, age standardized, for all causes of death by deprivation twentieth, ages 15–64 years, 1999-2003, United Kingdom (England and Wales).

Dashed lines are average mortality rates for men and women in some areas of the United Kingdom (England and Wales).

Table 2.1

Male life expectancy, between- and within-country inequities, selected countries

Place	Life expectancy at birth
United Kingdom, Scotland, Glasgow (Calton)[b]	54
India[a]	62
United States, Washington DC (black)[c]	63
Philippines[a]	64
Lithuania[a]	65
Poland[a]	71
Mexico[a]	72
United States[a]	75
Cuba[a]	75
United Kingdom[a]	77
Japan[a]	79
Iceland[a]	79
United States, Montgomery County (white)[c]	80
United Kingdom, Scotland, Glasgow (Lenzie N.)[b]	82

a) Country data: 2005 data from World Health Statistics (WHO, 2007c).

b) Pooled data 1998-2002 (Hanlon, Walsh & Whyte, 2006).

c) Pooled data from 1997-2001 (Murray et al., 2006).

Health inequity, as the data above illustrate, is a concern for all, in all countries worldwide. The urgency of that concern is compounded by the fact that the pattern of the health problems confronting countries, and requiring solutions, is converging. While the poorest countries have a high burden of communicable disease as well as non-communicable disease and injury, in all other regions of the world non-communicable diseases predominate (WHO, 2005c). The causes of heart disease, cancer, and diabetes are the same wherever these diseases occur. The action needed to combat them is likely, therefore, to be similar in rich and poor countries alike. The global picture of non-communicable and communicable disease dictates the need for a coherent framework for global health action.

IS CLOSING THE HEALTH GAP IN A GENERATION POSSIBLE?

The differences in health that we have illustrated above are so large that it may strain credibility to envisage closing the health gap in one generation. The fact is that health can change dramatically in a remarkably short time. With health equity, what can worsen can improve. The data show this. Child mortality of 50 per 1000 is unacceptably high. That was the situation in Greece and Portugal 40 years ago (Fig. 2.4). The latest figures show them to be just above the levels for Iceland, Japan, and Sweden. Egypt provides perhaps the most striking example of rapid change – from 235 to 35 per 1000 in 40 years. The figures for Egypt are lower now than those of Greece or Portugal 40 years ago.

But just as things can improve with remarkable speed, they can also deteriorate fast. In the 30-year period between 1970 and 2000, infant mortality was falling in both Russian Federation and Singapore. LEB, however, rose by 10 years in Singapore and fell by 4 years in Russian Federation. The divergence arose because of the rise in adult mortality in Russian Federation, a rise itself associated with 'shock therapy' changes in political, economic, and social systems in the country from 1992 onwards. Fig. 2.5 shows how quickly the magnitude of the

Figure 2.4: Under-5 mortality rates per 1000 live births, selected countries, 1970 and 2006

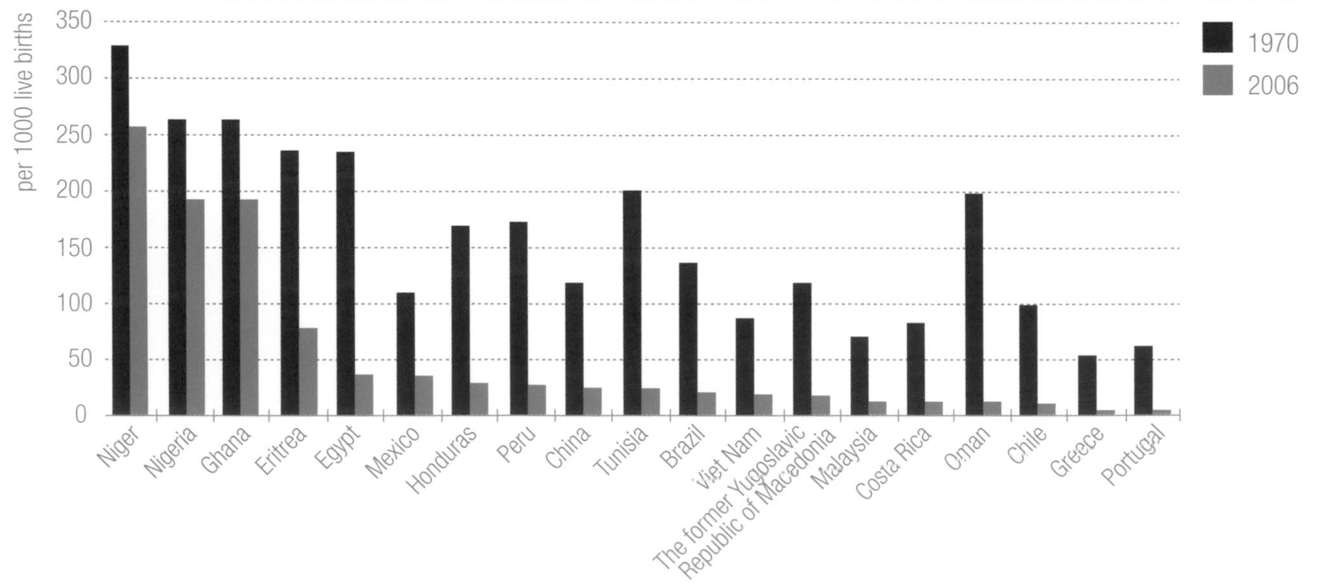

But just as things can improve with remarkable speed, they can also deteriorate fast. In the 30-year period between 1970 and 2000, infant mortality was falling in both Russian Federation and Singapore, LEB, however, rose by 10 years in Singapore and fell by 4 years in Russian Federation. The divergence arose because of the rise in adult mortality in Russian Federation, a rise itself associated with 'shock therapy' changes in political, economic, and social systems in the country from 1992 onwards. Fig. 2.5 shows how quickly the magnitude of the social gradient in health can change for the worse, too, related to the level of educational attainment.
Source: (UNICEF, 2007c).

social gradient in health can change for the worse, too, related to the level of educational attainment.

BUILDING ON SOLID FOUNDATIONS: HISTORICAL EXPERIENCE

Bringing together global action for health equity under the rubric of social determinants of health is new. The ideas behind it are not. By one name or another, there is long experience relevant to our present concerns. Over centuries, collective actions, such as the emancipation of women, universal franchise, the labour movement, and the civil rights movement, have contributed to the improved living and working conditions of millions of people worldwide. Although not explicitly concerned with health, such movements have advanced people's ability, globally, to lead a flourishing life.

The good health of the Nordic countries has long attracted attention. Analysis of the Nordic health improvements since the latter part of the 19th century emphasized the importance of civil rights, political rights, and social rights (Lundberg et al., 2007). Important features of the Nordic experience include commitment to universalist policies based on equality of rights to benefits and services, full employment, gender equity, and low levels of social exclusion. These are related to a relatively compressed income distribution and the absence of large differences in living standards between individuals and population groups.

Some low-income countries, Costa Rica, China, India (State of Kerala), and Sri Lanka, have achieved a level of good health out of all proportion to expectation based on their level of national income. This suggests strongly that good and equitable health do not depend on a relatively high level of national wealth. Cuba is another example. The lessons to be learned from these countries emphasize the importance of five shared political factors (Irwin & Scali, 2005):

- historical commitment to health as a social goal;

- social welfare orientation to development;

- community participation in decision-making processes relevant to health;

- universal coverage of health services for all social groups;

- intersectoral linkages for health.

Founded in 1948, WHO embodied a new vision of global health, defining health as, "a state of complete physical, mental and social well being and not merely the absence of disease or infirmity". Thirty years later, in 1978, the community of nations came together again in Alma Ata, where then Director-General Halfdan Mahler advanced his vision that "Health for All" implied removing the obstacles to health quite as much as it did the solution of purely medical problems. The Alma Ata declaration (WHO & UNICEF, 1978) promoted Primary Health Care (PHC) as its central means towards good and fair global health – not simply health services at the primary care level (though that was important), but rather a health system model that acted also on the underlying social, economic, and political causes of poor health.

In the decades that followed, though, a social model of health was not often seen in practice (Irwin & Scali, 2005). Neither intersectoral action (ISA) nor comprehensive PHC were really put into practice. Under the pressure of an ascendant global package of market-oriented economic policies, including significant reduction in the role of the state and levels of public spending and investment, a different development model was pursued from the 1980s. That model has been the target of a great deal of deserved criticism. Structural adjustment programmes, following the Washington consensus, had – and continue to have, in other policy and programme forms – an overreliance on markets to solve social problems that proved damaging. It has been noted, too, that the set of economic

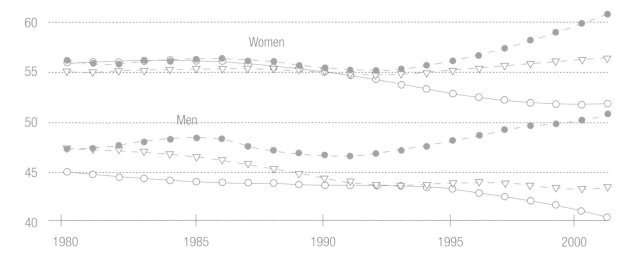

Figure 2.5: Trends in male and female life expectancy at age 20, by educational attainment, Russian Federation.

Educational attainment: ○ elementary (open circles), ▽ intermediate (triangles), and ● university (filled circles).
Reprinted, with permission of the publisher, from Murphy et al. (2006).

principles being promoted in low-income countries were not the same as those being followed in high-income countries (Stiglitz, 2002; Stiglitz, 2006).

The proponents of health for all did not disappear. They remain numerous and vocal around the world. The PHC movement has its strong advocates. Indeed, PHC plays a central role in WHO's current agenda and is the focus of the 2008 World Health Report. The 1986 Ottawa Charter on Health Promotion, and its renewal in Bangkok in 2005, embraced a global vision of public health action and the importance of a social determinants approach (WHO, 1986; Catford, 2005). The Latin American social medicine movement, Community-Oriented Primary Care that started in pre-apartheid South Africa (Kark & Kark, 1983) and spread to Canada, Israel, the United States, and United Kingdom (Wales) (Abramson, 1988), the community health movement in the United States (Geiger, 1984; Geiger, 2002; Davis et al., 1999), Canada (Hutchison, Abelson & Lavis, 2001), and Australia (Baum, Fry & Lennie, 1992; Baum, 1995), the Village Health worker (Sanders, 1985) and the People's Health Movement, the General Comment on the Right to Health, and the broad social vision of the MDGs all reaffirm the central importance of health, the need for social and participatory action on health, and the core human value of equity in health (Tajer, 2003; PHM, 2000; UN, 2000a; UN, 2000b). The Commission acknowledges a great debt to these movements, and builds on their achievements and continuing vision.

CHAPTER 3
Causes and solutions

There is no question that differences in health within and between countries can change quickly. It is our judgement that this process can be encouraged by better economic and social arrangements.

SOCIAL POLICIES, ECONOMICS, AND POLITICS THAT PUT PEOPLE AT THE CENTRE

At the heart of our concern is creating the conditions in which people can lead flourishing lives. People need good material conditions to lead a flourishing life; they need to have control over their lives; and people, communities, and countries need political voice (Sen, 1999). Governments can create conditions for good and equitable health through careful use of social and economic policy and regulation. Achievement of health equity will take action across the whole range of government supported by an international policy environment that values holistic social development as well as economic growth. Money, while by no means the whole solution, is critical. The minister of finance may have more influence over health equity than the minister of health, the global financial architecture more influence than international assistance for health care.

But it is not just government that must act. Where government lacks capacity or political will, there must be technical and financial support from outside, and a push from popular action. When people organize – come together and build their own organizations and movements – governments and policy-makers respond with social policies.

INEQUITY IN CONDITIONS OF DAILY LIVING

Of the 3 billion people who live in urban settings, about 1 billion live in slums. In most African countries, the majority of the urban population live in slums. In Kenya, for example, 71% of the urban population live in slums; in Ethiopia, 99%. It takes only 10-20 years for the urban population to double in many African countries (World Bank, 2006b).

Half of the rural population in Mozambique has to walk for longer than 30 minutes to get water; only 5% of the rural population have access to piped water (DHS, nd).

Around 126 million children aged 5-17 are working in hazardous conditions (UNICEF, nd,a).

In India, 86% of women and 83% of men employed in areas outside the agricultural sector are in informal employment (ILO, 2002).

In the African region, coverage for old-age income protection is lower than 10% of the labour force (ILO, nd).

Over 900 doctors and 2200 nurses trained in Ghana are working in high-income countries. Ghana has 0.92 nurse per 1000 population; the United Kingdom has over 13 times as many (WHO, 2006).

There will, of course, need to be a partnership with the health sector in both disease control programmes and the development of health systems. It is likely that paying attention to the social determinants of health, including health care, will make health services more effective. The health sector will also play a leadership and advocacy role in the development of policies to deal with the social determinants of health. But lack of health care is not the cause of the huge global burden of illness: water-borne diseases are not caused by lack of antibiotics but by dirty water, and by the political, social, and economic forces that fail to make clean water available to all; heart disease is caused not by a lack of coronary care units but by the lives people lead, which are shaped by the environments in which they live; obesity is not caused by moral failure on the part of individuals but by the excess availability of high-fat and high-sugar foods. The main action on social determinants of health must therefore come from outside the health sector.

Seeing health and its fair distribution as a marker of social and economic development has profound implications. Where policies – in whichever field of action – aim to improve well-being in the population, health is a measure of success of those policies. Health equity is a measure of the degree to which those policies are able to distribute well being fairly.

One set of the Commission's recommendations deals with the circumstances in which people are born, grow, live, work, and age. But people's lives are shaped by a wider set of forces: economics, social policies, and politics. These, too, must be addressed and much of the report and its recommendations do this.

We stated that a toxic combination of poor social policies, unfair economics, and bad politics is responsible for much of health inequity. In low-income countries and some poor communities in rich countries, this translates into material deprivation: lack of the material conditions for a decent life. No one who has experienced the slums that house 1 billion of the world's people, no one who has witnessed the lack of opportunities for economic livelihood of the world's rural poor, can doubt the importance of combating poverty. The toxic combination is also responsible for the social gradient in health in those who are above the level of material deprivation but still lack the other goods and services that are necessary for a flourishing life.

STRUCTURAL DRIVERS OF HEALTH INEQUITIES

The top fifth of the world's people in the richest countries enjoy 82% of the expanding export trade and 68% of foreign direct investment – the bottom fifth, barely more than 1% (UNDP, 1999).

In 1999, the developing world spent US$ 13 on debt repayment for every US$ 1 it received in grants (World Bank, 1999).

Of the population in the developed nations, 20% consume 86% of the world's goods (UNDP, 1998).

In 1997, the East Asian financial crisis was triggered by a reversal of capital flows of around US$ 105 billion, a relatively small amount in global terms, but equivalent to 10% of the combined gross domestic product (GDP) of the region. Similar shocks have since affected Russia and Brazil (ODI, 1999).

Since 1990, conflicts have directly killed 3.6 million people, (UNICEF, 2004). Sudan has 5.4 million internally displaced people, Colombia 3 million, Uganda 2 million, Congo 1.7 million, and Iraq 1.3 million (UNHCR, 2005).

Many countries spend more on the military than on health. Eritrea, an extreme example, spends 24% of GDP on the military and only 2% on health. Pakistan spends less on health and education combined than on the military (UNDP, 2007).

Each European cow attracts a subsidy of over US$ 2/day, greater than the daily income of half the world's population. These subsidies cost the European Union (EU) taxpayer about 2.5 billion per year. Half of this money is spent on export subsidies, which damage local markets in low-income countries (Oxfam, 2002).

BOX 3.1: INEQUITY AND INDIGENOUS PEOPLES – THE EFFECTS OF A TOXIC COMBINATION OF POLICIES

Indigenous People worldwide are in jeopardy of irrevocable loss of land, language, culture, and livelihood, without their consent or control – a permanent loss differing from immigrant populations where language and culture continue to be preserved in a country of origin. Indigenous Peoples are unique culturally, historically, ecologically, geographically, and politically by virtue of their ancestors' original and long-standing nationhood and their use of and occupancy of the land. Colonization has de-territorialized and has imposed social, political, and economic structures upon Indigenous Peoples without their consultation, consent, or choice. Indigenous

Peoples' lives continue to be governed by specific and particular laws and regulations that apply to no other members of civil states. Indigenous People continue to live on bounded or segregated lands and are often at the heart of jurisdictional divides between levels of government, particularly in areas concerning access to financial allocations, programmes, and services. As such, Indigenous Peoples have distinct status and specific needs relative to others. Indigenous Peoples' unique status must therefore be considered separately from generalized or more universal social exclusion discussions.

ECONOMIC GROWTH AND SOCIAL POLICIES

Wealth is important for health. The relation of national income to LEB is shown in Fig. 3.1 – the Preston curve (Deaton, 2003; Deaton, 2004). At low levels of national income there is a steep relation between income and LEB. This is consistent with the benefits of economic growth improving life chances and health. But there are two important caveats. First, at higher levels of income, above about US$ 5000 at purchasing power parity[2], there is little relation between national income and LEB. Second, there is great variation around the line. As described earlier, there are notable examples – Costa Rica, India (Kerala), Sri Lanka – of relatively poor countries and states achieving excellent health without the benefit of great national wealth. Among the lessons from those countries is the importance of good social policy emphasizing education, particularly for girls and women.

Economic growth gives the opportunity to provide resources to invest in improvement of people's lives. But growth per se, without appropriate social policies, brings no benefit to health. Economist Angus Deaton warns, "Economic growth is much to be desired because it relieves the grinding material poverty of much of the world's population. But economic growth, by itself, will not be enough to improve population health, at least in any acceptable time. ... As far as health is concerned, the market, by itself, is not a substitute for collective action" (Deaton, 2006a; Deaton, 2006b). Growth with equitable distribution of benefits across populations is the key. Collective action may involve building social institutions and adopting regulations that both deliver people's needs for housing, education, food, employment protection, environmental protection and remediation, and social security, and correct for market failure (Stiglitz, 2006).

ECONOMIC GROWTH AND ITS DISTRIBUTION

For any country – arguably most pressingly for countries with low incomes – economic growth brings the possibility of great benefit. But there has, to date, already been enormous global growth in wealth, technology, and living standards. The issue for the world is not whether it needs further economic growth in order to relieve poverty and achieve the MDGs. To do that, there is wealth and income in abundance. The question is how it is distributed and used.

First, the benefits of economic growth over the last 25 years – a period of rapid globalization – have been shared most unequally among countries. Table 3.1 shows that in 1980 the richest countries, containing 10% of the world's population, had gross national income 60 times that of the poorest countries, containing 10% of the world's population. By 2005 this ratio had increased to 122.

Table 3.1

Increasing income inequality among countries

	Gross national income per capita in nominal US$		
Year	Richest countries*	Poorest countries*	Ratio
1980	US$ 11 840	US$ 196	60
2000	US$ 31 522	US$ 274	115
2005	US$ 40 730	US$ 334	122

*Containing 10% of the world's population. Data derived from Table 1 in the World Bank's World Development Reports for 1982, 2002, and 2007, respectively, and market exchange rates in the relevant years. The ratios among these nominal US$ figures are comparable across years.

Reprinted, with permission of the publisher, from Pogge (2008).

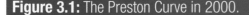

Figure 3.1: The Preston Curve in 2000.

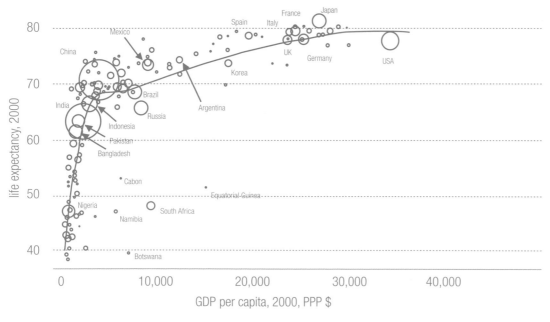

Circles have a diameter proportional to population size. GDP per capita is in purchasing power parity (PPP) dollars.

[2]A purchasing power parity exchange rate equalizes the purchasing power of different currencies in their home countries for a given basket of goods.

Second, international flows of aid – grossly inadequate in themselves, and well below the levels promised by Organization for Economic Cooperation and Development (OECD) donor countries in 1970 – are dwarfed by the scale of many poor countries' debt repayment obligations (UNDESA, 2006). The result is that, in many cases, there is a net financial outflow from poorer to richer countries – an alarming state of affairs. These financial flows are themselves small in comparison with the massive volumes of capital flowing through global financial markets – at a rate of US$ 3.2 trillion per day in 2007 (HIFX, 2007) – with enormous potential, through capital flight, to disrupt the socioeconomic development of low- and middle-income countries.

It has been calculated that the annual cost of bringing the 40% of the world's population currently below the US$ 2/day line up to it would be US$ 300 billion – less than 1% of the gross national income of the high-income countries (Pogge, 2008). We will make the point throughout this report that money alone is not the central point. More important is the way the money is used for fair distribution of goods and services and building institutions within low-income countries. But this simple calculation shows that there is no global shortage of money.

Third, income inequality applies not only between but also within countries. The trend over the last 15 years has been for the poorest quintile of the population in many countries to have a declining share in national consumption (MDG Report, 2007). There has been a vigorous debate as to whether income inequality itself is a major contributor to the level of health of a country (Wilkinson, 1996; Deaton, 2003). However,

income inequality is one marker of the unequal distribution of goods and services. There is therefore strong empirical justification for a concern with growing income inequalities. Governments have the power to reduce the effects of pre-tax income inequality. Fig. 3.2 shows, for a number of high-income countries, the effects of policy on poverty (Lundberg et al, 2007). It takes a relative definition of poverty as below 60% of median income and shows that in Nordic countries fiscal policy leads to a much lower prevalence of poverty than in the United Kingdom or the United States. Policy matters.

For countries at lower levels of national income, it should be obvious that greater economic growth will have a much smaller effect on income poverty the greater the income inequalities. The United Nations Development Programme (UNDP) has calculated that in Kenya, for example, at current economic growth rates, and with the present level of income inequality, the median family in poverty would not cross the poverty line until 2030. Doubling the share of income growth enjoyed by the poor means that reduction in poverty would happen by 2013. In other words, the MDG for reduction in poverty implies attention to the distribution of income not just economic growth.

Figure 3.2: Proportion relatively poor pre- and post-welfare state redistribution, various countries.

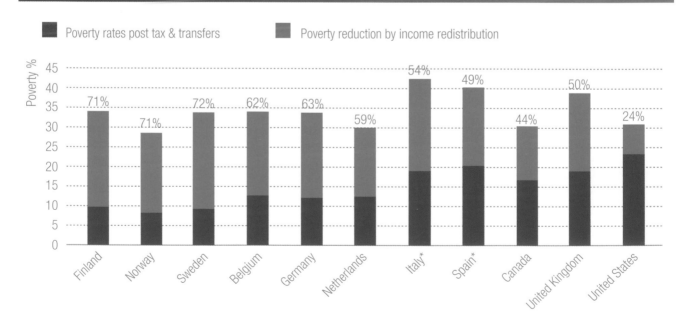

Poverty threshold = 60% of median equivalent disposable income.
*For these countries, the poverty threshold before redistribution is calculated on incomes net income taxes.
Data from the Luxembourg Income Study.
Reprinted, with permission of the authors, from Lundberg et al. (2007) citing Ritakallio & Fritzell (2004).

RETURNS FROM INVESTING IN HEALTH

Just as economic growth, and its distribution, is vitally important for health, investment in health and its determinants is an important strategy for boosting economic development (CMH, 2001). Raising the health status of people lower down the social hierarchy even to the population median level of health would have a major impact on overall health and should improve a nation's productivity (Box 3.2) (Health Disparities Task Group, 2004; Mackenbach, Meerding & Kunst, 2007).

BOX 3.2: INVESTING FOR HEALTH AND ECONOMIC RETURN, CANADA

A study in Canada shows that reducing health disparities has the potential for major economic benefits resulting from a reduction both in health-care needs and in the costs of lost productivity.

Health-care spending in Canada is about 120 billion Canadian dollars per year (with the institutionalized population accounting for 26 billion Canadian dollars and the household population accounting for 94 billion Canadian dollars). The lowest income quintile of the household population accounts for approximately 31% of the 94 billion Canadian dollars, approximately double the utilization of the highest-income quintile. The study reported that if the health status and utilization patterns of those in the lower-income groups equalled those with middle income, significant savings on health-care costs could be possible.

In addition, the study reported that better health enables more people to participate in the economy. Reducing the costs of lost productivity by only 10-20% could add billions of dollars to the economy.

Source: Health Disparities Task Group, 2004

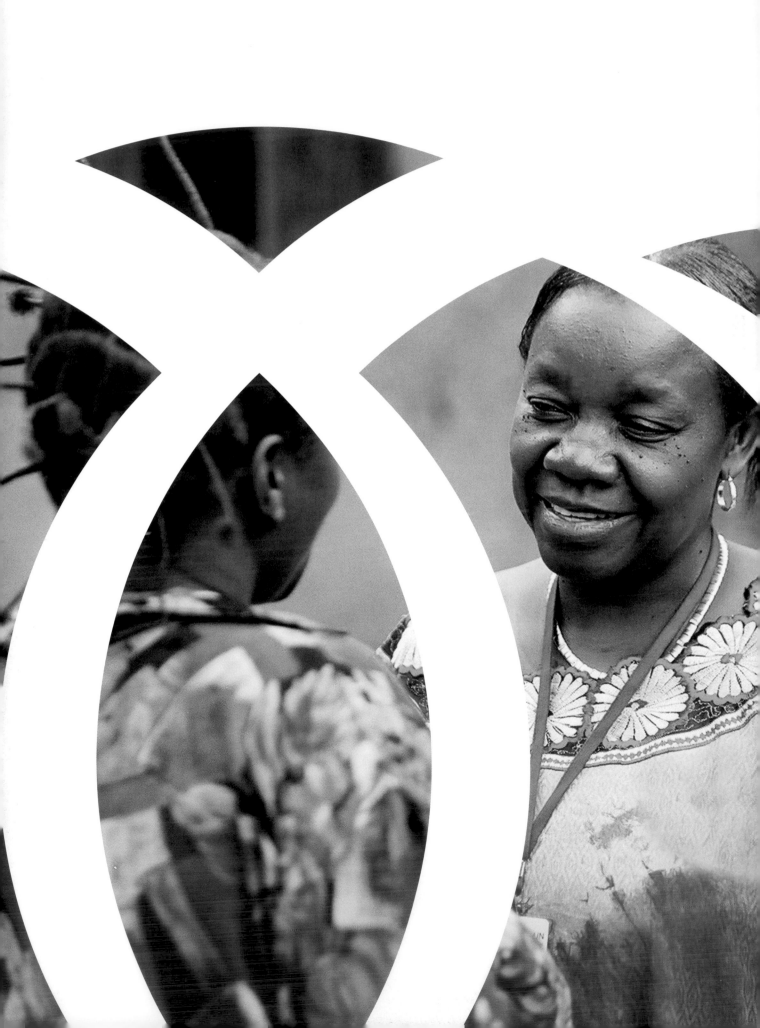

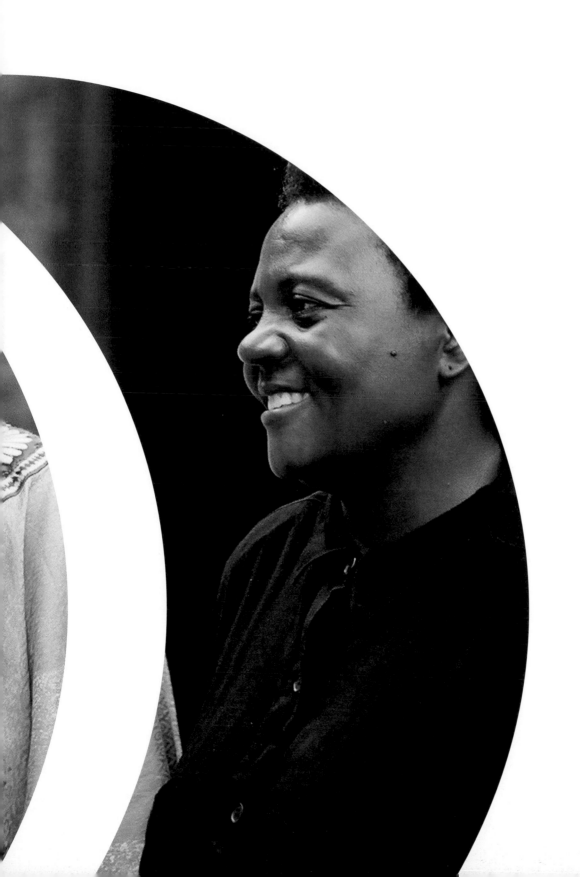

CHAPTER 4
The nature of evidence and action

ASSEMBLING THE EVIDENCE

The values that inform the Commission's approach to its task were set out in Part 1: the importance of health and social justice and the view that all individuals should be treated with equal dignity. For policy, however important an ethical imperative, values alone are insufficient. There needs to be evidence on what can be done and what is likely to work in practice to improve health and reduce health inequities.

An early decision was necessary on what constituted evidence. In the medical care arena the hierarchy of evidence is fairly clear. Does a new medical intervention work better than existing therapies? Subject it to the benchmark randomized controlled trial, which provides an unbiased estimate of effects under carefully controlled conditions.

When it comes to the social determinants of health there are two linked problems that make this an unrealistic ideal: the nature of the intervention and the lack of evidence in areas where it matters. In our judgement, as set out in this report, global and national economic arrangements and social policies are critical to people's living and working conditions and hence to health equity. For many of these areas it is difficult to see how randomized controlled trials could be possible. Countries do not lend themselves to randomization. Interventions such as the development and implementation of laws that protect gender equity, for instance, cannot be randomized across countries. Had the Commission made a decision to rely on evidence solely from well-controlled experiments, this would be a short report with only biomedical evidence-based recommendations and the conclusion that more research is needed. Equity and social justice, even health, would not have progressed much.

More research is needed. Although given the nature of the interventions that this report considers in Parts 3-5, little of it will look like a medical randomized controlled trial. But this lack cannot be a barrier to making judgements with the current evidence. The Commission took a broader view of what constituted evidence (Kelly et al., 2006). In this report the reader will find evidence that comes from observational studies (including natural experiments and cross-country studies), case studies, and field visits, from expert and lay knowledge, and from community intervention trials where available. While the Commission endeavoured to assemble globally representative evidence, there are inevitably gaps, particularly in low- and middle-income countries, possibly because the information does not exist, was not published in an accessible manner, or is not available in English, which has been the working language of the Commission.

THE COMMISSION'S CONCEPTUAL FRAMEWORK

Strengthening health equity – globally and within countries – means going beyond contemporary concentration on the immediate causes of disease. More than any other global health endeavour, the Commission focuses on the 'causes of the causes' – the fundamental global and national structures of social hierarchy and the socially determined conditions these create in which people grow, live, work, and age. Fig. 4.1 shows the conceptual framework that was developed for the Commission (Solar & Irwin, 2007). This framework suggests that interventions can be aimed at taking action on:

The circumstances of daily life:

- differential exposures to disease-causing influences in early life, the social and physical environments, and work, associated with social stratification. Depending on the nature of these influences, different groups will have different experiences of material conditions, psychosocial support, and behavioural options, which make them more or less vulnerable to poor health;

- health-care responses to health promotion, disease prevention, and treatment of illness;

And the structural drivers:

- the nature and degree of social stratification in society – the magnitude of inequity along the dimensions listed;

- biases, norms, and values within society;

- global and national economic and social policy;

- processes of governance at the global, national, and local level.

By their nature many of the social determinants considered by the Commission are relatively distant, spatially and temporally, from individuals and health experience. This is challenging, both conceptually and empirically, when trying to attribute causality and demonstrate effectiveness of action on health equity. In choosing the range of social determinants on which to focus, the Commission's selection was based on coherence in the global evidence base – that is, a mixture of conceptual plausibility, availability of supporting empirical evidence, and consistency of relationship between and among populations – and the demonstration that these determinants were amenable to intervention. In addition, a few determinants were identified that, while they had a strong plausible relationship with health inequities, still lacked evidence on what could be done to effect change.

On this basis, and underpinned by the conceptual framework, the knowledge work stream of the Commission was established primarily around nine Knowledge Networks whose themes incorporated global issues, health systems level issues, and a lifecourse approach to health. The Knowledge Networks focused on early child development (ECD) (ECDKN), employment conditions (ECOMNET), urban settings (KNUS), social exclusion (SEKN), women and gender equity (WGEKN), globalization (GKN), health systems (HSKN), priority public health conditions (PPHCKN), and measurement and evidence (MEKN). Gender issues have been systematically considered in each of the other themes. Other issues including food and nutrition, rural factors, violence and crime, and climate change did not have a dedicated Knowledge Network but are recognized as important factors for health equity. The Commission deals with these in subsequent chapters, providing some general recommendations but without outlining the more specific steps of exactly how action could happen.

JUDGING THE EVIDENCE

Formulating the Commission's recommendations about what should be done in order to improve global health equity has involved balancing the use of different types of evidence, considering the scope and completeness of the evidence, and assessing the degree to which action in these social determinants of health has been shown to be possible and effective. The recommendations made by the Commission are: a) underpinned by an aetiological conceptual framework, b) supported by a vast global evidence base that demonstrates an impact of action on these social determinants of health and health inequities (effectiveness), c) supported by evidence on feasibility of implementation in different scenarios, and d) supported by evidence showing consistency of effects of action in different population groups and countries with different levels of national economic development.

THE COMMISSION'S KEY AREAS FOR ACTION AND RECOMMENDATIONS

Globally it is now understood better than at any moment in history how social factors affect health and health equity. While information is always partial and the need for better evidence remains, we have the knowledge to guide effective action. By linking our understanding of poverty and the social gradient, we now assert the common issues underlying health inequity. By recognizing the nature and scale of both non-

communicable and communicable diseases, we demonstrate the inextricable linkages between countries, rich and poor. Action is needed on the determinants of health – from structural conditions of society to the daily conditions in which people grow, live, and work at all levels from global to local, across government and inclusive of all stakeholders from civil society and the private sector.

As we have pursued our work we have become convinced that it is possible to close the health gap in a generation. It will take a huge effort but it can be done. The chapters that follow in Parts 3-5 show that there is urgent need for change – in how we understand the causes of health inequities, in the way we accept and use different types of evidence, in the way we work together, and in the different types of action that is taken to tackle global- and national-level health inequities. Action to effect these interventions will be at global, national, local, and individual levels.

In Chapter 1 we stated that the Commission's analysis leads to three principles of action:

1. Improve the conditions of daily life – the circumstances in which people are born, grow, live, work, and age.

2. Tackle the inequitable distribution of power, money, and resources – the structural drivers of those conditions of daily life – globally, nationally, and locally.

3. Measure the problem, evaluate action, expand the knowledge base, develop a workforce that is trained in the social determinants of health, and raise public awareness about the social determinants of health.

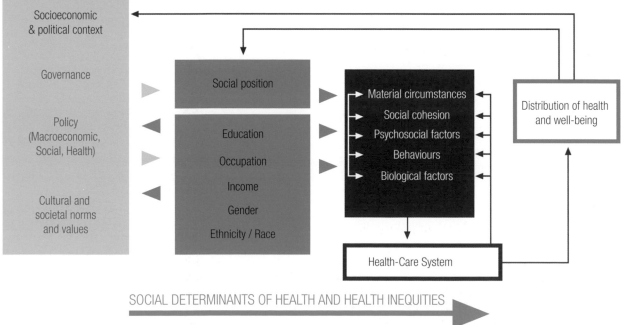

Figure 4.1 Commission on Social Determinants of Health conceptual framework.

Socioeconomic & political context

Governance

Policy (Macroeconomic, Social, Health)

Cultural and societal norms and values

Social position

Education
Occupation
Income
Gender
Ethnicity / Race

Material circumstances
Social cohesion
Psychosocial factors
Behaviours
Biological factors

Distribution of health and well-being

Health-Care System

SOCIAL DETERMINANTS OF HEALTH AND HEALTH INEQUITIES

Source: Amended from Solar & Irwin, 2007

The three principles of action identified by the Commission are embodied in the three overarching recommendations below. If action is taken in accordance with these recommendations, and with the more detailed recommendations in subsequent chapters, it will be possible to achieve a more equitable realization of the rights to the conditions necessary to achieve the highest attainable standard of health.

THE COMMISSION'S OVERARCHING RECOMMENDATIONS

1. Improve Daily Living Conditions

Improve the well-being of girls and women and the circumstances in which their children are born, put major emphasis on early child development and education for girls and boys, improve living and working conditions and create social protection policy supportive of all, and create conditions for a flourishing older life. Policies to achieve these goals will involve civil society, governments, and global institutions.

2. Tackle the Inequitable Distribution of Power, Money, and Resources

In order to address health inequities, and inequitable conditions of daily living, it is necessary to address inequities – such as those between men and women – in the way society is organized. This requires a strong public sector that is committed, capable, and adequately financed. To achieve that requires more than strengthened government – it requires strengthened governance: legitimacy, space, and support for civil society, for an accountable private sector, and for people across society to agree public interests and reinvest in the value of collective action. In a globalized world, the need for governance dedicated to equity applies equally from the community level to global institutions.

3. Measure and Understand the Problem and Assess the Impact of Action

Acknowledging that there is a problem, and ensuring that health inequity is measured – within countries and globally – is a vital platform for action. National governments and international organizations, supported by WHO, should set up national and global health equity surveillance systems for routine monitoring of health inequity and the social determinants of health and should evaluate the health equity impact of policy and action. Creating the organizational space and capacity to act effectively on health inequity requires investment in training of policy-makers and health practitioners and public understanding of social determinants of health. It also requires a stronger focus on social determinants in public health research.

Parts 3-5 of the report are structured according to these three principles. While the Commission's recommendations as a whole are aimed at addressing both the conditions of daily living and the structural drivers that shape the distribution of these, within each of the thematic chapters (5-16 within Parts 3-5), recommendations are made relating to action that tackles the structural drivers and immediate causes of inequities in these themes. The recommendations range in character from governance and policy matters to community action – a combination of top-down and bottom-up approaches at the global, regional, national, and sub-national levels.

IMPLICATIONS FOR DIFFERENT ACTORS

While the Commission advocates strongly the central role of government and the public sector in taking action on the social determinants of health for health equity, it also recognizes the plurality of actors across the field – global institutions and agencies, governments themselves (national and local), civil society, research and academic communities, and the private sector. Each of these actors should be able to see themselves clearly in the chapters that follow in Parts 3-5, and in the implications of the recommendations for action. An overview of the key areas for action and recommendations for each actor is given below, pointing towards the specific recommendations that can be found in each of the subsequent thematic chapters.

Multilateral agencies

An overarching Commission recommendation is the need for intersectoral coherence – in policy-making and action – to enhance effective action on the social determinants of health and achieve improvements in health equity. Multilateral specialist and financing agencies can do much to strengthen their collective impact on the social determinants of health and health equity, including:

- *Coherent global monitoring and action:* Adopt health equity as a fundamental shared goal, and use a common global framework of indicators to monitor development progress; collaborate in multi-agency thematic working groups for coherent social determinants of health action.

- *Coherent and accountable financing:* Ensure that increases in aid and debt relief support coherent social determinants of health policy-making and action among recipient governments, using health equity and social determinants of health performance indicators as core conditions of recipient accountability.

- *Improved participation of UN Member States in global governance:* Support equitable participation of Member States and other stakeholders in global policy-making fora.

WHO

WHO is the mandated leader in global health. It is time that WHO's leadership role is enhanced through the agenda for action on the social determinants of health and global health equity. This involves a range of actions, including:

- *Policy coherence globally and nationally:* Adopt a stewardship role supporting social determinants of health capacity-building and policy coherence across partner agencies in the multilateral system; strengthen technical capacity globally and among Member States for representation of public health in all major multilateral fora; and support Member States in developing mechanisms for coherent policy and ISA for social determinants of health.

- *Measurement and evaluation:* Support goal setting on health equity and monitor progress on health equity between and within countries as a core developmental objective through a global health equity surveillance system; support the establishment of national health equity surveillance systems in Member States, and build necessary technical capacities in countries; support Member States in development and use of health equity impact assessment tools and other health equity-related tools such as a national equity gauge; and convene a global meeting as part of a periodic review of the global situation.

- *Enhancing WHO capacity:* Build internal social determinants of health capacity across WHO, from headquarters, through the Regional Offices, to Country Programmes.

National and local government

Underpinning action on the social determinants of health and health equity is an empowered public sector, based on principles of justice, participation, and intersectoral collaboration. This will require strengthening of the core functions of government and public institutions, nationally and sub-nationally, particularly in relation to policy coherence, participatory governance, planning, regulation development and enforcement, and standard setting. It also depends on strong leadership and stewardship from the ministry of health, supported by WHO. Government actions include:

- *Policy coherence across government:* Place responsibility for action on health and health equity at the highest level of government, and ensure its coherent consideration across all ministerial and departmental policy-making.

- *Strengthening action for equity:* Commit to progressive building of universal health-care services; establish a central gender unit to promote gender equity across government policy-making; improve rural livelihoods, infrastructure investment, and services; upgrade slums and strengthen locally participatory health urban planning; invest in full employment and decent labour policy and programmes; invest in ECD; build towards universal provision in vital social determinants of health services and programmes regardless of ability to pay, supported by a universal programme of social protection; and establish a national framework for regulatory control over health-damaging commodities.

- *Finance:* Streamline incoming international finance (aid, debt relief) through a social determinants of health action framework, with transparent accountability; strengthen revenue through improved progressive domestic taxation; and collaborate with other Member States in the development of regional and/or global proposals for new sources of international public finance.

- *Measurement, evaluation, and training:* Build towards universal birth registration; set cross-government performance indicators for health equity through the establishment of a national health equity surveillance system; build capacity to use health equity impact assessment as a standard protocol in all major policy-making; ensure training of practitioners and policy-makers on the social determinants of health; and raise public awareness about the social determinants of health.

Civil society

Being included in the society in which one lives is vital to the material, psychosocial, and political aspects of empowerment that underpin social well-being and equitable health. As community members, grassroots advocates, service and programme providers, and performance monitors, civil society actors from the global to the local level constitute a vital bridge between policies and plans and the reality of change and improvement in the lives of all. Helping to organize and promote diverse voices across different communities, civil society can be a powerful champion of health equity. Many of the actions listed above will be, at least in part, the result of pressure and encouragement from civil society; many of the milestones towards health equity in a generation will be marked – achieved or missed – by the attentive observation of civil society actors. Civil society can play an important role in action on the social determinants of health through:

- *Participation in policy, planning, programmes, and evaluation:* Participate in social determinants of health policy-making, planning, programme delivery, and evaluation from the global level, through national intersectoral fora, to the local level of needs assessments, service delivery, and support, and monitor service quality, equity, and impact.

- *Monitoring performance:* Monitor, and report and campaign on, specific social determinants of health, such as upgrading of and services in slums, formal and non-formal employment conditions, child labour, indigenous rights, gender equity, health and education services, corporate activities, trade agreements, and environmental protection.

Private sector

The private sector has a profound impact on health and well-being. Where the Commission reasserts the vital role of public sector leadership in acting for health equity, this does not imply a relegation of the importance of private sector activities. It does, though, imply the need for recognition of potentially adverse impacts, and the need for responsibility in regulation with regard to those impacts. Alongside controlling undesirable effects on health and health equity, the vitality of the private sector has much to offer that could enhance health and well-being. Actions include:

- *Strengthening accountability:* Recognize and respond accountably to international agreements, standards, and codes of employment practice; ensure employment and working conditions are fair for men and women; reduce and eradicate child labour, and ensure compliance with occupational health and safety standards; support educational and vocational training opportunities as part of employment conditions, with special emphasis on opportunities for women; and ensure private sector activities and services (such as production and patenting of life-saving medicines, provision of health insurance schemes) contribute to and do not undermine health equity.

- *Investing in research:* Commit to research and development in treatment for neglected diseases and diseases of poverty, and share knowledge in areas (such as pharmaceuticals patents) with life-saving potential.

Research institutions

Knowledge – of what the health situation is, globally, regionally, nationally, and locally; of what can be done about that situation; and of what works effectively to alter health inequity through the social determinants of health – is at the heart of the Commission and underpins all its recommendations. Research is needed. But more than simply academic exercises, research is needed to generate new understanding and to disseminate that understanding in practical accessible ways to all the partners listed above. Research on and knowledge of the social determinants of health and ways to act for health equity will rely on continuing commitments among academics and practitioners, but it will rely on new methodologies too – recognizing and utilizing a range of types of evidence, recognizing gender bias in research processes, and recognizing the added value of globally expanded knowledge networks and communities. Actions in this field of actors include:

- *Generating and disseminating evidence on the social determinants of health:* Ensure research funding is allocated to social determinants of health work; support the global health observatory and multilateral, national, and local cross-sectoral working through development and testing of social determinants of health indicators and intervention impact evaluation; establish and expand virtual networks and clearing houses organized on the principles of open access, managed to enhance accessibility from sites in all high-, middle-, and low-income settings; contribute to reversal of the brain drain from low- and middle-income countries; and address and remove gender biases in research teams, proposals, designs, practices, and reports.

CONTEXTUALIZING THE RECOMMENDATIONS

A central challenge for the Commission arises from the pervasive nature of health inequities. To be sure, they are bigger in scale in some countries than in others but they are remarkably widespread. As will be seen from the subsequent chapters in Parts 3-5, there are general principles that will apply in all countries. There will need to be differences in policies for low- and middle-income countries. The chapters go some way to dealing with this issue. Experience suggests that, although there are general principles, the precise nature of policy solutions needs to be worked out in national and local context.

Changes are required in the global economic environment if the Commission's proposals are to be beneficial to health in the poorest countries and thus to global health equity. It will require action to alleviate external economic pressures, expand national policy space to act on health equity, redress public sector financial constraints, improve national infrastructure and human capacity, and solidify and upgrade women's educational gains. Implementing the Commission's recommendations requires changes in the operation of the global economy to prevent market pressures and international commitments from impeding implementation or giving rise to unintended adverse effects.

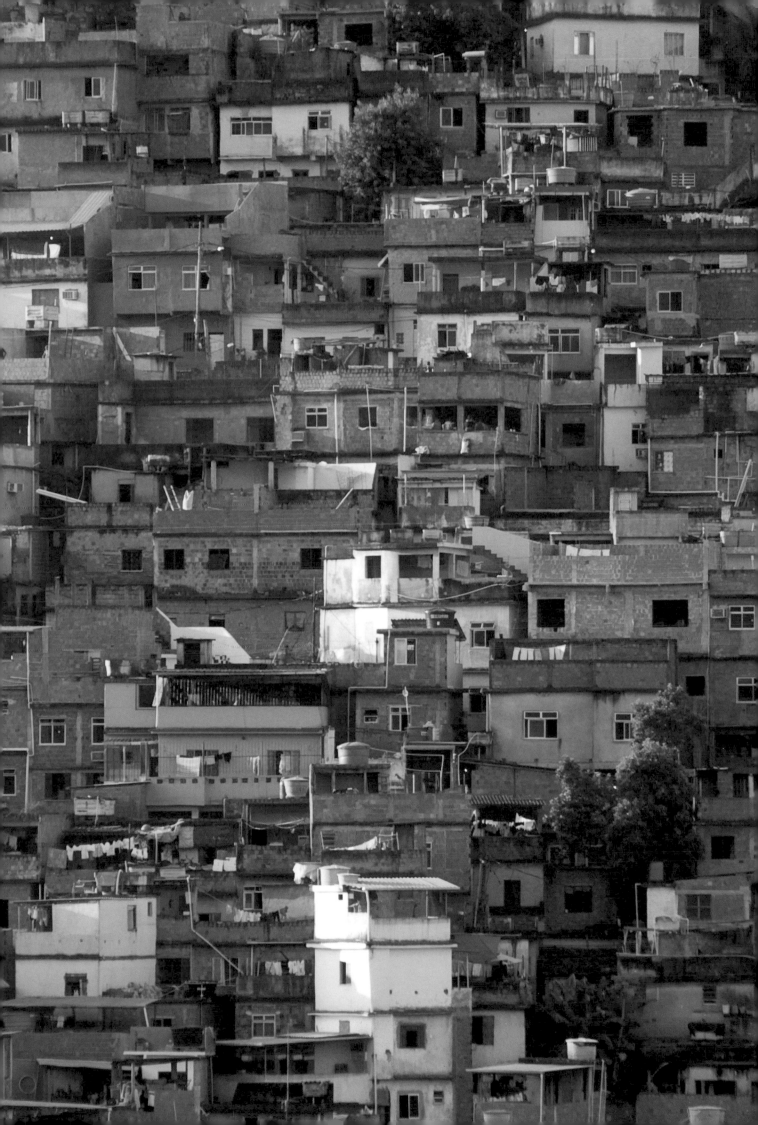

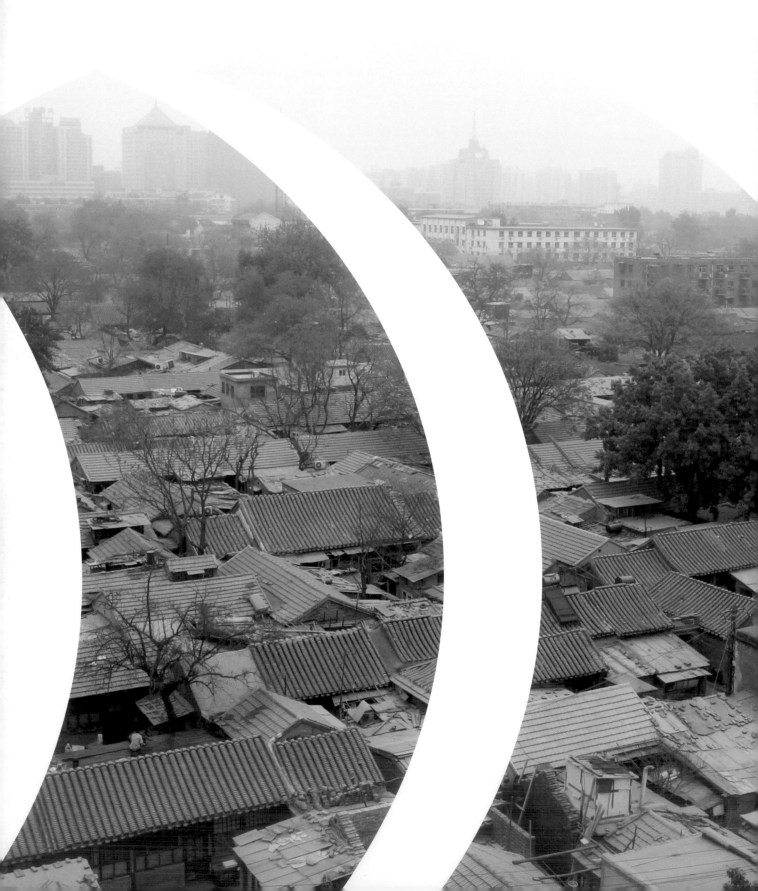

IMPROVE DAILY LIVING CONDITIONS

The first of the Commission's three principles of action is:

Improve the conditions of daily life – the circumstances in which people are born, grow, live, work, and age.

Inequities in how society is organized mean that freedom to lead a flourishing life and to enjoy good health is unequally distributed between and within societies. This inequity is seen in the conditions of early childhood and schooling, the nature of employment and working conditions, the physical form of the built environment, and the quality of the natural environment in which people reside. Depending on the nature of these environments, different groups will have different experiences of material conditions, psychosocial influences, and behavioural options that make them more or less vulnerable to poor health. Social stratification likewise determines differential access to and utilization of health care, with consequences for the inequitable promotion of health and well-being, disease prevention, and illness recovery and survival.

Implicit in the work of the Commission is a lifecourse perspective on how the social determinants of health operate at every level of development – pregnancy and childbirth, early childhood, childhood, adolescence, and adulthood – both as an immediate influence on health and to provide the basis for health or illness later in life.

The following chapters, Chapters 5–9, focus on the conditions of daily life and make recommendations for action, sequentially, relating to the conditions of early life and through the school years, the social and physical environment with a focus on cities, and the nature of both employment and working conditions. The nature of social protection, and in particular income protection, is considered here as an essential resource for daily living. The final chapter in Part 3 relates to the health-care system.

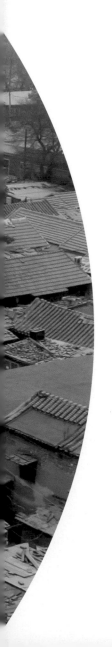

CHAPTER 5
Equity from the start

"Each one of you is your own person, endowed with rights, worthy of respect and dignity. Each one of you deserves to have the best possible start in life, to complete a basic education of the highest quality, to be allowed to develop your full potential and provided the opportunities for meaningful participation in your communities."

Nelson Mandela and Graça Machel (UNICEF, 2000)

EARLY CHILD DEVELOPMENT AND EDUCATION – POWERFUL EQUALIZERS

Worldwide, 10 million children die each year before their fifth birthday (Black, Morris & Bryce, 2003). The vast majority of these deaths occur among children born in low- or middle-income countries, and within these countries, among children of more disadvantaged households and communities (Houweling, 2007). Even in high-income countries such as the United Kingdom, infant mortality is higher among disadvantaged groups (Department of Health, 2007). There is an urgent need to address these mortality inequities. Equally important, at least 200 million children are not achieving their full developmental potential, with huge implications for their health and for society at large (Grantham-McGregor et al., 2007). The figure of 200 million is certainly an underestimate, as it is based on a definition of poverty at US$ 1/day, whereas there is a stepwise effect of wealth on child development (ECDKN, 2007a). Experiences in early childhood (defined as prenatal development to 8 years of age), and in early and later education, lay critical foundations for the entire lifecourse (ECDKN, 2007a). It is better for the individual child, and for society – in rich and poor countries alike – to provide a positive start, rather than having to resort to remedial action later on. Building on the child survival agenda, governments can make major and sustained improvement in population health and development, while fulfilling their obligations under the UN Convention on the Rights of the Child, by using a more comprehensive approach to the early years of life (ECDKN, 2007a).

A more comprehensive approach to the early years in life

The science of ECD shows that brain development is highly sensitive to external influences in early childhood, starting in utero, with lifelong effects. The conditions to which children are exposed, including the quality of relationships and language environment, literally 'sculpt' the developing brain (Mustard, 2007). Raising healthy children means stimulating their physical, language/cognitive, and social/emotional development (ECDKN, 2007a). Healthy development during the early years provides the essential building blocks that enable people to lead a flourishing life in many domains, including social, emotional, cognitive, and physical well-being (ECDKN, 2007a).

Education, preschool and beyond, also fundamentally shapes children's lifelong trajectories and opportunities for health. Yet despite recent progress, there are an estimated 75 million children of primary-school age not in school (UIS, 2008). Educational attainment is linked to improved health outcomes, partly through its effects on adult income, employment, and living conditions (Ross & Wu, 1995; Cutler & Lleras-Muney, 2006; Bloom, 2007). There are strong intergenerational effects – educational attainment of mothers is a determinant of child health, survival, and educational attainment (Caldwell, 1986; Cleland & Van Ginneken, 1988).

Many challenges in adult society have their roots in the early years of life, including major public health problems such as obesity, heart disease, and mental health problems. Experiences in early childhood are also related to criminality, problems in literacy and numeracy, and economic participation (ECDKN, 2007a).

Social inequities in early life contribute to inequities in health later on, through ECD and educational attainment. Children from disadvantaged backgrounds are more likely to do poorly in school and subsequently, as adults, are more likely have lower incomes and higher fertility rates and be less empowered to provide good health care, nutrition, and stimulation to their own children, thus contributing to the intergenerational transmission of disadvantage (Grantham-McGregor et al., 2007). The seeds of adult gender inequity are also sown in early childhood. Gender socialization and gender biases in the early years of life have impacts on child development, particularly among girls. Early gender inequity, when reinforced by power relations, biased norms, and day-to-day experiences, go on to have a profound impact on adult gender inequity (ECDKN, 2007a).

Much of child survival and development depends on factors discussed in other chapters of this report. In the early years, the health-care system has a pivotal role to play (ECDKN, 2007a). Mothers and children need a continuum of care from pre-pregnancy, through pregnancy and childbirth, to the early days and years of life (WHO, 2005b) (see Chapter 9: *Universal Health Care*). Children need to be registered at birth (see Chapter 16: *The Social Determinants of Health: Monitoring, Research, and Training*). They need safe and healthy environments – good-quality housing, clean water and sanitation facilities, safe neighbourhoods, and protection against violence (see Chapter 6: *Healthy Places Healthy People*). Good nutrition is crucial and begins in utero with adequately nourished mothers, underlining the importance of taking a lifecourse perspective in tackling health inequities (ECDKN, 2007b). It is important to support the initiation of breastfeeding within the first hour of life, skin to skin contact immediately after birth, exclusive breastfeeding in the first 6 months of life, and continued breastfeeding through the second year of life, as is ensuring the availability of and access to healthy diets for infants and young children through improving food security (PPHCKN, 2007a; Black et al., 2008; Victora et al., 2008).

More distally, child survival and development depend on how well and how equitably societies, governments, and international agencies organize their affairs (see Chapters 10 and 14: *Health Equity in All Policies, Systems, and Programmes; Political Empowerment – Inclusion and Voice*). Gender equity, through maternal education, income, and empowerment, plays an important role in child survival and development (see Chapter 13: *Gender Equity*). Children benefit when national governments adopt family-friendly social protection policies that allow an adequate income for all (see Chapter 8: *Social Protection Across the Lifecourse*) and allow parents and caregivers to balance their home and work life (see Chapter 7: *Fair Employment and Decent Work*). Political leaders, nationally and internationally, should play a key role in averting acute threats to the development of young children, including war and violence, child labour, and abuse (WHO, 2005a). Yet global inequities in power influence the ability of poor countries in particular to enact policies that are optimal for child development (ECDKN, 2007a) (see Chapters 11, 12, and 15: *Fair Financing; Market Responsibility; Good Global Governance*).

Children need supporting, nurturing, caring, and responsive living environments. And they need opportunities to explore their world, to play, and to learn how to speak and listen to others. Schools, as part of the environment that contributes to children's development, have a vital role to play in building children's capabilities and, if they are truly inclusive, in achieving health equity. Well-designed ECD programmes can help to smooth the transition of children to primary school, with benefits for subsequent schooling (UNECSO, 2006b).

Creating the conditions for all children to thrive requires coherent policy-making across sectors. Parents and caregivers can do a lot, but support is needed from government, civil society organizations, and the wider community. The neglect of children worldwide has occurred largely in the watch of governments. Civil society organizations therefore have an important role to play in advocating and improving the conditions for healthy child development.

While environments strongly influence ECD, children are social actors who shape, and are shaped by, their environment (ECDKN, 2007b). The appreciation of the relational nature of the child and the environment has implications for action and research, with the need to recognize the importance of giving children greater voice and agency (Landon Pearson Resource Centre for the Study of Childhood and Children's Rights, 2007).

Early child development: a powerful equalizer

Investments in ECD are one of the most powerful that countries can make – in terms of reducing the escalating chronic disease burden in adults, reducing costs for judicial and prison systems, and enabling more children to grow into healthy adults who can make a positive contribution to society, socially and economically (ECDKN, 2007a; Engle et al., 2007; Schweinhart, Barnes & Weikart, 1993; Schweinhart, 2004; Lynch, 2004). Investment in ECD can also be a powerful equalizer, with interventions having the largest effects on the most deprived children (Scott-McDonald, 2002; Young, 2002;

Engle et al., 2007). If governments in rich and poor societies were to act while children were young by implementing quality ECD programmes and services as part of their broader development plans, these investments would pay for themselves many times over (Schweinhart, Barnes & Weikart, 1993; Schweinhart, 2004; Lynch, 2004). Unfortunately, most investment calculus in health and other sectors discounts such future benefits and values disproportionately those benefits seen in the immediate to short term.

Reducing health inequities within a generation requires a new way of thinking about child development. An approach is needed that embraces a more comprehensive understanding of the development of young children, including not just physical survival but also social/emotional and language/cognitive development. Recognizing the role of ECD and education offers huge potential to reduce health inequities within a generation. It provides a strong imperative for action early in life, and to act now. Inaction has detrimental effects that can last more than a lifetime.

ACTION TOWARDS A MORE EQUITABLE START IN LIFE

The Commission argues that a comprehensive approach to child development, encompassing not just child survival and physical development but also social/emotional and language/cognitive development, needs to be at the top of the policy agenda. This requires commitment, leadership, and policy coherence at the international and national level. It also requires a comprehensive package of ECD interventions for all children worldwide.

Changing the mindset

The Commission recommends that:

5.1. **WHO and UN Children's Fund (UNICEF) set up an interagency mechanism to ensure policy coherence for early child development such that, across agencies, a comprehensive approach to early child development is acted on (see Rec 15.2; 16.8).**

The development of young children is influenced by actions across a broad range of sectors, including health, nutrition, education, labour, and water and sanitation. Similarly, many players within and outside the UN system have a bearing on ECD. These include UNDP, Office of the UN High Commissioner for Refugees (UNHCR), UNICEF, UN Population Fund (UNFPA), World Food Programme (WFP), UN Human Settlements Programme (UN-HABITAT), International Labour organization (ILO), the Food and Agriculture Organization of the UN (FAO), UN Educational, Scientific, and Cultural Organization (UNESCO), WHO, Joint UN Programme on HIV/AIDS (UNAIDS), the World Bank, International Monetary Fund (IMF), and International Organization for Migration (IOM), as well as civil society

---

EQUITY FROM THE START : ACTION AREA 5.1

Commit to and implement a comprehensive approach to early life, building on existing child survival programmes and extending interventions in early life to include social/emotional and language/cognitive development.

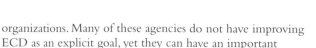

organizations. Many of these agencies do not have improving ECD as an explicit goal, yet they can have an important bearing on it, positively or negatively.

An interagency mechanism should be set up to ensure a comprehensive, coherent approach to ECD. The interagency mechanism can take various forms. A good model is a so-called sub-committee, such as the UN System Standing Committee on Nutrition (SCN) (Box 5.1). Such a committee would bring together not only relevant UN agencies and government actors, but also civil society organizations and professional ECD networks (see Chapter 15: *Good Global Governance*).

Following the SCN model, key activities of the interagency mechanism could include: (i) the development and implementation of a strategy for high-level advocacy and strategic communication, (ii) tracking and reporting on progress towards a healthy start in life for all children, (iii) facilitating the integration of ECD into MDG-related activities at the country level through the UN coordination system, (iv) mainstreaming human rights approaches – in particular, the rights in early childhood as embodied in General Comment 7 on Implementing Child Rights in Early Childhood (UN, 2006a) – into the work of the interagency mechanism, and (v) identifying key scientific and operational gaps (Standing Committee on Nutrition, nd,b). At the country level, the interagency group can promote an approach in which policy makers, practitioners, researchers, and civil society actors form integrated ECD networks to ensure open-access sharing and dissemination of research and practice findings.

Ensuring policy coherence for ECD, nationally and internationally, requires that international organizations, WHO and UNICEF in particular, strengthen their leadership on and institutional commitment to ECD. Within these organizations, many programmes have a bearing on child development, including programmes on child survival, immunization, reproductive health, and HIV/AIDS. ECD should explicitly be taken into account in these programmes. This requires dedicated staff and financing for ECD, in order to:

- play a critical role in advocacy for ECD as a key social determinant of health;

- provide technical support for inclusion of ECD in national-level policies and international development frameworks (such as the Poverty Reduction Strategy Papers [PRSP]);

- provide technical support to regions, countries, and partners for integration of simple ECD interventions (such as Integrated Management of Childhood Illness [IMCI] Care for Development, see Box 5.7) in health services and community health initiatives;

- take responsibility for gathering evidence on the effectiveness of ECD interventions, especially those that are connected to the health-care system;

- support countries in gathering national statistics on and setting up monitoring systems for ECD.

Ensuring a comprehensive approach to ECD requires that international organizations and donors support national governments in building capacity and developing financing mechanisms for implementation of such an approach. A global funding strategy needs to be established to assist countries that are signatories of the Convention of the Rights of the Child to truly implement the UN Committee on the Rights of the Child's General Comment 7, regarding child rights in early childhood.

A comprehensive approach to early childhood in practice

The Commission recommends that:

5.2. Governments build universal coverage of a comprehensive package of quality early child development programmes and services for children, mothers, and other caregivers, regardless of ability to pay (see Rec 9.1; 11.6; 16.1).

An integrated policy framework for early child development

A healthy start for all children is best served by an integrated policy framework for ECD, designed to reach all children. This requires interministerial coordination and policy coherence, with a clear articulation of the roles and responsibilities of each sector and how they will collaborate. Better collaboration between the welfare and education sector, for example, can facilitate the transition from pre-primary programmes to primary education (OECD, 2001). ECD should be integrated into the agendas of each sector to ensure that it is considered routinely in decision-making (see Chapter 10: *Health Equity in all Policies, Systems, and Programmes*).

BOX 5.1: EXAMPLE OF AN INTERAGENCY MECHANISM – THE UN SYSTEM STANDING COMMITTEE ON NUTRITION

The mandate of the SCN is to promote cooperation among UN agencies and partner organizations in support of community, national, regional, and international efforts to end malnutrition in all of its forms in this generation. It will do this by refining the direction, increasing the scale, and strengthening the coherence and impact of actions against malnutrition worldwide. It will also raise awareness of nutrition problems and mobilize commitment to solve them at global, regional, and national levels. The SCN reports to the Chief Executives Board of the UN. The UN members are the Economic Commission for Africa, FAO, International Atomic Energy Agency, International

Fund for Agricultural Development, ILO, UN, UNAIDS, UNDP, UN Environment Programme, UNESCO, UNFPA, UNHCR, UNICEF, UN Research Institute for Social Development, UN University, WFP, WHO, and the World Bank. The International Food Policy Research Institute and Asian Development Bank (ADB) are also members. From the outset, representatives of bilateral partners have participated actively in SCN activities, as have nongovernmental organizations (NGOs).

Reproduced, with permission of the UN, from Standing Committee on Nutrition (nd,a).

Implementing a more comprehensive approach to early life includes extending quality interventions for child survival and physical development to incorporate social/emotional and language/cognitive development. ECD programmes and services should comprise, but not be limited to, breastfeeding and nutrition support, comprehensive support to and care of mothers before, during, and after pregnancy – including interventions that help to address prenatal and postnatal maternal mental health problems (Patel et al., 2004) (see Chapter 9: *Universal Health Care*) – parenting and caregiver support, childcare, and early education starting around age 3 (see Action area 2, below) (ECDKN, 2007a). Also, services are needed for children with special needs, including those with mental and physical challenges. Such services include early detection, training caretakers to play and interact with their children at home, community-based early intervention programmes to help children reach their potential, and community education and advocacy to prevent discrimination against children with disabilities (UNICEF, 2000; UNICEF, 2007a). Interventions are most effective when they provide a direct learning experience to the children and their caretakers and are high intensity, high quality, of longer duration, targeted towards younger and disadvantaged children, and built onto established child survival and health programmes to make ECD programmes readily accessible (Engle et al., 2007).

Implementing an integrated policy framework for ECD requires working with civil society organizations, communities, and caregivers. Civil society can advocate and initiate action on ECD, and can be instrumental in organizing strategies at the local level to provide families and children with effective delivery of ECD services, to improve safety and efficacy of residential environments, and to increase the capacity of local and relational communities to better the lives of children (ECDKN, 2007a).

Most countries do not have an integrated policy framework for ECD. At the same time, there are examples of interventions from around the world that illustrate what can be done.

From single to comprehensive packages of ECD services

The implementation of programmes and services that seek to improve the development of young children can follow a number of models. Some are directed to single issues, such as early literacy (Box 5.2), while others deal with ECD more comprehensively (see Boxes 5.3 and 5.4).

Interventions that integrate the different dimensions of child development, among others by incorporating stimulation (interaction between caregivers and children, which is related to brain development) and nutrition, are particularly successful (Engle et al., 2007). They tend to result in sustained improvements in physical, social/emotional, and language/cognitive development, while simultaneously reducing the immediate and future burden of disease, especially for those who are most vulnerable and disadvantaged (ECDKN, 2007a). This is illustrated in Fig. 5.1, which shows that the mental development of stunted children who were given both food supplementation and psychosocial stimulation was about as good as that of non-stunted children (Fig. 5.1).

BOX 5.2: STIMULATING READING OUT LOUD – UNITED STATES

Reach Out and Read is a United States national non-profit organization that promotes early literacy by giving books to children and advice to parents attending paediatric examinations about the importance of reading aloud for child development and school readiness. At every check-up, doctors and nurses encourage parents to read aloud to their young children, and offer age-appropriate tips and encouragement. Parents who may have difficulty reading are encouraged to invent their own stories to go with picture books and spend time naming objects with their children. Also, providers give every child between the ages of 6 months and 5 years developmentally appropriate children's books to keep. In literacy-rich waiting-room environments, often with volunteer readers, parents and children learn about the pleasures and techniques of looking at books together. Parents who have received the intervention were significantly more likely to read to their children and have more children's books at home. Most importantly, children who received the interventions showed significant improvements in preschool language scores – a good predictor of later literacy success.

Source: ECDKN, 2007a

Even more integrated packages of services can be provided, including stimulation, nutrition, parental education, and various forms of family support (Box 5.3).

Starting early in life, using a lifecourse approach

Younger children tend to benefit more from ECD interventions than older children, emphasizing the importance of providing programmes and services as early in life as possible (Engle et al., 2007). Some factors need to be addressed before birth – even before conception. Box 5.4 illustrates how child development and nutrition problems can be addressed through a lifecourse perspective, including not just children, but also pregnant and lactating mothers and adolescent girls.

Prioritizing the provision of interventions to the socially most disadvantaged

Within a framework of universal access, special attention to the socially disadvantaged and children who are lagging behind in their development will help considerably to reduce inequities in ECD. An important reason is that ECD interventions tend to show the largest effect in these disadvantaged groups (Scott-McDonald, 2002; Young, 2002; Engle et al., 2007).

Unfortunately, children in the poorest households and communities are usually least likely to have access to ECD programmes and services (UNESCO, 2006b). When new interventions are introduced, the better off tend to benefit

Figure 5.1: Effects of combined nutritional supplementation and psychosocial stimulation on stunted children in a 2-year intervention study in Jamaica.[a]

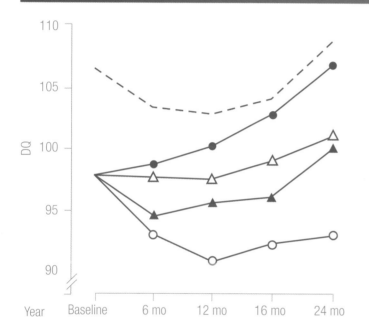
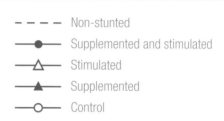

[a]Mean development scores (DQ) of stunted groups adjusted for initial age and score compared with a non-stunted group adjusted for age only, using Griffiths Mental Development Scales modified for Jamaica. Reprinted, with permission of the publisher, from Grantham-McGregor et al. (1991).

BOX 5.3: A COMPREHENSIVE APPROACH TO ADDRESSING EARLY CHILD DEVELOPMENT CHALLENGES IN JAMAICA

Young children in poor Jamaican communities face overwhelming disadvantages, among others of poverty. The Malnourished Children's Programme addresses the nutritional and psychosocial needs of children admitted to the hospital for malnutrition. Hospital personnel observed that, before initiation of their outreach programme, many children who recovered and were sent home from the hospital had to be readmitted for the same condition shortly after. To address this, follow-up home visits were set up to monitor children discharged from hospital. During home visits, staff focus on stimulation, environmental factors potentially detrimental to the child's health,

the child's nutritional status, and the possible need for food supplementation. Parents participate in an ongoing weekly parenting education and social welfare programme. They are helped to develop income-generating skills, begin self-help projects, and find jobs or shelter. Unemployed parents are also provided with food packages, bedding, and clothing. In addition, there is an outreach programme in poor communities, including regular psychosocial stimulation of children aged 3 and under, supported by a mobile toy-lending library.

Adapted, with permission of the publisher, from Scott-McDonald (2002).

first (Victora et al., 2000; Houweling, 2007). This seems to be the case for the Integrated Management of Childhood Illness programme which, when implemented under routine conditions, does not preferentially reach the poor (PPHCKN, 2007a). On the other hand, examples from, among others, the Philippines illustrate that reaching disadvantaged children is feasible (Box 5.5). In countries where resources are limited, priorities must be set such that the most vulnerable children are reached first, while universal coverage should remain the longer-term goal (ECDKN, 2007a).

Reaching all children

A core objective should be universal coverage for quality ECD interventions (Box 5.6), with special attention to the most deprived. Universal access must include equal access for girls and boys as a matter of course. Low-income countries should strive to progressive realization of universal coverage, starting with the most vulnerable. Governments need to develop strategies for scaling up effective programmes from the local to the national level, without sacrificing the characteristics of the programme that made it effective. It is important that implementation integrity and accountability at the local level are sustained, even when programmes are scaled up to the national level (ECDKN, 2007a).

BOX 5.4: STARTING INTERVENTIONS BEFORE CONCEPTION – THE INTEGRATED CHILD DEVELOPMENT SERVICES (ICDS), INDIA

The ICDS is one of the largest child development and child nutrition programmes in the world, currently serving more than 30 million children. The services include support for pregnant and lactating mothers and adolescent girls, among others through improving their access to food. They also include childcare centres, preschool education, growth monitoring for children aged 0-5 years, supplementary feeding for malnourished children, assistance for child immunization, and some emergency health care (Engle et al., 2007). The results of the programme appear to be mixed, with positive results on malnutrition and child motor and mental development in some states (Engle et al., 2007; Lokshin et al., 2005). Within states, poorer villages were more likely to be served. However, states with high levels of child malnutrition have lowest programme coverage and lowest budgetary allocations from the central government (Das Gupta et al., 2005). An evaluation by the World Bank found "only modest positive effects, probably because of low funding, work overload of community workers, and insufficient training"

(Engle et al., 2007).

BOX 5.5: REACHING MARGINALIZED COMMUNITIES IN THE PHILIPPINES

"A programme in the Philippines provides health, nutrition and early education services to young children in marginalized communities. Involving various ministries at the national level, and extension agents and Child Development Officers at the community level, the programme helps track every child's growth; monitors access to iodized salt, micronutrients, clean water and a toilet; and counsels parents on nutrition and child development."

Reprinted, with permission of the author, from UNICEF (2001).

BOX 5.6: UNIVERSAL CHILD DEVELOPMENT SERVICES IN CUBA

Cuba's Educa a Tu Hijo (Growing-up with your child) programme is generally thought to be an important factor in Cuba's educational achievements at the primary school level (UNICEF, 2001). The programme, introduced in 1985, is a non-formal, non-institutional, community-based, family-centred ECD service under the responsibility of the Ministry of Education (Preschool Education). The programme operates with the participation of the Ministries of Public Health, Culture, and Sports, the Federation of Cuban Women, the National Association of Small Farmers, the National Committee for the Defence of the Revolution, and student associations. This extended network includes 52 000 Promotres (teachers, pedagogues, physicians, and other trained professionals), 116 000 Executors (teachers, physicians, nurses, retired professionals, students, and volunteers), and more than 800 000 families. During the 1990s the programme was extended, reaching 99.8% of children aged 0-5 years in 2000 – probably the highest enrolment rate in the world.

Source: CS, 2007

Building onto established child survival and health programmes to make early child development interventions readily accessible

Health-care systems are in a unique position to contribute to ECD (see Chapter 9: *Universal Health Care*). Given the overlap in underlying determinants of survival/physical development and social/emotional and language/cognitive development, the health-care system can be an effective site for promoting development in all domains. The health-care system is a primary contact for many child-bearing mothers and, in many instances, health-care providers are the only professionals with whom families come into contact in the early years of the child's life (ECDKN, 2007a). Health-care systems can serve as a platform for information and support to parents around ECD, and they can link children and families to existing community-based ECD services. When ECD programmes and services become integral components of established health-care services, such as the IMCI (Box 5.7), they can become a highly effective way of promoting ECD (ECDKN, 2007a).

Acting on gender inequities

An important aspect of the quality of ECD programmes and services is the promotion of gender equity. Early gender socialization, the learning of cultural roles according to one's sex and norms that define 'masculine' and 'feminine', can have large ramifications across the lifecourse. Girls, for example, may be required to care for their younger siblings, which can prevent them from attending school. Preschool programmes that take care of the younger siblings can contribute to solving this problem.

An important strategy in promoting positive gender socialization for young boys and girls is through developmentally appropriate, gender-sensitive, and culturally relevant parenting programmes (Koçak, 2004; UNICEF, 1997; Landers, 2003). These seek to raise awareness among parents and caregivers of their role in helping their children to develop self-esteem and confidence as a boy or girl from the beginning of their lives. Gender-biased expectations of boys and girls can be brought up during group discussions with fathers and mothers as well as other caregivers and preschool teachers.

Involving fathers in child-rearing from their children's birth is another important strategy for improving child health and developmental outcomes, while promoting gender equity.

Fathers can enjoy their fatherhood roles while establishing a positive and fulfilling relationship with their children and can be a positive role model for both their daughters and sons. Parenting programmes in, for example, Bangladesh, Brazil, Jamaica, Jordan, South Africa, Turkey, and Viet Nam include specific activities to engage fathers more actively in the upbringing of their children (Koçak, 2004; UNICEF, 1997; Landers, 2003).

Involving communities

The involvement of communities, including mothers, grandmothers, and other caregivers, is key to the sustainability of action on ECD. This includes involvement in the development, implementation, monitoring, and reviewing of ECD policies, programmes, and services (ECDKN, 2007a). It can build a common purpose and consensus regarding outcomes related to the needs of the community, foster partnership among the community, providers, parents, and caregivers, and enhance community capacity through active involvement of families and other stakeholders (ECDKN, 2007a). Box 5.8 shows how an ECD project in the Lao People's Democratic Republic was community driven, at all stages, from identification of need to implementation. Community participation and community-based interventions do not absolve governments from their responsibilities. However, they can ensure stronger relationships between government, providers, the community, and caretakers (ECDKN, 2007a) (see Chapter 14: *Political Empowerment – Inclusion and Voice*).

The scope of education

While the Commission has not investigated education through a dedicated Knowledge Network, broad areas for attention have emerged from the Commission's work. The Commission recognizes the critical importance of education for health equity. Education, formal and informal, is understood as a lifelong process starting at birth. The focus in this section is on education from pre-primary to the end of secondary school, with an emphasis on extending the comprehensive approach to education that incorporates attention to children's physical, social/emotional, and language/cognitive development.

BOX 5.7: BUILDING EARLY CHILD DEVELOPMENT ONTO EXISTING HEALTH PROGRAMMES AND SERVICES

In partnership with UNICEF, WHO has developed a special early childhood development component, called Care for Development, intended to be incorporated into existing IMCI programmes. Care for Development aims to enhance awareness among parents and caregivers of the importance of play and communication with children by providing them with information and instruction during children's clinical visits. Evidence has shown that Care for Development is an effective method of supporting parents' and caregivers' efforts to provide a stimulating environment for their children by building on their existing skills. Health-care professionals are encouraged to view children's visits for acute minor illnesses as opportunities to spread the messages of Care for Development, such as the importance of active and responsive feeding to improve children's nutrition and growth, and the importance of play and communication activities to help children move to the next stages in their development.

Sources: ECDKN, 2007a; WHO, nd,d

The Commission recommends that:

5.3. Governments provide quality education that pays attention to children's physical, social/emotional, and language/cognitive development, starting in pre-primary school.

In every country children, particularly those from the poorest communities, would benefit immensely from early education programmes. Expanding and improving early childcare and education is part of the UNESCO Education for All strategy (UNESCO, 2006b; UNESCO, 2007a). The Commission supports the UNESCO Education for All goals (summarized in Box 5.9).

Providing quality pre-primary education

Extending the availability of quality pre-primary school, which adopts the principles of ECD, to all children and making special efforts to include those from socially disadvantaged backgrounds requires a commitment from the highest level

of government and from ministries responsible for care and education of young children. It requires joint working across health and education sectors, and review of existing pre-primary provision involving broad consultation with families, communities, nongovernmental and civil society organizations, and preschool providers to identify needs and develop a comprehensive strategy. Areas to be addressed in strategy development include: levels of funding, infrastructure (including buildings and facilities), support for children with special educational needs, ratio of staff to children, recruitment, support and training of preschool staff, and the nature of the preschool programme.

BOX 5.8: VILLAGE-BASED EARLY CHILD DEVELOPMENT CURRICULUM DEVELOPMENT IN THE LAO PEOPLE'S DEMOCRATIC REPUBLIC

The Women's Development Project worked to promote various development initiatives for women in five Lao provinces. After 5 years, interest developed and a need was identified to address child development issues more directly. The Early Childhood and Family Development Project grew out of this. Project-planning workshops were organized in villages in the initial steps of development and implementation. Village-level planning resulted in agreement on needs and objectives, an understanding of overall design, assessments of resources and constraints, activity planning, setting up the project committee, and criteria for selecting village volunteers. The community-based curriculum-development process focused on participatory input at the local level to create a curriculum that could be adapted to the particular needs of different ethnic groups. The process focused on village data collection and needs assessment. Analysis of existing traditional knowledge was used as a basis for curriculum development. One of the notable activities was a village engagement agreement signed by village members and the village development committee. It was based on a child rights framework and included actions that could be taken immediately while waiting for needed external assistance.

Source: ECDKN, 2007a

PROVISION AND SCOPE OF EDUCATION : ACTION AREA 5.2

Expand the provision and scope of education to include the principles of early child development (physical, social/emotional, and language/cognitive development).

BOX 5.9: UNESCO EDUCATION FOR ALL GOALS

Expand and improve early childcare and education.	Achieve a 50% improvement in adult literacy rates.
Provide free and compulsory universal primary education by 2015.	Eliminate gender disparities in primary and secondary education by 2005 and at all levels by 2015.
Ensure equitable access to learning and life-skills programmes.	Improve all aspects of the quality of education.
	Source: UNESCO, 2007a

Quality primary and secondary education

There is emerging evidence that integrating social and emotional learning in curricula in primary and secondary schools as well as attention to the children's physical and cognitive/language development improves school attendance and educational attainment (CASEL, nd), and potentially would have consequent long-term gains for health. Social and emotional learning comes under the broad umbrella of life-skills education, which is incorporated into UNICEF's definition of quality education (UNICEF, nd,b). The Education for All goals include equitable access to 'life skills' as a basic learning need for young people, to be addressed either through formal education or non-formal settings (UNESCO, 2007a). The Commission endorses increased attention to life skills-based education in all countries as a way of supporting healthy behaviours and empowering young people to take control of their lives. UNICEF has highlighted the importance of life-skills education for HIV/AIDS prevention and a comprehensive approach to quality education that responds to learners' needs and is committed to gender equity (UNICEF, nd,c).

Making schools healthy for children is the basis for the FRESH (Focusing Resources on Effective School Health) Start approach (Partnership for Child Development, nd), a joint initiative by WHO, UNICEF, UNESCO, the World Bank, and other partners to coordinate action to make schools healthy for children and improve quality and equity in education, contributing to the development of child friendly schools (Box 5.11).

Innovative, context-specific, school-based interventions can be developed to tackle health challenges faced by young people. For example, in Australia the MindMatters programme (Curriculum Corporation, nd) has been developed to promote mental health in schools, and in the United States the Action for Healthy Kids programme addresses the growing obesity epidemic (Action for Healthy Kids, 2007). These programmes demonstrate how working across sectors and involving a range of both governmental and NGOs can address health challenges in the school setting. Out-of-school programmes in non-formal settings can also be developed to achieve similar objectives using the same approach.

Barriers to education

The Commission recommends that:

5.4   Governments provide quality compulsory primary and secondary education for all boys and girls, regardless of ability to pay, identify and address the barriers to girls and boys enrolling and staying in school, and abolish user fees for primary school (see Rec 6.4; 13.4).

Barriers to education include issues of access to education and quality and acceptability of education. In many countries, but particularly low-income countries, it is children from families on low incomes and with parents with little education who are less likely to attend school and more likely to drop out of school. Poverty relief and income-generating activities (discussed in Chapters 7 and 8: *Fair Employment and Decent Work; Social Protection across the Lifecourse*) together with measures to reduce family out-of-pocket expenditure on school attendance, school books, uniforms, and other expenses are critical elements of a comprehensive strategy to make access to quality education a reality for millions of children.

Other policies aimed at encouraging parents to send their children to school vary by country but include provision of free or subsidized school meals (Bajpai et al., 2005) and providing cash incentives conditional on school attendance, removal of school fees (Glewwe, Zhao & Binder, 2006), and provision of free deworming tablets or other health interventions, for example, the Malawi School Health Initiative (Pasha et al., 2003). Context-specific analyses are needed to identify barriers to education and to develop and evaluate policies that encourage parents to enrol and keep children in school.

BOX 5.10: COUNTRY APPROACHES TO PRE-PRIMARY EDUCATION

In Chile, the expansion of pre-primary education for socially disadvantaged children began by extending provision first for ages 5-6, then ages 4-5, then ages 3-4. The programme focuses on integrating quality education, care, nutrition, and social attention for the child and his or her family care (JUNJI, nd).

Expansion of preschool education in Sweden was achieved with a government commitment that preschool education should have an emphasis on play, children's natural learning strategies, and their comprehensive development. It was a policy goal to integrate this comprehensive approach to education into the entire education system (Choi, 2002).

BOX 5.11:CHILD FRIENDLY SCHOOLS

UNICEF has developed a framework for child friendly schools that takes a rights-based approach to education. Child friendly schools create a safe, healthy, gender-sensitive learning environment, with parent and community involvement, and provide

quality education and life skills. This model or similar models are now developed or being developed in more than 90 countries, and adapted as national quality standard in 54 countries.

Source: UNICEF, nd,d

Of note, there has been rapid expansion of primary education in low-income countries over recent years, a trend attributed, in part, to the abolition of school fees in a number of countries. As the Kenyan experience highlights (Box 5.12), abolishing primary school fees needs to be complemented by hiring and training teachers, building more schools and classrooms, and providing educational materials. Increased access to primary school needs to be accompanied by attention to quality of education. In addition, expansion of primary education will require investments in secondary education to increase capacity for the new entrants, assuming they reach secondary level. The transition from primary to secondary school is a critical point for girls and for gender equity (Grown, Gupta & Pande, 2005).

A major investment is required by national governments – allocating sufficient funds to school infrastructure development, the recruitment, training, and remuneration of staff, and the provision of educational materials. Supporting low- and middle-income countries to do this requires donor countries to fulfil their aid commitments (see Chapter 11: *Fair Financing*). The annual external financing requirement to meet the 'Education for All' goals is estimated to be about US$ 11 billion per annum (UNESCO, 2007a).

Educating girls

There needs to be a particular effort in securing primary and secondary education for girls, especially in low-income countries (UNESCO, 2007a, Levine et al., 2008). Abolishing user fees for primary education is a critical step. In response to continued challenges to gender equity in education, Task Force 3 on Education and Gender Equality of the UN Millennium Project identified the need to strengthen opportunities for secondary education for girls while simultaneously meeting commitments to universal primary education as key to achieving MDG 3 – promote gender equality and empower women (Grown, Gupta & Pande, 2005).

Strategies for promoting secondary education for girls include increasing access and retention. Interventions to improve both the physical and social environment (Rihani, 2006) include building functional toilets/latrines for girls and female teachers and creating a safe environment for girls (WHO, 2005a) by

introducing and enforcing codes of conduct. Measures to improve the relevance and quality of schooling (Rihani, 2006) include teacher training and curriculum reform to reduce gender biases and introducing frameworks for participation of girls in decisions about their schooling. Other interventions include targeted scholarships for girls, such as the Bangladesh's Female Secondary School Assistance Programme (WGEKN, 2007; SEKN, 2007), and programmes that address the needs of pregnant schoolgirls, such as the Botswana Diphalana Initiative (WGEKN, 2007).

Early childhood offers huge opportunities to reduce health inequities within a generation. The importance of early child development and education for health across the lifecourse provides a strong imperative to start acting now. Inaction will have detrimental effects that can last more than a lifetime. A new approach is needed that embraces a more comprehensive understanding of early child development and includes not just physical survival but also social/emotional and language/cognitive development. This approach should be integrated into lifelong learning.

BOX 5.12: KENYA – ABOLITION OF SCHOOL FEES

When Kenya abolished school fees in 2003, there was an immediate influx of 1.3 million children into the school system, overwhelming school infrastructure and teachers. School enrolments since 2002 increased by 28% while the total number of teachers increased by only 2.6% between 2002 and 2004; in some areas the ratio rose to one teacher for 100 pupils.

Source: Chinyama, 2006

BOX 5.13: DEMAND FOR QUALITY EDUCATION, SUB-SAHARAN AFRICA

The total fertility rate in sub-Saharan Africa is 5.5 (UNDP, 2007); Niger and Uganda have particularly high fertility rates (Niger 7.4, Uganda 6.7). Nearly 44% of the total population of sub-Saharan Africa is under 15 years old, compared with approximately 18% in high-income OECD countries. With so many children of school age, some countries in sub-Saharan Africa face particular challenges in ensuring high-quality education for all.

CHAPTER 6
Healthy places – healthy people

"Rapid and chaotic urbanisation is being accompanied by increasing inequalities which pose enormous challenges to human security and safety"

Anna Tibaijuka, Executive Director UN-HABITAT (UN-HABITAT, 2007b)

WHY PLACE MATTERS FOR HEALTH EQUITY

Where people live affects their health and chances of leading flourishing lives. Communities and neighbourhoods that ensure access to basic goods, that are socially cohesive, that are designed to promote good physical and psychological well-being, and that are protective of the natural environment are essential for health equity.

The growth of urbanization

The year 2007 saw, for the first time, the majority of human beings living in urban settings (WorldWatch Institute, 2007), and almost 1 billion people living in life-threatening conditions in urban slums[3] and informal settlements. By 2010 it is expected that 3.48 billion people worldwide will live in urban areas. The growth of the 'megacity', massive urban agglomerations of 10 million inhabitants and upwards, is an issue of importance for global health and health equity. But a very real challenge for the future is the growth of around 500 'smaller' cities of 1-10 million people – cities that are characterized by outward sprawl.

The regions of the world with the fastest growing urban populations are also the regions with the highest proportion of slum dwellers (Table 6.1). Data from around 2003 show that almost half of all urban dwellers in developing regions live in slums, and this rises to four out of five urban dwellers in the poorest countries. But slums are not only a problem of low- and middle-income countries; 6% of urban dwellers in high-income regions live in slums.

In Nairobi, where 60% of the city's population live in slums, child mortality in the slums is 2.5 times greater than that in other areas of the city.

In Manila's slums, up to 39% of children aged between 5 and 9 are already infected with TB – twice the national average.

The push from rural to urban living

While urban living is now the dominant form globally, the balance of rural and urban dwelling varies enormously across areas – from less than 10% urban in Burundi and Uganda to 100% or close to it in Belgium, Kuwait, Hong Kong SAR,

and Singapore. Policies and investment patterns reflecting the urban-led growth paradigm (Vlahov et al., 2007) have seen rural communities worldwide, including Indigenous Peoples (Indigenous Health Group, 2007), suffer from progressive underinvestment in infrastructure and amenities, with disproportionate levels of poverty and poor living conditions (Ooi & Phua, 2007; Eastwood & Lipton, 2000), leading ultimately to out-migration to unfamiliar urban centres. This, combined with population growth and stagnant agricultural productivity, saw sub-Saharan Africa experience one of the highest rates of urban growth internationally between the 1960s and 1990s (140%), with rural-urban migration accounting for roughly half of this (Barrios et al., 2006). These major inequities, to the disadvantage of rural conditions, contribute to the stark health inequities between urban and rural dwellers in many low-income countries (Houweling et al., 2007).

Vulnerability in urban settings

Following the current trajectory of urban growth, city populations will age and there will be more urban sprawl and greater numbers of people living in poverty, slums, and squatter settlements (Campbell & Campbell, 2007). The proportion of the older adult population residing in cities in high-income countries matches that of younger age groups and will rise at the same pace. In low- and middle-income countries, however, the share of older people in urban communities will multiply 16 times from about 56 million in 1998 to over 908 million in 2050 (WHO, 2007d). Similarly, people with disabilities are vulnerable to health threats, particularly in urban areas due to the challenges of a high population density, crowding, unsuitable living design, and lack of social support (Frumkin et al., 2004).

"A warmer world with a more intense water cycle and rising sea levels will influence many key determinants of wealth and wellbeing, including water supply, food production, human health, availability of land, and the environment" (Stern, 2006)

The current model of urbanization poses significant environmental challenges, particularly climate change – the impact of which is greater in low-income countries and among vulnerable subpopulations (McMichael et al., 2008; Stern, 2006) (Fig. 6.1). At present, greenhouse gas emissions are determined mainly by consumption patterns in cities of high-income countries. However, rapid development and concurrent urbanization in poorer regions means that low- and middle-income countries will be both vulnerable to health hazards from climate change and an increasing contributor to the problem (Campbell-Lendrum & Corvalan, 2007).

---

[3] The general definition of slums used by UN-HABITAT denotes 'a wide range of low-income settlements and/or poor human living conditions.' These areas generally share four characteristics: buildings of poor quality; overcrowding (in, for instance, the number of persons per room); inadequate provision of infrastructure and services; and relatively low price. In many, there is a fifth characteristic – insecurity – because of some aspects of illegality (especially for squatters) or no legal protection for the inhabitants (those who rent).

Table 6.1: Urban and slum-dwelling households, circa 2003

	Total urban population (millions)	Urban populations as % of total population	Urban slum population (millions)	Slum population as % of total urban population
World	**2923**	**47.7%**	**924**	**31.6%**
Developed regions	**902**	**75.5%**	**54**	**6.0%**
Europe	534	73.6%	33	6.2%
Other	367	78.6%	21	5.7%
Developing regions	**2022**	**40.9%**	**870**	**43.0%**
Northern Africa	76	52.0%	21	28.2%
Sub-Saharan Africa	231	34.6%	166	71.9%
Latin America and the Caribbean	399	75.8%	128	31.9%
Eastern Asia	533	39.1%	194	36.4%
Eastern Asia excluding China	61	77.1%	16	25.4%
South-central Asia	452	30.0%	262	58.0%
South-East Asia	203	38.3%	57	28.0%
Western Asia	125	64.9%	41	33.1%
Oceania	2	26.7%	0	24.1%
Transition countries	**259**	**62.9%**	**25**	**9.6%**
Commonwealth of Independent States	181	64.1%	19	10.3%
Other Europe	77	60.3%	6	7.9%
Least developed countries	**179**	**26.2%**	**140**	**78.2%**

UN-HABITAT 2003 and other UN data: Reproduced from KNUS (2007).

Figure 6.1: Deaths from climate change.

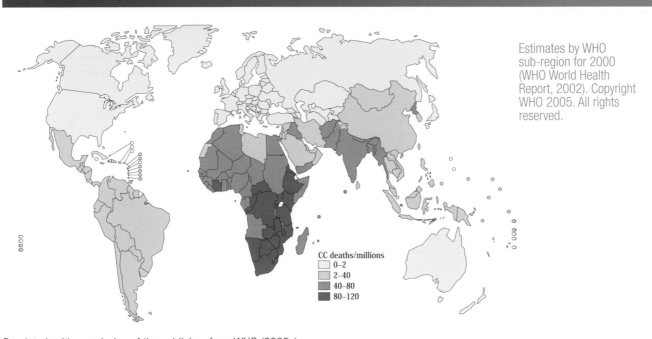

Estimates by WHO sub-region for 2000 (WHO World Health Report, 2002). Copyright WHO 2005. All rights reserved.

CC deaths/millions
- 0–2
- 2–40
- 40–80
- 80–120

Reprinted, with permission of the publisher, from WHO (2005e).

Transport and buildings contribute 21% to CO2 emissions – a major contributor to climate change (IPCC, 2007). Rural agriculture poses a major challenge. Crop yields, which feed rural and urban dwellers alike, depend in large part on prevailing climate conditions. Worldwide, agricultural activity accounts for about one fifth of global greenhouse gas emissions (McMichael et al., 2007).

New urban health

Infectious diseases and undernutrition will continue in particular regions and groups around the world. However, urbanization itself is re shaping population health problems, particularly among the urban poor, towards non-communicable diseases and injuries, alcohol- and substance-abuse, and impact from ecological disaster (Campbell & Campbell, 2007; Yusuf et al., 2001).

Obesity is one of the most challenging health concerns to have arisen in the past couple of decades. It is a pressing problem, particularly among socially disadvantaged groups in many cities throughout the world (Hawkes et al., 2007; Friel, Chopra & Satcher, 2007). The shift in population levels of weight towards obesity is related to the 'nutrition transition' – the increasing consumption of fats, sweeteners, energy-dense foods, and highly processed foods. This, together with marked reductions in energy expenditure, is believed to have contributed to the global obesity epidemic. The nutrition transition tends to begin in cities. This is due to a variety of factors including the greater availability, accessibility, and acceptability of bulk purchases, convenience foods, and 'supersized' portions (Dixon et al., 2007). Physical activity is strongly influenced by the design of cities through the density of residences, the mix of land uses, the degree to which streets are connected and the ability to walk from place to place, and the provision of and access to local public facilities and spaces for recreation and play. Each of these plus the increasing reliance on cars is an important influence on shifts towards physical inactivity in high- and middle-income countries (Friel, Chopra & Satcher, 2007).

Violence and crime are major urban health challenges. Of the 1.6 million violence-related deaths worldwide (including those from conflict and suicide) that occur each year, 90% happen in low- and middle-income countries (WHO, 2002a). In the informal settlements of large cities, social exclusion and threat of violence are highly prevalent (Roberts & Meddings, 2007). In North American and European cities, and increasingly in the cities of other high-income countries, violence and crime have become concentrated problems in urban neighbourhoods, especially those with large-scale housing estates in suburbs. Alcohol is implicated in injury and violence in low-, middle-, and high-income countries – figures from WHO suggest that of the large number of deaths associated with alcohol globally, 32% are from unintentional injuries and 14% are from intentional injuries (Roberts & Meddings, 2007). The highest burden of alcohol-related disease in the world is in the region of the former Soviet Union and Central Asia, where it amounts to 13% of the total disease burden (PPHCKN, 2007b).

Urban areas are by far the most affected by road-traffic injuries and vehicle-related air pollution, with approximately 800 000 annual deaths from ambient urban air pollution and 1.2 million from road-traffic accidents (Roberts & Meddings, 2007; Prüss-Üstün & Corvalán, 2006). The decline in road-traffic deaths between 1987 and 1995 in highly motorized countries (Fig. 6.2) offers hope for other countries where motorization is on a steep upward slope – illustrating the positive effects of policy initiatives such as traffic planning, safer roads and cars, and safer driving due to, for example, compulsory and enforced seat-belt wearing and punishment for driving under the influence of alcohol.

About 14% of the global burden of disease has been attributed to neuropsychiatric disorders, mostly due to depression and

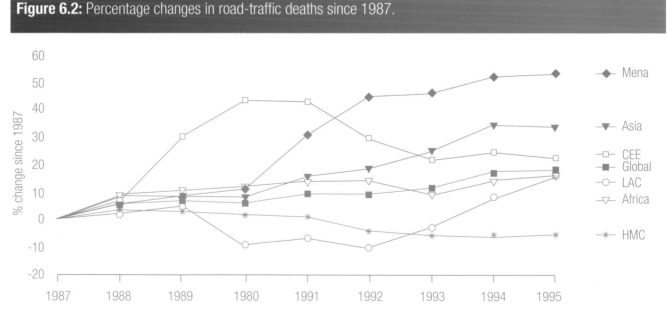

Figure 6.2: Percentage changes in road-traffic deaths since 1987.

HMC = highly motorized countries: North America, Australia, New Zealand, Japan, and Western Europe; CEE = Central and Eastern Europe; LAC = Latin/Central America and the Caribbean; Mena = Middle East and North Africa.
Reprinted, with permission of the publisher, from Jacobs et al. (2000).

other common mental disorders, alcohol- and substance-use disorders, and psychoses (Prince et al., 2007). The burden of major depression is expected to rise to be the second leading cause of loss of disability-adjusted life years in 2030 and will pose a major urban health challenge.

These emerging health problems, in countries with different levels of infrastructure and health system preparedness, pose significant health equity challenges in the 21st century. Improvements over the last 50 years in mortality and morbidity in highly urbanized countries such as Japan, the Netherlands, Singapore, and Sweden, are testimony to the potential of modern cities to promote health. They also show that this is only achievable as long as there are supportive political structures, financial resources applied in an appropriate manner, and social policies that underpin the equitable provision of the conditions in which people are able to thrive (Galea & Vlahov, 2005).

ACTION TO BUILD A FLOURISHING LIVING ENVIRONMENT

If urbanization continues unabated along its current path, it will present humanity, within a generation, with social, health, and environmental challenges on a scale unprecedented in human history. There is urgent need for a new approach to urbanization and a new paradigm of urban public health, with action in three key areas:

- Within cities, new models of governance are required to plan cities that are designed in such a way that the physical, social, and natural environments prevent and ameliorate the new urban health risks, ensuring the equitable inclusion of all city dwellers in the processes by which urban policies are formed.

- Sustained investment in rural areas – making them viable places for flourishing living – must balance investment in cities in national development plans.

- Underpinning these areas of action is the development of adaptation and mitigation strategies for environmental change that take into account the social and health equity dimensions.

While the Commission did not consider rural health issues in detail, it recognizes the need for a sustainable development strategy based on balanced rural-urban growth. An overarching recommendation to this effect is made in this chapter. Similarly, climate change was outside the remit of the Commission, but there are clear opportunities for simultaneously improving health equity and cutting greenhouse gas emissions through action in the urban and rural sectors. A general recommendation in relation to climate change and health equity is made at the end of this chapter and picked up again in Part 6: *Building a Global Movement*.

Guiding urban development in a manner that places the well-being of all people and environmental sustainability at its core will require strategic participatory planning, including city, county, and regional planning policy, embracing the dimensions of transport, housing, employment, social cohesion, and environmental protection.

The Commission recommends that:

6.1. **Local government and civil society, backed by national government, establish local participatory governance mechanisms that enable communities and local government to partner in building healthier and safer cities (see Rec 14.3).**

Participatory urban governance

Despite the evidence of the importance of community participation in addressing urban living conditions (Box 6.1), the resources and control over decision-making processes often remain beyond the reach of people normally excluded at the local and community level.

'Healthy Settings' refers to places and social contexts that promote health. In particular, the Healthy Cities movement is an existing local governance model that may be adapted worldwide to promote health equity (WHO Healthy Cities, nd; Alliance for Healthy Cities, nd; PAHO, 2005). The Healthy Settings approach has been applied not only to cities but municipalities, villages, islands, marketplaces, schools, hospitals, prisons, restaurants, and public spaces. More recently, the Healthy Cities principles have been used to develop initiatives that recognize the shifting demographic towards an ageing population (The Age-Friendly Cities initiative). At its best, the Healthy Cities model provides a 'neutral game board' where all parties in a city can come together to negotiate healthy outcomes in relation to a diverse range of city activities including planning, housing, environmental protection, style of health services, and responses to issues such as injury prevention and drug and alcohol control. Some evaluation and assessment of Healthy Settings has been conducted at city and regional levels, but there has been no systematic review at the global level. It is important that researchers and government evaluate, where possible, the health equity impacts of Healthy Cities/Settings type programmes, formal or otherwise, in order to build evidence for relevant and effective local government actions.

Improving urban living conditions

Applying healthy urban design principles, a city would be designed for a dense, residentially mixed population with easy access to services, including designated commercial and non-commercial land use, with land also set aside for protection of natural resources and recreation. Such an urban development agenda also considers the supply of basic amenities and sufficiently developed infrastructure (Devernman, 2007). Low- and middle-income countries are not likely, in the near future, to be able to provide all the funds needed to create an entirely healthy living environment. Funding from more affluent countries will be required to support the plans made by peoples and governments in less affluent countries (Sachs, 2005).

HEALTH AND EQUITY : ACTION AREA 6.1

Place health and health equity at the heart of urban governance and planning.

Shelter/housing

One of the biggest challenges facing cities is access to adequate shelter for all. Not only is the provision of shelter essential, but the quality of the shelter and the services associated with it, such as water and sanitation, are also vital contributors to health (Shaw, 2004).

The Commission recommends that:

6.2. **National and local government, in collaboration with civil society, manage urban development to ensure greater availability of affordable quality housing. With support from UN-HABITAT where necessary, invest in urban slum upgrading including, as a priority, provision of water and sanitation, electricity, and paved streets for all households regardless of ability to pay (see Rec 15.2).**

Many cities in rich and poor countries alike are facing a crisis in the availability of, and access to, affordable quality housing. This crisis will worsen social inequities in general, and in health in particular. In the United States, for example, inequities are being exacerbated by neighbourhoods that have adopted low-density-only zoning as a way to control growth. These have become more exclusionary, leading to fewer African American and Hispanic residents (NNC, 2001).

It is important therefore that local government regulates land development for urban regeneration, ensuring reserved urban land for low-income housing. Creating more equitable housing development means reversing the effects of exclusionary zoning through regional fair-share housing programmes, inclusionary zoning, and enforcement of fair housing laws. Taking an integrated approach, local authorities could use criteria for distribution of affordable housing tax credits to stimulate production of new affordable housing in proximity to transit, schools, and commercial areas (Box 6.2) (NNC, 2001).

There is a role for local government to monitor the health and health-equity impacts of housing, building, and infrastructure standards. Domestic energy inefficiencies and related fuel poverty[4] have a number of effects on health and are very socially patterned (Box 6.3). It is shocking that in an economically rich country such as the Republic of Ireland, a remarkable 17% of households are fuel poor (Healy, 2004).

The situation for slum dwellers needs immediate attention. The improvement of slums is a huge investment but is nevertheless affordable in most countries (Mitlin, 2007). The central goal of UN-HABITAT, under the Economic and Social Council, is to promote socially and environmentally sustainable towns and cities with the goal of providing adequate shelter for all (UN-HABITAT, 2007a). An integrated strategic plan between UN-HABITAT and WHO would provide the mandate and

---

BOX 6.1: IMPROVING LIVING CONDITIONS AND SECURING TENURE IN THAILAND

Approximately 62% of Thailand's slum population lives in Bangkok and 1.6 million (20%) of Bangkok's population lives in slums. Nine communities along the Bangbua canal in north Bangkok initiated a slum upgrade project in the wake of a threatened eviction due to a proposed highway construction project. Through public hearings, it was decided that the communities wanted to negotiate legal tenure and upgrade the communities. The communities worked with a governmental agency, the Community Organization Development Institute (CODI), and an NGO, the Chumthonthai Foundation, both of which work within the national Baan Man Kong (secure tenure) housing programme, in addition to the Treasury Department, district offices, and local universities.

This project required action on two levels. The operations level was primarily led by the community. A working group was established to coordinate the project overall. This working group conducted workshops and action planning with each community to develop the housing scheme and master plan with the community. A network committee linked the nine communities and encouraged participation. Individual community committees communicated with community members and gathered information for planning and implementation. A community savings group encouraged participation in a savings scheme

that was transparent and included a community-auditing system. The policy level was primarily led by governmental agencies. CODI provided loans for urban poor housing and worked with other concerned institutions on land tenure, capacity building, housing design, and housing construction. The Treasury Department was the landlord and landowner and had provided 30-year leases to the participating communities. The local district office provided building permissions and coordinated with higher government authorities. The local university provided technical and support staff with knowledge about improving the physical and social environment.

Housing units have been built in the pilot community and construction began in January 2006 in three other communities. Several lessons have been learned from the Bangbua experience. At the institutional level, there is recognition of the need for community participation through community networks. At the community level, the network demonstrated the ability to engage the community in housing development, to build community capacity, and to assure other stakeholders of the communities' commitment to housing development, which in turn moved the process of securing land tenure forward.

Source: KNUS, 2007

---

[4] Fuel poverty is defined here as the inability to heat one's home to an adequate (i.e. comfortable and safe) temperature, owing to low household income and low household energy efficiency.

technical support for many low- and middle-income countries worldwide to tackle these urban issues and, in doing so, help work towards the MDGs (see Chapter 15: *Good Global Governance*).

Based on previous estimates (Garau et al., 2005), global slum upgrading would cost less than US$ 100 billion. A 'Marshall plan for the world's urban slums' could be financed on a shared basis, for instance by international agencies and donors (45%), national and local governments (45%), and concerned households themselves (10%), in the latter case helped by micro-credit schemes.

"A slum dweller in Nairobi or Dar es Salaam, forced to rely on private water vendors, pays 5 to 7 times more for a liter of water than an average North American citizen" (Tibaijuka, 2004)

Enabling slum upgrading will require the political recognition of informal settlements, supported by regularization of tenure in slum settlements in order to allow official (public or private) utilities to extend infrastructure and services there (Box 6.5). Such action will help to empower women and improve their health by increasing access to basic resources such as water and sanitation (WGEKN, 2007).

BOX 6.2: CALIFORNIA TAX CREDIT PROGRAMME

In June 2000, the state of California reformed its tax credit programme for affordable rental housing. The new programme establishes a point system that prioritizes projects meeting sustainable development goals (such as walking distance to transit and schools) and projects in neighbourhoods where housing is an integrated part of a comprehensive revitalization effort.

Source: NNC, 2001

BOX 6.3: SOUTH COAST OF ENGLAND: A RANDOMIZED TRIAL OF HOUSING UPGRADING AND HEALTH

Although outwardly affluent, the city of Torquay in the south of England has pockets of deprivation. Watcombe is an estate of former council-owned properties with much higher levels of deprivation than the regional average and the highest out-of-hours visiting rate by family doctors in the town – 15% above the town average. Half the estate population was receiving benefits and 45% of children under 5 years old were living in single-parent households. A randomized-to-waiting list design was agreed with residents and the Council. The intervention comprised upgrading houses (including central heating, ventilation, rewiring, insulation, and re-roofing) in two phases, a year apart.

Evaluation of the intervention was positive. The interventions succeeded in producing warmer, drier houses that were more energy efficient as measured by changes in the indoor environment and energy rating of the house. Residents appreciated the improvements and felt their health and well-being had improved as a result. Greater use of the whole house, improved relationships within families, and a greater sense of self-esteem were all mentioned as benefits. For those living in intervention houses, non-asthma-related chest problems and the combined asthma symptom score for adults diminished significantly compared with those living in control houses.

Source: Barton et al., 2007

BOX 6.4: SLUM UPGRADING IN INDIA

Slum upgrading, providing the conditions necessary for a decent quality of life for the urban poor in Ahmadabad, India, cost only US$ 500/household. This included community contributions of US$ 50/household. Following the investment in these slums, there was improvement in the health of the community, with a decline in waterborne diseases, children started going to school, and women were able to take paid work, no longer having to stand in long lines to collect water.

Air quality and environmental degradation

A significant urban health issue is the pollution generated from the increased use of motorized transport. Pollution from transport contributes to total air pollution, which is estimated to be responsible for 1.4% of all deaths worldwide (WHO, 2002b). Transport accounts for 70–80% of total emissions in cities in low- and middle-income countries and this is increasing (Schirnding, 2002). There is a vicious cycle of growing car dependence, land-use change to facilitate car use, and increased inconvenience of non-motorized modes, leading to further rises in car ownership, with its knock-on effects on air quality, greenhouse gas emissions, and physical inactivity (NHF, 2007).

In order to address what is becoming a public health disaster, it is important that national and local government, with private sector collaboration, control air pollution and greenhouse gas emissions from vehicles, primarily through investment in improved technology, improved mass transport systems, and congestion charges on private transport use. For example, experiences from London (Box 6.6), Stockholm, and Singapore show that introduction of congestion charges has an immediate impact on the volume of car traffic, and subsequently on air pollution.

Urban planning and design that promotes healthy behaviours and safety

The nature of the urban environment has a major impact on health equity through its influence on behaviour and safety. Indeed, many of the risks for the urban health trajectory that is escalating towards non-communicable diseases and injuries are behaviour related. This chapter concentrates primarily on the role of urban design in relation to physical activity, diet, and violence. Clearly, the nature of different places and settings is also very influential on other behaviours such as smoking and alcohol consumption. Recommendations relating to the regulatory control of alcohol and tobacco are described in Chapter 12: Market Responsibility.

The Commission recommends that:

6.3. **Local government and civil society plan and design urban areas to promote physical activity through investment in active transport; encourage healthy eating through retail planning to manage the availability of and access to food; and reduce violence and crime through good environmental design and regulatory controls, including control of the number of alcohol outlets (see Rec 12.3).**

BOX 6.5: CITY-WIDE UPGRADING IN THE UNITED REPUBLIC OF TANZANIA

In 1972, the United Republic of Tanzania Government recognized the importance of slums in shelter delivery and subsequently endorsed Cabinet Papers 81 and 106 on National Urban Housing Policy and Squatter Improvement Schemes, respectively. These initiatives paved the way for the World Bank-funded Sites and Services and Squatter Upgrading projects of the early 1970s.

In the United Republic of Tanzania, except for slum dwellers who live on hazardous lands, compensation is paid if permanent properties are demolished. Besides compensation, the 1995 Land Policy and the subsequent 1999 Land Act provide room for the regularization of slums. Land in the United Republic of Tanzania is owned by the government and is issued under leasehold. Recently, the Ministry of Lands and Human Settlements Development embarked on a project to formalize properties in selected slums by issuing housing/property licences for two years. In parallel to this, the Property and Business Formalization Programme is under way. The two projects are aimed at reducing urban poverty. This needs to be seen in the broad framework of the National Strategy for Growth and Reduction of Poverty, which is organized in three clusters: 1) growth and reduction of income poverty, 2) good governance and accountability, and 3) improved quality of life and social well-being.

Residents of 2 out of 17 wards of Arusha City in the north part of the United Republic of Tanzania were selected to pilot the Cities Without Slums Arusha initiative. The two wards registered 20 Community Development Committees (CDCs). Subsequently, the CDCs identified the key environmental issues affecting their areas – those that they could solve themselves with minimal assistance from the government (e.g. plot subdivision and issuance of land titles, solid waste management, social services improvement) and those that needed technical and financial assistance from the city authority such as water supply and major roads. While the CDCs were prioritizing environmental problems and identifying the resources within their reach, they also elected members (from among their leaders) to represent them in restructured City Council upgrading organs, which included two ward planning committees, the Municipal Team, and the Project Steering Committee. The CDCs and these committees were specifically incorporated into the traditional set-up of the local government administrative structure in order to broaden community participation at grassroots level and improve good governance.

The Arusha City Council has started to upgrade some of the identified major roads using its own resources, particularly the road fund. The project cost for the two wards (with a population of 60 993) is estimated to be US$ 19 141 (approximately US$ 32/person).

Source: Sheuya et al., 2007

Planning tools to develop the local environment for health purposes are beginning to emerge internationally and provide guiding principles that may be adapted elsewhere (Box 6.7).

Diet and physical activity

Addressing the escalating problem of obesity in rich and poor countries alike cannot be left to market forces, but requires national and local government intersectoral approaches involving agriculture, urban planning, health, and sustainable development sectors. It is important that urban planning prioritizes cycling and walking and provides affordable and convenient mass transport and design spaces for recreation and play – in all neighbourhoods – while paying careful attention to the implications for violence and crime reduction. As highlighted in the recent United Kingdom Building Health report (NHF, 2007), a key mechanism to achieve this is through transport ministries requiring local authorities not only to adopt the policy of prioritizing pedestrians and cyclists in their

---

BOX 6.6: THE LONDON CONGESTION CHARGE (LCC) SCHEME

The primary objective of the LCC was to address the ever-increasing congestion problem that was hampering business and damaging London's status as a world city. A major strength of the LCC is its long-term incremental nature. The LCC area was widened and the cost level raised 2.5 years after its implementation. This is fundamental to a behaviour-change programme, as it means that the public can take decisions about their future behaviour based on a firm expectation that the balance of financial advantage will continue to move away from the car.

Key outcomes were:

Between 35 000 and 40 000 car trips/day switched to public transport, creating an average 6 minutes' additional physical activity per trip compared with private motor transport.

Between 5000 and 10 000 car trips switched to walking, cycling, motorcycle, taxi, or car share.

Cycling mileage within the zone rose by 28% in 2003 and by a further 4% in 2004.

Survey respondents reported improvement in comfort and overall quality of walking and public transport systems.

A large portion of the scheme revenues were reinvested in improvements in public transport, walking, cycling, and safe routes to schools.

Source: NHF, 2007

BOX 6.7: HEALTHY BY DESIGN, MELBOURNE, AUSTRALIA: AN INNOVATIVE PLANNING TOOL FOR THE DEVELOPMENT OF SAFE, ACCESSIBLE, AND ATTRACTIVE ENVIRONMENTS

The Heart Foundation in Victoria, Australia, developed Healthy by Design to assist local government and associated planners in the implementation of a broader set of Supportive Environments for Physical Activity guidelines.

Healthy by Design presents design considerations that facilitate 'healthy planning', resulting in healthy places for people to live, work, and visit. Healthy by Design provides planners with supporting research, a range of design considerations to promote walking, cycling, and public transport use, a practical design tool, and case studies. The 'Design Considerations' demonstrate ways planners can improve the health of communities through their planning and design. This is encouraged by providing:

well-planned networks of walking and cycling routes;

streets with direct, safe, and convenient access;

local destinations within walking distance of homes;

accessible open spaces for recreation and leisure;

conveniently located public transport stops;

local neighbourhoods fostering community spirit.

Traditionally, planners consider a range of guidelines that have an impact on health, safety, and access, often in isolation from each other. The Healthy by Design matrix has been developed as a practical tool that demonstrates the synergies between the different guidelines that influence built environment design, all of which contribute to positive health outcomes.

Source: KNUS, 2007

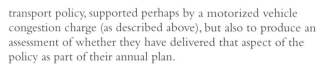

transport policy, supported perhaps by a motorized vehicle congestion charge (as described above), but also to produce an assessment of whether they have delivered that aspect of the policy as part of their annual plan.

There are a small number of examples of local planning policy that considers community-based and small-scale-retailer-oriented solutions to the problems of equitable access to healthy food. The city of Sam Chuk in Thailand restored its major food and small goods market with the assistance of local ISA that included architects. The markets are now designed not only to provide greater availability of foodstuffs, but also to be more welcoming and accessible to city residents. The London Development Agency plans to establish a sustainable food distribution hub to supply independent food retailers, restaurants, and city-based institutions (Dixon et al., 2007). One regulatory action that local government can effectively adopt in order to reduce access to foods high in fats and salt is the utilization, or strengthening, of planning regulations to manage the proliferation of fast food outlets in particular areas, for example, near schools and in socially disadvantaged neighbourhoods.

Undernutrition often sits alongside obesity among the urban poor. It is necessary to establish food security policies and programmes supported by national and/or local government and civil society actors (Box 6.8).

Violence and crime

Ensuring that all groups in society live in safety and are secure from crime and violence poses a major societal challenge. Reducing the prevalence of violent behaviour involves integrated strategies that target key domains for violence prevention such as nurturing and safe relationships between children and parents; reducing violence in the home; reducing access to alcohol, drugs, and lethal means (Villaveces et al., 2000); enhancing the life skills and opportunities of children and youth; and improving criminal justice and social welfare

systems (WHO, 2008c). Newer approaches to violence prevention include regulatory control – including alcohol sales designed so that harmful drinking is reduced (Voas et al., 2006) – conflict transformation, crime prevention through environmental design, and community-based approaches to social capital (WHO, 2007e; Roberts & Meddings, 2007).

The Commission points to the need for national and local government to invest in street lighting, early closing of nightclubs and bars, gun control, establishment of neighbourhood watch initiatives, and educational and recreational activities (including job training opportunities). The WHO Safe Communities programmes concerned with injury reduction (**http://www.phs.ki.se/csp/index_ en.htm**) have been utilized with some success in various cities throughout the world. It is recommended that these be adapted in different contexts and monitored for their effectiveness for health equity.

The Brazilian example (Box 6.9) illustrates the need for integrated efforts, attentive to both national and local specificities. A continuous dialogue with civil society and authorities at different levels was a precondition for the success of this initiative. The provision of financial support by local government to local communities to develop and deliver crime-prevention and dispute-resolution services will go a long way to help rebuild trust and social capital within communities and between communities and local authorities.

Helping to counter nationally inequitable consequences of urban growth requires sustained investment in rural development. Governments, national and local, are more likely to meet these rural challenges if the challenges are integrated into the broader context of economic and social policies aimed at development and poverty reduction; these policies should be included in documents such as the PRSP.

BOX 6.8: THE NAIROBI AND ENVIRONS FOOD SECURITY, AGRICULTURE AND LIVESTOCK FORUM (NEFSALF)

Achieving food security is imperative in poor urban settings. To eradicate the problem of food insecurity, there is a need to focus on the development of policies covering enhanced productivity, increased levels of employment, and improved access to food and the market. The importance of urban and peri-urban agriculture and livestock keeping in sustaining the urban poor as well as social, economic, and recreational values is being recognized and appreciated globally. NEFSALF, initiated in January

2004, represents a mix of actors from the community, government, and market sectors whose aim is to promote urban and peri-urban agriculture. The forum provides access to an elementary training course on urban agriculture and livestock keeping. Farmers are trained in farming as a business, group dynamics, basic skills in crop and animal husbandry, and environmental management.

Source: KNUS, 2007

HEALTH AND EQUITY : ACTION AREA 6.2

Promote health equity between rural and urban areas through sustained investment in rural development, addressing the exclusionary policies and processes that lead to rural poverty, landlessness, and displacement of people from their homes.

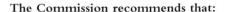
The Commission recommends that:

6.4. National and local government develop and implement policies and programmes that focus on: issues of rural land tenure and rights; year-round rural job opportunities; agricultural development and fairness in international trade arrangements; rural infrastructure including health, education, roads, and services; and policies that protect the health of rural-to-urban migrants (see Rec 5.4; 9.3).

Land rights

For most of the poor in low- and middle-income countries, land is the primary means of generating a livelihood. Redistributive land reform has positive impacts on poverty reduction and employment (Quan, 1997). An important advance in favour of gender equity, in countries such as Brazil, Colombia, Costa Rica, the Dominican Republic, Guatemala,

Honduras, and Nicaragua, has been legislation that contains provisions for the mandatory joint adjudication and titling of land to couples and/or that give priority to female household heads or specific groups of women (Deere & Leon, 2003). It is critical that national and local governments, in collaboration with international agencies, enhance and enforce processes of land tenure and land rights claims for rural communities, particularly focusing on marginalized and landless groups.

Rural livelihoods

Wider investment in agriculture, support, and services is needed to ensure viable rural communities (Montgomery et al., 2004). Lessons from the Green Revolution highlight the need for a multifaceted approach to sustainable agriculture and livelihood support. These issues have been reflected in recent recommendations from the Indian farmers representative body (Box 6.10). A central element of a comprehensive approach to rural health equity is an increase in rural household income,

---

BOX 6.9: COMMUNITY MOBILIZATION AGAINST VIOLENCE IN BRAZIL

Brazil has one of the highest homicide rates in the world. Between 1980 and 2002, the national homicide rate more than doubled, from 11.4 to 28.4 per 100 000 population. In São Paulo city, the homicide rate more than tripled during the same period, from 17.5 to 53.9 per 100 000 population. Jardim Angela is a conglomerate of slums located in the southern region of São Paulo city, with about 250 000 inhabitants. In July 1996, Brazil's Veja magazine reported an average homicide rate of 111 per 100 000 population, ranking this region as one of the most violent in the world. Jardim Angela was experiencing what has been termed the urban penalty, which was characterized in this case by structural violence, mistrust, and lack of social cohesion.

In 1996, a community integrated effort of 200 institutions called Fórum de Defesa da Vida (Life Defense Forum) was created. Parallel to the creation of this alliance, a social protection network involving civil society was organized, capitalizing on community capacity, social movements, and formal and informal health and social services. This network engaged in a broad range of community interventions ranging from

providing assistance to recently incarcerated children to a collective initiative for rebuilding community spaces. As a result of the investment in community space, abandoned spaces such as squares, clubs, and schools were rebuilt, providing space for sports, complementary school activities, and alcohol- and drug-abuse programmes. The community and police also established a coalition aimed at securing community welfare through surveillance of violence, criminality, and drug traffic. A range of policies and services were also implemented with community input including closing times for bars, a programme for victims of domestic violence, and health promotion interventions aimed at reducing teen pregnancy.

In 2005, the homicide rate for the City and State of São Paulo was 24 per 100 000 population and 18 per 100 000 population, respectively, reflecting a 51% reduction in homicide for the State. More recently, from January to July 2006, Jardim Angela experienced a more than 50% reduction in reports of muggings, assaults, pick pocketing, and car thefts compared with previous years.

Source: KNUS, 2007

BOX 6.10: INDIA – SUSTAINABLE AGRICULTURE

The Indian National Commission on Farmers and others have outlined an agriculture renewal programme that consists of the following five integrated and reinforcing action plans: soil health enhancement; irrigation water supply augmentation and demand management; credit and insurance; technology (bridging the know-how-do-how gap); and farmer-friendly markets. Overseeing the agriculture renewal programme could be an Indian Trade

Organization to complement and challenge the World Trade Organization (WTO). An underlying principle of such an organization would be the recognition of the need to ensure support for livelihood saving and balanced support for commodities that can be considered trade distorting in the global market and damaging to health and health equity.

Source: Swaminathan, 2006

with particular focus on adequate household nutrition, through strengthened support to agricultural development and rural on- and off-farm job creation. In doing so, it is important to ensure that local agriculture is not threatened by international trade agreements and agriculture protection in rich countries (World Bank, 2008) (see Chapter 12: *Market Responsibility*).

While safe, secure, year-round work is by far the preferred option to help lift rural dwellers out of poverty, micro-credit schemes, as a short-term measure, can empower impoverished groups. The Bangladesh example (Box 6.11) highlights how an integrated approach decreased levels of poverty by 30% in three years.

Poverty and hunger in poor rural populations are inextricably linked. Addressing widespread hunger and food security in rural populations cannot be done without linking it with work security and social security. This link has been well recognized by Indian policy-makers who have designed Food-for-Work and Employment Guarantee schemes with a food security component (Dreze, 2003); in Ghana where food for education initiatives are being expanded to help develop the

local agricultural economy (SIGN, 2006); and through the Millennium Villages Project, which uses an integrated approach to tackle the social determinants of health in African villages (Millennium Villages Project, nd).

Rural infrastructure and services

The provision of infrastructure and access to quality and culturally acceptable services are major health issues for rural dwellers. Progress towards MDG 3 will be made by addressing these issues through the improvement of rural women's access to time-saving technologies, particularly access to water. Redressing the urban bias in infrastructure and services investment requires investment in the rural sector to provide: quality compulsory primary and secondary school education regardless of ability to pay (see Chapter 5: *Equity from the Start*); electricity; comprehensive primary health care (see Chapter 9: *Universal Health Care*); usable roads and accessible public transport; and access to modern electronic communication. The example from Thailand (Box 6.12) illustrates government commitment to rural health through budget allocation and regionally appropriate service development.

BOX 6.11: BANGLADESH RURAL ADVANCEMENT COMMITTEE (BRAC) AND MICRO-CREDIT

With funding from the Canadian International Development Agency (CIDA), United Kingdom Department for International Development (DFID), EU, NOVIB (the Dutch affiliate of Oxfam), and WFP, the BRAC is undertaking a multi-dimensional social and economic development project focusing on the ultra-poor – typically people who are too poor to participate in micro-finance initiatives. Launched in 2002, this project provides income-generation skills training, access to health services, a monthly stipend (US$ 0.17/day) for subsistence, social development training to promote greater awareness of rights and social justice issues, and mobilization of local elites for programme support. Evaluation found that 55% of the 5000 poorest households from the poorest districts

in the country were able to gain sufficient resources to benefit from joining a micro-credit programme. The proportion of people in these areas living on less than US$ 1/day decreased from 89% to 59% during the first three years of the project and chronic food deficit fell from 60% to around 15% for project households. Factors contributing to the success of this project include: work with local elite to create an enabling environment for the programme; the provision of health education and identity cards to facilitate access to local health facilities; the provision of training and refresher training for income-generating skills; and the installation of latrines and tube-wells to improve sanitation.

Source: Schurmann, 2007

BOX 6.12: THAI RURAL HEALTH SERVICES

Since 1983, the Thai government health budget allocation to rural district hospitals and health centres has been greater than that given to urban hospitals. As a result, there was extensive geographical coverage of health services to the most peripheral level. Today, a typical health centre and district hospital cover populations of 5000 and 50 000, respectively. Health centres are staffed by a team of 3-5 nurses and paramedics, while a 30-bed district hospital is staffed by 3-4 general physicians, 30 nurses, 2-3 pharmacists, a dentist, and other paramedics – acceptable numbers of qualified staff to provide health services. In addition,

there were integrations of public health programmes (prevention, disease control, and health promotion) at all levels of care. As all public health and medicine graduates are produced by publicly funded medical colleges, students are heavily subsidized by the government. In return, mandatory rural service by new graduates, notably at district hospitals, is enforced. This plays a significant role in the functioning of district hospitals. The programme started with medical graduates in 1972; it later extended to other groups including nurses, dentists, and pharmacists.

Source: HSKN, 2007

Rural-urban migration

Displacement from rural areas, either forced through war and conflict or due to continual lack of rural resources, has resulted in rural-urban migration on a massive scale. For example, more than 40 years of armed conflict has given Colombia the largest number of displaced people in the western hemisphere (UNHCR, 2007) and the second highest proportion of displaced people after Sudan (IDMC, 2007). Consequently, a massive health burden is imposed on these populations. It is important therefore that national and local governments, in collaboration with international agencies, establish supportive policies for rural-urban migrants, ensuring maintained rights of access to essential services such as education and health.

Successful policies need to place services within reach of migrant populations. For example, the use of outreach clinics can ensure the provision of health services in areas where internal migrants are found (IOM, 2006). However, for this to be effective, migrants must be aware of the services available to them. Governments should therefore promote these services to internal migrants through advertisements in migrants' languages and by adapting their practices – most notably their opening hours and providing training for staff in multicultural health-care delivery – to meet the needs of the particular ethnic communities (Ingleby et al., 2005).

The natural environment

The disruption and depletion of natural environmental systems, including the climate system, and the task of reducing health inequities around the world go hand in hand. Ecological damage is affecting the lives of everyone in society but it has the greatest impact on the most vulnerable groups, including Indigenous Peoples who are now surviving in fragile ecologies due to unsustainable deforestation and intensive exploration for minerals and other resource-based industries (Indigenous Health Group, 2007). It is critical that the erosion of natural resources through further environmental degradation is stopped. In particular, there is an urgent need to reduce greenhouse gas emissions (McMichael et al., 2008). Highly related to the areas of action in this report is the development of adaptation and mitigation strategies for environmental change that take into account the social and health equity dimensions. There is still a need for much research into the type of action most likely to affect the triangulated relationships between social factors, environmental change, and health equity.

To begin with, the Commission recommends that:

6.5. **International agencies and national governments, building on the Intergovernmental Panel on Climate Change recommendations, consider the health equity impact of agriculture, transport, fuel, buildings, industry, and waste strategies concerned with adaptation to and mitigation of climate change.**

As noted earlier, the detailed consideration and analysis of specific policy options and development models to counter climate change was outside the remit of the Commission. The call, from the Stern Report (Stern, 2006) and others, has been for international funding to support improved regional information on climate change impacts. This offers a unique opportunity, led by WHO, to integrate the climate change and health equity agendas, ensuring information systems and policy development go through a health equity filter.

HEALTH AND EQUITY : ACTION AREA 6.3

Ensure that economic and social policy responses to climate change and other environmental degradation take into account health equity.

CHAPTER 7
Fair employment and decent work

"it is an absurdity to call a country civilized in which a decent and industrious man, laboriously mastering a trade which is valuable and necessary to the common weal, has no assurance that it will sustain him while he stands ready to practice it, or keep him out of the poorhouse when illness or age makes him idle"

HL Mencken (nd)

THE RELATIONSHIP BETWEEN WORK AND HEALTH INEQUITIES

Employment and working conditions have powerful effects on health and health equity. When these are good they can provide financial security, social status, personal development, social relations and self-esteem, and protection from physical and psychosocial hazards – each important for health (Marmot & Wilkinson, 2006). In addition to the direct health consequences of tackling work-related inequities, the health equity impacts will be even greater due to work's potential role in reducing gender, ethnic, racial, and other social inequities. This has major implications for the achievement of MDG 3.

Work and health inequities

Employment conditions

A number of employment-related conditions are associated with poorer health status, including unemployment and precarious work – such as informal work, temporary work, contract work, child labour, and slavery/bonded labour. Evidence indicates that mortality is significantly higher among temporary workers compared to permanent workers (Kivimäki et al., 2003). Poor mental health outcomes are associated with precarious employment (e.g. informal work, non-fixed term temporary contracts, and part-time work) (Artazcoz et al., 2005; Kim et al., 2006). Workers who perceive work insecurity experience significant adverse effects on their physical and mental health (Ferrie et al., 2002).

Working conditions

The conditions of work also affect health and health equity. Poor work quality may affect mental health almost as much as loss of work (Bartley, 2005; Muntaner et al., 1995; Strazdins et al., 2007). Adverse conditions that expose individuals to a range of health hazards tend to cluster in lower-status occupations. Work-related fatalities through hazardous exposures remain an extremely serious problem (ILO, 2005) (Fig. 7.1). Stress at work is associated with a 50% excess risk of coronary heart disease (Marmot, 2004; Kivimäki et al., 2006), and there is consistent

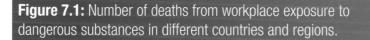

Figure 7.1: Number of deaths from workplace exposure to dangerous substances in different countries and regions.

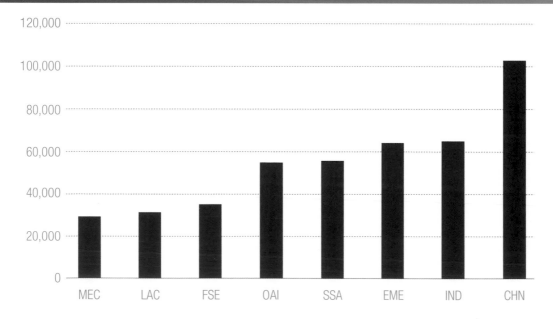

MEC = Middle East Crescent; LAC = Latin America and the Caribbean; FSE = Formerly Socialist Economies; OAI = Other Asia and Islands; SSA = sub-Saharan Africa; EME = Established Market Economies; IND = India; CHN = China.
Reprinted, with permission of the author, from ILO (2005).

evidence that high job demand, low control, and effort-reward imbalance are risk factors for mental and physical health problems (Stansfeld & Candy, 2006).

The nature of employment and working arrangements

Since the increase in global market integration began in the 1970s, there has been an emphasis on productivity and supply of products to global markets. Institutions and employers wishing to compete in this market argue the need for a flexible and ever-available global workforce. This brings with it a number of major health-related changes in employment arrangements and working conditions (Benach & Muntaner, 2007).

People's economic opportunity and financial security is primarily determined, or at least mediated, by the labour market. In 2007, there were 3 billion people aged 15 years and older in work. However, there are still 487 million workers in the world who do not earn enough to lift themselves and their families above the US$ 1/day poverty line and 1.3 billion workers do not earn above US$ 2/day (ILO, 2008). The regional variation in working poor is significant (Fig. 7.2).

The increasing power of large transnational corporations and international institutions to determine the labour policy agenda has led to a disempowerment of workers, unions, and those seeking work and a growth in health-damaging working arrangements and conditions (EMCONET, 2007). In high-income countries, there has been a growth in job insecurity and precarious employment arrangements (such as informal work, temporary work, part-time work, and piecework), job losses, and a weakening of regulatory protections (see Chapter 12: *Market Responsibility*). Most of the world's workforce, particularly in low- and middle-income countries, operates within the informal economy, which by its nature is precarious and characterized by a lack of statutory regulation to protect working conditions, wages, occupational health and safety (OHS), and injury insurance (EMCONET, 2007; ILO, 2008) (Fig. 7.3).

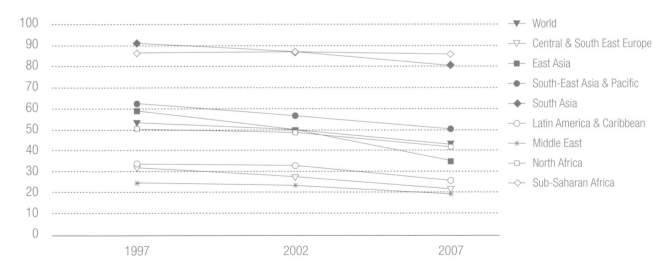

Figure 7.2: Regional variation in the percentage of people in work living on US$ 2/day or less.

2007 figures are preliminary estimates.
Reprinted, with permission of the author, from ILO (2008).

The formal economy, dominant in industrialized nations, previously tended to be characterized by progressive labour market policy-making, strong influence of unions, and often permanent full-time employment. This has undergone significant change (EMCONET, 2007). For example, Fig. 7.4 illustrates the increasing prevalence of temporary and part-time work since the early 1990s across the European Union.

Vulnerable populations

Analyses by Heymann and colleagues (2006) of nationally representative household surveys in Botswana, Brazil, Mexico, Russian Federation, South Africa, the United States, and Viet Nam found consistently that the protection and benefits provided by work are poorer for women than men (Fig. 7.5) (see also Chapter 13: *Gender Equity*).

Fair employment requires freedom from coercion – including all forms of forced labour such as bonded labour, slave labour, or child labour. Globally, it is estimated that there are about 28 million victims of slavery, and 5.7 million children are in bonded labour (EMCONET, 2007). Although major progress has been made towards the elimination of the worst forms of child labour (ILO, 2007a), there are still more than 200 million children globally aged 5-17 years who are economically active (ILO, 2006a). Increasing poor households' income and ensuring essential quality schooling will help to reduce the need for children to work. It is estimated that 70% of child labourers in India would go to school if it was available and free (Grimsrud, 2002).

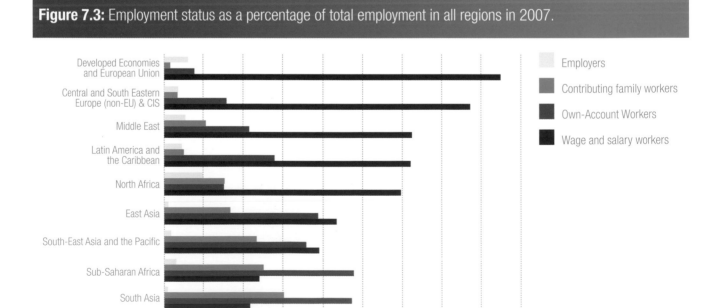

Figure 7.3: Employment status as a percentage of total employment in all regions in 2007.

Contributing family workers and own-account workers are, by their nature, forms of precarious work.
Reprinted, with permission of the author, from ILO (2008).

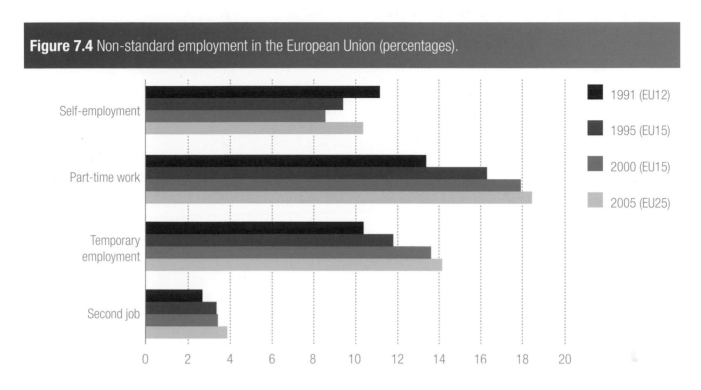

Figure 7.4 Non-standard employment in the European Union (percentages).

Reprinted, with permission of the author, from Parent-Thirion et al. (2007).

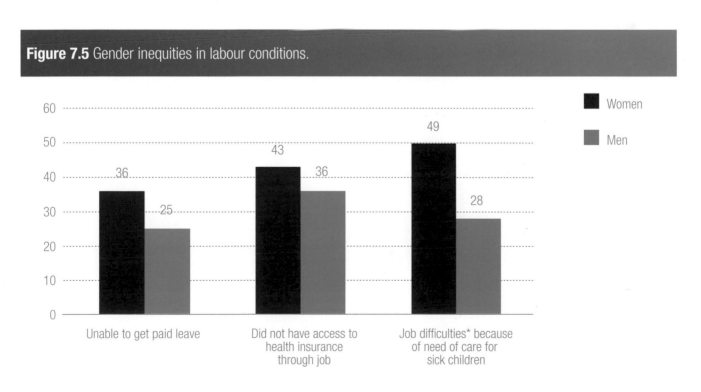

Figure 7.5 Gender inequities in labour conditions.

* Job difficulties: lost pay or lost job promotions or difficulty retaining jobs.
Adapted from Heymann (2006). Average percentages based on selected countries.

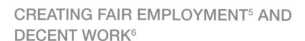
CREATING FAIR EMPLOYMENT[5] AND DECENT WORK[6]

It is good for both the economy and health equity to make the promotion of fair employment and decent work a central focus in countries' policy agendas and strategies for development. The development, implementation, and enforcement of laws, policies, standards, and working conditions to promote good health must involve government, employers, workers, and those seeking work. Such action at the national level will also require efforts to create a more conducive global economic environment.

The Commission recommends that:

7.1. **Full and fair employment and decent work be made a shared objective of international institutions and a central part of national policy agendas and development strategies, with strengthened representation of workers in the creation of policy, legislation, and programmes relating to employment and work (see Rec 10.2; 14.3; 15.2).**

A supportive international environment

The level and terms of work are increasingly determined by economic developments at the global level, particularly in low- and middle-income countries. Therefore, implementation of the Commission's recommendations is critically dependent upon changes in the functioning of the global economy, both to promote and sustain full employment globally and to foster and support economic policies at the national level that will contribute to the generation of fair and decent work. This indicates a need for changes in the interactions of national economies with global markets, and in the activities of international institutions, for example, WTO Agreements and IMF- and World Bank-supported programmes (see Chapters 12 and 15: *Market Responsibility; Good Global Governance*). It is critical that UN bodies and other international agencies dealing with the rights of workers have the power to influence the adoption of fair employment practices among Member States. While further consideration and analysis is needed of specific policy options and development models, measures that could potentially contribute to this process might include the following:

- Direct market constraints:
  - reduced dependence on external capital through effective financial sector regulation, appropriate use of capital controls, and measures to mobilize and retain domestic capital;
- Competitive constraints:
  - an end to 'dumping' of products in low- and middle-income country markets at prices below their cost of production;
  - graduation of required labour standards and upward convergence over time;
  - an end to tariff escalation against exports from low- and middle-income countries;
  - reduced reliance on export markets through promotion of the production of goods for the domestic market;
  - promotion of intraregional trade among low- and middle-income countries, including through the establishment and strengthening of regional trade agreements;
  - encouragement of shorter working hours in high-income countries;
- International agreements:
  - greatly increased emphasis on Special and Differential Treatment for low- and middle-income countries in future WTO Agreements;
  - stronger safeguard provisions in WTO Agreements (and bilateral and trade agreements) with respect to public health;
  - increased access by (particularly smaller) low- and middle-income countries to the WTO's Dispute Settlement Mechanism.

Most of these measures require action at the international level – either discretionary changes by individual governments (in the case of increases in, or changes in the conditions attached to, donor support) or collective action mediated by international institutions.

FAIR EMPLOYMENT AND DECENT WORK   **ACTION AREA 7.1**

Make full and fair employment and decent work a central goal of national and international social and economic policy-making.

---

[5] The term 'fair employment' complements the concept of decent work. It encompasses a public health perspective in which employment relations, as well as all the behaviours, outcomes, practices and institutions that emanate or impinge upon the employment relationship, need to be understood as a key factor in the quality of workers' health. Fair employment implies a just relationship between employers and employees.

[6] Decent work involves opportunities for work that is productive and delivers a fair income, security in the workplace, and social protection for families; better prospects for personal development and social integration; freedom for people to express their concerns, organize, and participate in the decisions that affect their lives; and equality of opportunity and treatment for all women and men.

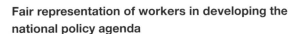
Fair representation of workers in developing the national policy agenda

To date, relatively few countries have integrated employment and working conditions into economic and social policies. To make this happen means redressing the power balance between private and public actors. Public sector leadership is critical, nationally and globally, and requires mechanisms that strengthen the representation of all workers and those seeking work in the creation of policy, legislation, and programmes relating to employment and work.

Historically, workers' participation has been positively associated with the development of collective labour rights, the labour movement, and the policies and labour market developed by modern welfare states (Box 7.1).

Unions are powerful vehicles through which protection for workers – nationally and internationally – can be collectively negotiated (see also Chapters 12 and 13: Market Responsibility; Gender Equity). It is important that governments take responsibility to ensure real participation of less powerful social actors through the provision of state guarantee of the right to collective action among formal and informal workers (Box 7.2).

BOX 7.1: WORK AND HEALTH AMONG THE LANDLESS AND SMALL LANDED FARMING POPULATION OF BRAZIL

In Brazil, 45% of agricultural land is held by around 1% of landowners, while around 50% of proprietors together own only roughly 2% of all arable land. About 31 million Brazilian people (18.8% of the total population) live in the countryside. These people, known as agregados, are extremely poor and suffer high rates of many psychosocial, educational, and health problems.

In 1984, landless families organized into the Movimento dos Trabalhadores Rurais Sem Terra (MST), or Movement of Rural Landless Workers. MST is probably the largest social movement in Latin America, with around 1.5 million members. Its fundamental success has been the increasing number of landless families being allocated their own piece of land, rising from a few thousand to more than 300 000 in 2000 settlements.

Research has shown that members of MST communities enjoy better health than other agricultural workers. The improved health of MST community members was attributed to a higher production of livestock, better nutrition (partly due to a greater diversity of produce), community support in case of need, and direct involvement in community decisions.

MST has limitations but, from its inception, it has acted as a catalyst for reform – not only agrarian reform, but also reform of health, with a direct impact on governmental decisions, influence on public policies, and a role in the civil society council of the Bolivarian Alternative for the Americas.

Source: EMCONET, 2007

BOX 7.2: NEPAL – CHILD LABOUR

Trade unions in Nepal have been collecting information and formulating policy, and have included the child labour issue in their workers' education programmes. One key issue in Nepal is bonded labour[7]. This affects children as well, as whole families are bonded under the kamaiya system. The unions, together with other civil society groups, persuaded the government that this system should be abolished and it was formally abolished in 2000. The government's decision wiped the slate clean – all debts that were the foundation for the bondage were declared illegal. In order to ensure

that former kamaiyas did not find themselves again in such levels of poverty and need, unions worked with the government to develop two important protective measures: the minimum wage for agricultural workers and the right for unions to organize in the informal economy, including the informal agricultural sector. These were two major steps that the unions did not feel they could have achieved without their strong position within the child labour movement.

Source: Grimsrud, 2002

---

[7] Kamaiya is a traditional system of bonded labour in Nepal. The people affected by this system are also called kamaiya or kamaiyas. Traditionally, people without land or work could get loans from landowners allowing them to feed themselves and survive. In exchange for this, they had to live and work on the landowner's land as quasi slaves. Debts were charged exorbitantly and whole families were forced into slave labour for years and even generations. The kamaiya system existed in particular in western Nepal and affected especially the Tharu people and Dalits ('untouchables').

The Commission recommends that:

7.2. National governments develop and implement economic and social policies that provide secure work and a living wage that takes into account the real and current cost of living for health (see Rec 8.1; 13.5).

Towards full employment

At the 2005 world summit of the UN General Assembly, governments reaffirmed their commitment to the generation of full employment and decent work as one of the critical pathways to addressing the challenge of persistent poverty around the world. Full and productive employment and decent work for all has also been introduced as a new target under MDG 1 as a way to halve the proportion of people living in extreme poverty by 2015. However, while governments resolved to make the creation of full employment and decent work for all a central objective of national and international policies (UN, 2005), this commitment has not appeared consistently.

Reaching this goal is complex, requiring integrated economic and social policy, and will require different mechanisms in different country contexts. This could include domestic action aimed directly at employment generation, for example, through labour-intensive public works, local procurement policies, expansion of income-generation programmes, and support to small and medium enterprises. A starting point is state provision of a quantum of jobs. This has different implications for countries at different levels of development.

In low-wage settings such as India, where the infrastructure and administrative capacity often exists, state-provided work guarantees can act to lift people above the national poverty line (Box 7.3).

In many OECD countries, where most of the workforce is formal and there is relatively low unemployment, governments are trying to reach full employment by first encouraging jobseekers to become more active in their efforts to find work – through job-search support, services such as job information and matching, individualized counselling, and vocational guidance and training – and second by requiring contact with employment services as well as participation in programmes after a certain period of unemployment (OECD, 2005).

Healthy living wage

Providing a living wage that takes into account the real and current cost of living for health requires supportive economic and social policy that is regularly updated and is based on the costs of health needs including adequate nutritious food, shelter, water and sanitation, and social participation (Morris & Deeming, 2004). In low-income countries, competitive advantage is heavily dependent on low labour costs, and this may be compromised if provision of a regularly updated decent living wage becomes a statutory requirement. It is timely that:

• governments, along with public health and social policy researchers, should explore mechanisms to estimate the cost of healthy living in order to calculate the living wage level in each country (Box 7.4);

• in order to reach healthful employment equitably between countries, as a first step, governments explore mechanisms to create cross-country wage agreements, initially at regional level.

BOX 7.3: INDIAN NATIONAL RURAL EMPLOYMENT GUARANTEE PROGRAMME

The National Rural Employment Guarantee Act of 2005 obliges the Indian government to provide a social safety net for impoverished rural households, through the guarantee of 100 days of work, at minimum wage, to one family member per household.

While its implementation is relatively recent and there have been procedural difficulties, there is evidence to show that it has had a positive impact in several states where it has been implemented properly. It has provided wage security for poor rural families, aided economic empowerment of women, and created public assets. In Rajasthan, where public awareness of the programme is high, 77 days of employment per rural household were provided in 2006/07. In Uttar Pradesh, major improvements in public works are observed as the scale of employment has increased; minimum wages are being paid and delays to payments have been reduced, and exploitation by private contractors is being pushed out.

This is not to say the programme does not have its difficulties, but transparency safeguards and the capacity to enforce procedures have been critical in making major progress. There is also a need to fairly revise the payment rates and extend the number of days and family members covered. To ensure social inclusion, worksite facilities are needed for women with children.

Source: The Hindu, 2008; Ganesh-Kumar et al., 2004

FAIR EMPLOYMENT AND DECENT WORK   ACTION AREA 7.2

Achieving health equity requires safe, secure, and fairly paid work, year-round work opportunities, and healthy work-life balance for all.

Training for work

A crucial part of a multifaceted policy approach to full and fair employment is ensuring that people who are not in work, or are changing work, are helped to gain the appropriate set of skills and attributes to participate in quality work. This requires the establishment of partnerships between government and NGOs to develop a comprehensive set of programmes that suit the needs of different populations such as people with a disability or the long-term unemployed. Vocational training content and delivery must meet the needs of the community and, particularly as the workforce ages, retraining opportunities are required that suit the needs of older people. Denmark's 'flexicurity' system has been among the most successful in training its workforce to ensure employability (Box 7.5).

BOX 7.4: ESSENTIAL INCOME FOR HEALTHY LIVING

An assessment was made of the cost of living among single healthy men in the United Kingdom, aged 18-30 years, living away from their family and on their own. Based on consensual evidence, a basket of commodities considered necessary for healthy day-to-day living was priced including food and physical activity, housing, household services, household goods, transport, clothing and footwear, educational costs, personal costs, personal and medical care, savings and non-state pension contributions, and leisure goods and leisure activities, including social relationships. The total cost was considered indicative of the minimum disposable income that is now essential for health.

The minimum cost of healthy living was assessed at £131.86/week (based on April 1999 prices).

Component costs, especially those of housing (which represents around 40% of this total), depend on geographical region and on several assumptions. In today's society, the disposable income that could meet this minimal cost may be posited as a necessary precondition of health. Pay from the national minimum wage (in April 1999), £3.00 an hour at 18-21 years and £3.60 at 22 years plus, translates into disposable weekly income of £105.84 and £121.12, respectively, for a 38-hour working week after statutory tax and social security deductions. At 18-21, 51 hours, and at 22 years plus, 42.5 hours would have to be worked to earn the income needed to meet the minimum costs of healthy living.

Source: Morris et al., 2000

BOX 7.5: FLEXICURITY AND LIFELONG LEARNING IN DENMARK

The Danish labour market is as flexible as the British while offering employees the same level of security as the Swedish. Flexible rules of employment, active labour market policies with the right and duty to training and job offers, relatively high benefits, and a favourable business cycle lasting a decade have repeatedly been offered as explanations for this development. There are four elements of flexicurity in the Danish context:

flexible labour market;

generous welfare schemes;

lifelong learning;

active labour market policy.

For lifelong learning, social partners are highly involved and institutionally committed to the planning and implementation of education policies, in particular continuing vocational training (CVT) policies. A specific institutional characteristic of the Danish CVT policy is that it provides services and training for both the employed and the unemployed. Under the formal responsibility of the Ministry of Labour (now Ministry of Education), but administered largely by the social partners, CVT for unskilled workers was established in 1960 and a similar system was established for skilled workers in 1965. From the late 1980s, collective agreements also included agreements on education, usually entitling the employees to 2 weeks leave per year to participate in job-relevant education.

The state is the main financer of the system. This financing system externalizes the costs of training and education from the firms, and indirectly serves as a government subsidy to the competitiveness of Danish industry. Partly as a result of this financing arrangement and the extensive rights of participation in CVT, Denmark has, for a number of years, ranked consistently among the top performers in Europe in relation to participation in CVT activities. Since the CVT system is predominantly financed by the public budget, CVT activities are more likely to provide general rather than firm-specific skills, which are transferable on the external labour market and improve the functional flexibility of internal labour markets.

Source: Madsen, 2006

Safe and decent work standards

The nature of employment and working conditions to which people are exposed has a major impact on health and its social distribution. Work must be fair and decent. The state plays a fundamental role in the reduction and mitigation of the negative health effects caused by inappropriate employment and working conditions.

The Commission recommends that:

7.3. Public capacity be strengthened to implement regulatory mechanisms to promote and enforce fair employment and decent work standards for all workers (see Rec 12.3).

Labour standards

The four core principles – freedom of association and the effective recognition of the right to collective bargaining; freedom from forced labour; the effective abolition of child labour; and non-discrimination in employment – behind many of the ILO standards provide the basis for fair employment and decent work. The enforcement by government agencies of internationally agreed labour standards and codes (ILOLEX, 2007) is an essential step towards health and health equity. In addition, if basic labour standards are enforced, such as equal remuneration for women and men, there is potential for significantly reducing gender inequity (see Chapter 13: *Gender Equity*).

The effects of transnational corporations on employment and working conditions and the cross-border nature of work and labour provide a strong argument for an international mechanism to support national governments to ratify and implement core labour standards (see Chapter 12: *Market Responsibility*). The development of administrative capacity, infrastructure, and financial support to undertake the recommendations must be supported in a coherent way by the ILO and WHO with donors and representation of formal and informal workers (see Chapter 15: *Good Global Governance*). The capacity of low-income countries to enforce labour standards may be relatively limited, particularly when considered in the context of the wider set of recommendations being made by the Commission. Labour standards should be graduated according to levels of economic development but with at least the four core principles being covered, and consideration should be given to the feasibility of implementation in a particular country of any international enforcement mechanism. Once the basic four are established, labour standards should be subject to a planned process of upward convergence over time, to avoid adverse effects.

A long-term goal for countries should be the progressive development and implementation of binding codes of practice in relation to labour and OHS of both domestic and international suppliers. Similarly, the establishment of domestic disclosure regulations for companies – clear identification of where products and their component parts are produced and under what working conditions (EMCONET, 2007) – as a long-term policy goal may contribute to equitable employment and working conditions globally.

While a number of multinational corporations have adopted voluntary codes of conduct and reportedly insist on the same labour practices at their companies throughout the world (http://www.jnj.com/community/policies/global_labor.htm), this represents a limited response to the huge task ahead. As a starting point, regular public sector monitoring of private sector voluntary codes of practice in relation to labour and OHS standards can help reinforce their impact and ensure accountability (see Chapter 12: *Market Responsibility*). Consideration could also be given to changes to company law to alter the objective function of publicly quoted companies from maximization of shareholder value to a broader set of social and environmental objectives, including employment. However, such measures would need to be coordinated internationally, to avoid companies migrating away from countries making such a change, or companies based in countries that retain the shareholder value maximization principle taking over those in countries that adopt a different objective function. In the same way that, during the past two decades, the environmental movement has succeeded in increasing the responsibility of private firms for environmental degradation, a similar effort is now needed to address fair employment and decent work.

Work-life balance

It is increasingly recognized that overwork and the resulting imbalance between work and private life has negative effects on health and well-being (Felstead et al., 2002). Rebalancing work and private life requires government policy and legislative support that provides parents the right to time to look after children and the provision of childcare regardless of ability to pay, plus work provisions such as flexible working hours, paid holidays, parental leave, job share, and long-service leave (Lundberg et al., 2007). This type of policy has begun to emerge, mainly in high-income countries. Informal workers, as with other protective legislation, are excluded from any such provisions. It is timely therefore that government, with the participation of workers – both formal and informal – develop incentives to promote work-life balance policies and supportive social protection policy (see Chapter 8: *Social Protection Across the Lifecourse*), with clear mechanisms for financing and accountability.

Precarious work

The global dominance of precarious work, with its associated insecurities (Wilthagen et al., 2003), has contributed significantly to poor health and health inequities. The majority of the world's workforce is informal and is in an extremely precarious position. Given the connection between precarious jobs and poverty, women and their families will benefit from policies addressing the problems of work insecurity, low pay, and gender discrimination in informal work (see Chapter 13: *Gender Equity*). Also of note is the increasing number of migrant workers internationally. While many are in high-skilled work, large numbers of migrants, particularly illegal migrants, experience unprotected and poor conditions, often in the informal sector. Barriers are being erected to mobility between potential migrants and demand for foreign labour in host countries (see Chapter 9: *Universal Health Care*). This, plus the lack of economic opportunity within countries, has led to the smuggling and trafficking of people as a highly profitable enterprise at the expense of gross violations of basic human rights (ILO, 2006b).

The Commission recommends that:

7.4. Governments reduce insecurity among people in precarious work arrangements including informal work, temporary work, and part-time work through policy and legislation to ensure that wages are based on the real cost of living, social security, and support for parents (see Rec 8.3).

Regulation to protect precarious workers

Government policy and legislation are needed to create more security in different working arrangements, progressively working towards greater stability within the different dimensions of work. Some governments internationally are exploring ways to strengthen the regulatory controls on downsizing, subcontracting, and outsourcing (including supply chain regulation) and developing laws that limit the use of precarious work (Box 7.6).

The informal economy's contribution to health equity

The informal sector has the potential to impact health equity over and above the effects due to improvements in working conditions. Bringing informal enterprises into the tax system would provide governments with revenue that could be used for public goods and therefore health benefits (Gordon & Lei, 2005). Government-led action such as the following may help informal enterprises contribute to the development of the nation at large:

- development of legislation and regulation to protect working conditions, wages, OHS, and other benefits among informal workers;

- extension of labour standards, and their enforcement by government, employers, and workers organizations, to all informal workers;

- development by national and local government of policies targeted at the inclusion of informal businesses in the formal sector, such as special taxation gradients that would encourage small and home-based firms to register.

For many low- and middle-income countries, working towards each of these labour standard recommendations must be done while recognizing that, in general, the informal sector exists because even the burden of existing taxation and regulation is a serious constraint on the size of the formal sector. In the absence of effective social protection mechanisms, people need to earn incomes to survive, and are therefore driven into the informal sector. The informal sector is able to operate outside the reach of regulation and taxation because administrative capacity is often inadequate to apply them effectively to the tens or hundreds of thousands of micro-enterprises and individuals that it comprises. In many of the poorest countries, it is also likely that a large proportion of entrepreneurs in the informal sector will have minimal levels of education or literacy, severely limiting their ability to conform to regulatory requirements. Addressing the regulatory issues as described above must be part of a coherent economic and social policy approach that includes social protection, education, and public sector strengthening (see also Chapters 5, 8, 10, 11, 15, and 16: *Equity from the Start; Social Protection Across the Lifecourse; Health Equity in All Policies, Systems, and Programmes; Fair Financing; Good Global Governance; Social Determinants of Health: Monitoring, Research, and Training*).

The role of workers and civil society in achieving better employment conditions

Workers' organizations play a critical role in the protection of informal workers, and have become increasingly structured. For example, since 1998, informal workers have been

---

BOX 7.6: STRENGTHENING GOVERNMENT CONTROL ON SUBCONTRACTING

Production in the global economy is composed of an increasingly complex network of contractual arrangements or supply chains. Modern business practice, especially among large corporations, depends heavily on the outsourcing of production of goods and services to other firms or distant locations (including internationally). Outsourcing occurs through a variety of subcontracting arrangements, including the provision of labour-only services and partial or complete supply of services and goods. Subcontracting can be multi-tiered, involving numerous steps between the producer of a good or service and the ultimate client. Subcontractors include other firms, small businesses, and self-employed workers. International studies have overwhelmingly found that subcontracting leads to a deterioration of OHS. The OHS risks linked to subcontracting include financial/cost-cutting pressures on subcontractors, disorganization/fracturing of OHS management, and inadequate regulatory controls.

The legal framework and government and industry response to these issues varies widely and has generally been fragmented and inadequate. Governments have recently begun to explore supply chain regulation as a means of addressing the risk-shifting associated with complex subcontracting networks. The organization at the pinnacle of the

supply chain often exercises substantial control over the parties it engages to perform tasks. This control manifests itself in the financial dependence of subcontractors (for future work) and in the terms of contractual arrangements between the outsourcing firm and its suppliers to secure quantity, quality, timeliness, and price, and to allocate regulatory risks. Unlike social protection laws, this private regulatory control effectively spans international borders. Nonetheless, governmental regulation of these contractual arrangements, covering each step and focusing responsibility at the top of the supply chain, could establish the conditions, including OHS, under which work is performed. This would need to be supported internationally.

In Australia, laws integrating labour (pay, hours) and OHS standards and workers' compensation entitlements and entailing mechanisms (including mandatory codes) for transmitting legal responsibilities to the head of the supply chain have been introduced to protect home-based clothing workers and truck drivers. A statutory licensing system covering labour supply agencies (gang masters) in agriculture, horticulture, and food processing has been introduced in the United Kingdom.

Source: EMCONET, 2007

---

represented in Senegal by an autonomous federation, the Informal and Rural Workers' Federation. Unions in Ecuador and Panama have established departments for rural and indigenous workers. In Benin and Ghana, full-time officials are responsible for the informal economy. In Canada, unions have appointed both male and female Special Programme Union Representatives with the mandate to organize atypical workers. The example from the United States (Box 7.7) illustrates how community action can act as an important adjunct and impetus to government measures. Particularly where workers are disempowered from influencing employers or market-related issues, civil society in collaboration with unions can be powerful.

Improving working conditions

Improvements in employment arrangements need to be dovetailed with a more proactive approach to work quality (EFILWC, 2007) through the improvement of working conditions.

The Commission recommends that:

7.5. OHS policy and programmes be applied to all workers – formal and informal – and that the range be expanded to include work-related stressors and behaviours as well as exposure to material hazards (see Rec 9.1).

Protection for all

The health sector has a role and responsibility to lead occupational health policy and programme development to reach the formal and informal sectors. This could include:

- developing and strengthening occupational health legislation, policy, and services to provide basic OHS coverage to all workers;

- developing occupational training programmes targeting informal workers and relevant social movements;

- establishing workers' health as part of the primary health-care function of the health-care system.

BOX 7.7: FAIR-WEAR – WORKERS AND CIVIL SOCIETY ACTION

Over the past decade, the political antisweatshop movement has become a major political claim maker and transnational advocacy network. Large garment corporations are vulnerable targets for antisweatshop activism. Their buyer-driven character forces them to survive in highly competitive markets. To make a profit, they must compete with other sellers over increasingly fickle (non-brand loyal) consumers looking for good-quality clothing at very affordable prices. To maintain and even improve their market shares and profit margins, they outsource their manufacturing to countries where labour is inexpensive and devote considerable resources to competitive logo and image marketing. In the weakly regulated setting of outsourced garment manufacturing, worker welfare is jeopardized by the fast and flexible production needed to keep up with fashion-craving consumers.

The antisweatshop movement has used the vulnerable and competitive image situation of the buyer-driven corporate world to push to improve garment workers' rights and social justice. Wanting profits and a good image among consumers, logo garment corporations are now forced to address sweatshop problems.

Two events in 1995 were crucial formative events in North America: the establishment of the amalgamated Union of Needle, Industrial, and Technical Employees (UNITE! and now UNITE HERE!) and the police raid of

domestic sweatshops in El Monte, California. UNITE! triggered a new union activism that used consumer power to pry open space for organizing workers. The El Monte raid was a wake-up call for civil society and created a media sensation with ripple effects far into the future. Shortly afterwards, the antisweatshop movement gained momentum. Internet-based advocacy groups such as Global Exchange used its media talents to focus public and media attention on celebrity corporate leaders. Old and new civil society teamed up in the antisweatshop cause – organizations representing church groups, student groups, think tanks, policy institutes, foundations, consumer organizations, international organizations, local to global labour unions, labour-oriented groups, specific antisweatshop groups, no-sweat businesses, business investors, and international humanitarian and human rights organizations, networks, and groups. Noteworthy is the less common cooperation between unions and consumers, as illustrated by the UNITE! and National Consumers League's Stop Sweatshop campaign that reached out to more than 50 million consumers globally. The antisweatshop campaign has had success. For example, in Indonesia, exporting and foreign textiles and footwear producers increased wages 20-25% faster than others.

Source: Micheletti & Stolle, 2007

FAIR EMPLOYMENT AND DECENT WORK : ACTION AREA 3

Improve working conditions for all workers to reduce exposure to material hazards, work-related stress, and health-damaging behaviours.

Development work by national government, employers, international agencies, and workers is needed to include an OHS component in employment creation programmes, subcontracting and outsourcing regulation, and trade agreements. Monitoring their implementation, particularly through strengthened enforcement of occupational health legislation and inspection, would be an initial step towards ensuring that policies and employment arrangements with major global reach are conducive to health and health equity.

The breadth of occupational health and safety

Many work-related OHS policies and programmes still concentrate on traditional workplace exposures. In Canada, for example, the Canadian Environmental Protection Act, 1999, is the main piece of legislation governing chemical substances in Canada. The Chemicals Management Plan, announced in December 2006 and the policy framework now being used, aims to assess risks to human and environmental health posed by both new and existing chemical substances (see **www. chemicalsubstances.gc.ca**). While such OHS policies remain of critical importance, particularly in low- and middle-income countries, the evidence suggests the need to expand the remit of OHS to include work-related stress and harmful behaviours. The example from the United Kingdom (Box 7.8) illustrates how employers working with workers' unions can develop workplace standards that recognize the psychosocial environment as a legitimate component of working conditions.

Through the assurance of fair employment and decent working conditions, government, employers, and workers can help to eradicate poverty, alleviate social inequities, reduce exposure to physical and psychosocial hazards, and enhance opportunities for health and well-being. And, of course, a healthy workforce is good for productivity.

BOX 7.8: NATIONAL-LEVEL ACTION TO TACKLE WORKPLACE STRESS

The Health and Safety Commission identified work stress as one of its main priorities under the Occupational Health Strategy for Britain 2000: Revitalising Health and Safety, which set out to achieve, by 2010, a 30% reduction in the incidence of working days lost through work-related illness and injury; a 20% reduction in the incidence of people suffering from work-related ill-health; and a 10% reduction in the rate of work-related fatal and major injuries.

In 2004, the United Kingdom Health and Safety Executive (HSE) introduced management standards for work-related stress. These standards cover six work stressors: demands, control, support, relationships, role, and change. A risk assessment tool was released at the same time as the management standards; this consists of 35 items on working conditions covering the six work stressors. The HSE management standards adopted a population-based approach to tackling workplace stress aimed at moving organizational stressors to more desirable levels rather than identifying individual employees with high levels of stress. Instead of setting reference values for acceptable levels of psychosocial working conditions that all employers should meet, the standards set aspirational targets that organizations can work towards.

The management standards are not in themselves a new law but can help employers meet their legal duty under the Management of Health and Safety at Work Regulations 1999 to assess the risk of stress-related ill-health activities arising from work.

As part of a 3-year implementation programme, in 2006/07 the HSE actively rolled out management standards to 1000 workplaces by providing support for both conducting risk assessments and making changes based on results of risk assessments. So far, evaluations in workplaces adopting the management standards approach have mostly been qualitative and good practice case studies are being made available on the HSE website (**www.hse.gov.uk/stress**). A national monitoring survey was conducted in 2004 before the introduction of the management standards, to provide a baseline for future monitoring of trends in psychosocial working conditions.

Source: EMCONET, 2007

CHAPTER 8
Social protection across the lifecourse

Everyone has the right to a standard of living adequate for the health and well-being of himself and of his family, including food, clothing, housing and medical care and necessary social services, and the right to security in the event of unemployment, sickness, disability, widowhood, old age or other lack of livelihood in circumstances beyond his control.

Article 25(a) of the United Nations Universal Declaration on Human Rights (UN, 1948)

THE RELATIONSHIP BETWEEN SOCIAL PROTECTION AND HEALTH

Four out of five people worldwide lack the back up of basic social security coverage (ILO, 2003). Extending social protection to all people, within countries and globally, will be a major step towards securing health equity within a generation. Not only is this a matter of social justice; social protection can be instrumental in realizing developmental goals, rather than being dependent on their achievement (McKinnon, 2007).

Social protection can cover a broad range of services and benefits, including basic income security, entitlements to non-income transfers such as food and other basic needs, services such as health care and education (Van Ginneken, 2003), and labour protection and benefits such as maternity leave, paid leave, and childcare. In this chapter, we concentrate on

income security. Income security typically provides protection in periods in the lifecourse in which individuals are most vulnerable (as children, when caring for children, and in old age) and in case of specific shocks (such as unemployment, sickness or disability, and loss of a main household income earner). Specific labour protection and work-related benefits are discussed in Chapter 7 (*Fair Employment and Decent Work*), while provision of and access to quality education and health care are discussed in Chapters 5 and 9 (*Equity from the Start; Universal Health Care*).

The importance of social protection across the lifecourse

Poverty and low living standards are powerful determinants of ill-health and health inequity. They have significant consequences for ECD and lifelong trajectories, among others, through crowded living conditions, lack of basic amenities, unsafe neighbourhoods, parental stress, and lack of food security. Child poverty and transmission of poverty from generation to generation are major obstacles to improving population health and reducing health inequity (see Chapter 5: *Equity from the Start*). The influence of living standards on lifelong trajectories is seen, for example, in the effect on self-rated health at age 50+ of accumulated socioeconomic risk factors across the lifecourse (Fig. 8.1).

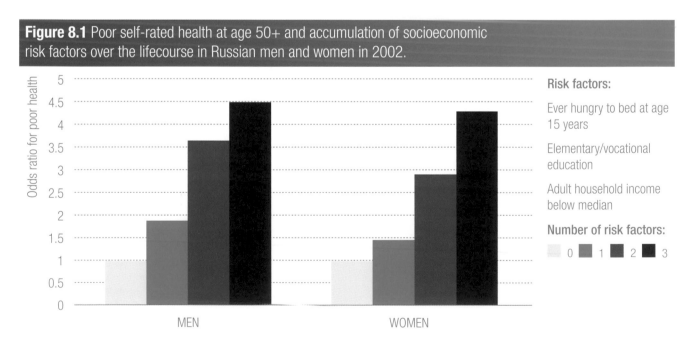

Figure 8.1 Poor self-rated health at age 50+ and accumulation of socioeconomic risk factors over the lifecourse in Russian men and women in 2002.

Risk factors:

Ever hungry to bed at age 15 years

Elementary/vocational education

Adult household income below median

Number of risk factors:
0 1 2 3

Source: Nicholson et al., 2005

Redistributive welfare systems, in combination with the extent to which people can make a healthy living through work, influence poverty levels (Lundberg et al., 2007). While evidence on the effects of these systems comes mainly from high-income countries, where data are available and policies are in place, it does show the potential effect of social protection policies more widely. In the Nordic countries, for example, poverty rates after taking into account taxes and transfers are substantially lower than in Canada, the United Kingdom, and the United States (although poverty rates are similar before taking taxes and transfers into account) (see Fig. 3.2, Chapter 3). If poverty levels among vulnerable groups are compared, variations between these countries in the prevalence of poverty become even more distinct. As Fig. 8.2 shows, the relative poverty rates among single parents, families with three or more children, and individuals aged 65+ in the Nordic countries are fairly low. It is important to highlight that this difference is not only caused by welfare state redistribution, but by a more indirect welfare state institution effect, namely, the extent to which one can make a healthy living on the labour market. Social security systems are vital; so is a minimum income that is sufficient for healthy living and labour protection (see Chapter 7: *Fair Employment and Decent Work*).

Countries with more generous social protection systems tend to have better population health outcomes, at least across high-income countries for which evidence is available (Lundberg et al., 2007). More generous family policies, for example, are associated with lower infant mortality rates (Fig. 8.3). Similarly, countries with a higher coverage and greater generosity of pensions and sickness, unemployment, and work accident insurance (taken together) have a higher LEB (Lundberg et al., 2007), and countries with more generous pension schemes tend to have lower old-age mortality (Lundberg et al., 2007). Data on the association between the magnitude of health inequities within countries and social protection policies remain scarce, however, and more investment in comparable data sources and methods is needed. The existing data from high-income countries show that while relative mortality inequities are not smaller in states with more generous, universal, social protection systems, absolute mortality levels among disadvantaged groups do appear to be lower (Lundberg et al., 2007).

Figure 8.2 Relative poverty rates for three 'social risk categories' in 11 countries, circa 2000.

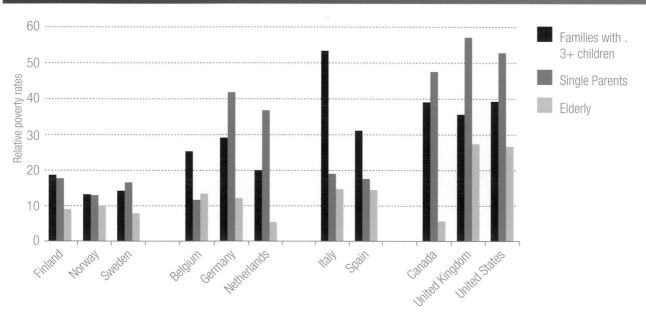

Poverty threshold = 60% of median equivalent disposable income. Equivalence scale; OECD scale.
Data source: the Luxembourg Income Study (LIS).
Reprinted, with permission of the authors, from Lundberg et al. (2007).

Protection in working life

Providing a decent wage and work-related protections and benefits including disability, employment injury, and occupational disease compensation, maternity leave, and pension benefits (EMCONET, 2007) will protect significant numbers of people worldwide. Yet only a small fraction of the world's workforce is covered by such protection schemes. For example, most workers receive no income during absences from work due to illness. Workers suffering long-term disability may also lose important skills and thus find it harder to find work in the future, or at least to continue in the work for which they have been trained. Also, the transformation of the composition of the workforce, with an increasing proportion of women working, often in precarious and informal forms of work that lack social protection, underscores the importance of universal social protection (EMCONET, 2007; WGEKN, 2007).

Vulnerability and older people

Global population ageing makes meeting social security needs an increasingly important challenge. In the next 45 years, the global population aged 60 years and over will triple. By 2050, one third of the European population will be aged 60 and over (UNDESA, Population Division, 2006). In low- and middle-income countries, the proportion of older people is growing even faster than in high-income countries. In these countries, contributory pension schemes play little role, as many people work in the informal sector. In sub-Saharan Africa and South Asia, less than 19% of older people have a contributory pension (HelpAge International, 2006a). At the same time, in many of these countries, traditional social security arrangements are weakening (McKinnon, 2007). Families are getting smaller, and older people may have no living adult children or no children willing or able to take care of them, for example, due to rural-urban migration. Older people, particularly grandmothers, are often carrying additional burdens, for example, taking care of children orphaned due to HIV/AIDS (McKinnon, 2007). Older women are often hit particularly hard. Although there is evidence that widowers are less able to care for themselves and manage their lives than widows, the absolute number of widows tends to be greater. Widowhood is when the cumulative effect of women's lower economic position throughout their lives is felt. Widows tend to be poorer, with higher rates of impoverishment and destitution, than widowers and many other subsets of the population (WGEKN, 2007). A number of low- and middle-income countries, including in Africa, have started to set up social pension systems.

Social protection in a globalizing world

Social protection systems should be created as a social right of all citizens. Yet, increasingly, large numbers of people are not bound by a country because they are international migrants, asylum seekers, or refugees. A concerted effort by donors, national governments, and international organizations, led by UNHCR, ILO and IOM, should be made to invest in

Figure 8.3: Total family policy generosity and infant mortality across 18 countries, circa 2000.

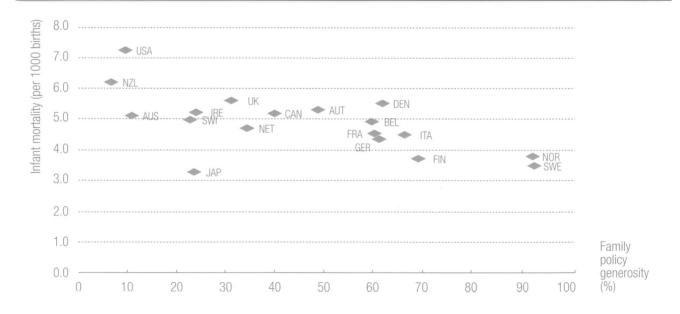

Net benefit generosity of transfers as a percentage of an average net production-worker's wage. Infant mortality expressed as deaths per 1000 live births.
AUS = Australia; AUT = Austria; BEL = Belgium; CAN = Canada; DEN = Denmark; FIN = Finland; FRA = France; GER = Germany; IRE = Ireland; ITA = Italy; JAP = Japan; NET = the Netherlands; NOR = Norway; NZL = New Zealand; SWE = Sweden; SWI = Switzerland; UK = the United Kingdom; USA = the United States of America.
Reprinted, with permission of the publisher, from Lundberg et al. (2007).

developing realistic solutions that enhance health equity, to address this growing problem.

Social protection is an important instrument to mitigate some of the negative impacts of globalization (Van Ginneken, 2003) such as trade liberalization-related economic insecurity and economy-wide shocks (GKN, 2007; Blouin et al., 2007). Under conditions of market integration, poor countries in particular have been losing important forms of public revenue (GKN, 2007), which raises issues regarding the fairness in global finance of public resources in low-income countries (see Chapters 12 and 15: *Market Responsibility; Good Global Governance*). Whereas trade liberalization and tax competition can erode the ability and/or willingness of governments to strengthen universal social protection systems, this is not universally the case. Indeed, some of the East Asian countries strengthened their social protection policies when faced with economic downturn (Box 8.1). The resources available may be further reduced by trade liberalization and tax competition (GKN, 2007).

Much can be done to protect people and support them in living flourishing lives. Social protection policies, particularly income protection, can be an important, sometimes the only, source of cash income for many households in poor and rich countries alike. In poor countries, even small cash benefits provided on a regular basis can have a large positive impact on well-being and can help combat social exclusion (McKinnon, 2007). And social protection policies are cost effective. Local economies benefit from the increase in disposable incomes (McKinnon, 2007). Evidence suggests that income redistribution, via taxes and transfers – the latter of which are key to social protection – are more efficient for poverty reduction than economic growth per se (Paes de Barros et al., 2002; de Ferranti et al., 2004; Woodward & Simms, 2006a). While limited institutional capacity remains an important barrier, it is feasible even for poor countries to start building social protection programmes, as shown by experience across the world (McKinnon, 2007).

ACTION TOWARDS UNIVERSAL SOCIAL PROTECTION

The Commission recommends that:

8.1 Governments, where necessary with help from donors and civil society organizations, and where appropriate in collaboration with employers, build universal social protection systems and increase their generosity towards a level that is sufficient for healthy living (see Rec 7.2, 11.1).

Universal social protection systems across the lifecourse

It is important for population health in general, and health of lower socioeconomic groups in particular, that social protection systems are designed such that they are universal in scope. Universality means that all citizens have equal rights to social protection. In other words, social protection is provided as a social right (Marshall, 1950), rather than given to just the poor out of pity (Lundberg et al., 2007). Universal approaches are important for the dignity and self-respect of those who need social protection the most. And because everybody benefits, rather than just one group that is singled out, universal social protection systems can enhance social cohesion (Townsend, 2007) and social inclusion (SEKN, 2007), and can be politically

---

BOX 8.1: STRENGTHENING SOCIAL PROTECTION IN CASE OF ECONOMIC CRISIS – THE CASE OF REPUBLIC OF SOUTH KOREA

Before the economic crisis, Republic of South Korea already had a social protection system that was far ahead of those of other East Asian countries. In response to rising unemployment rates due to the economic crisis, the Tripartite Commission (business-labour-government) launched legislation extending unemployment insurance to all sections of the labour force. Eligibility for this Temporary Livelihood Protection Program provided four main benefits to the newly unemployed: direct cash transfer (US$ 70/month), tuition fee waiver and lunch subsidies for their children who were students, and a 50% reduction in medical insurance premiums for 1 year. The success of this programme and its significance in cushioning the impact of the economic shock is evident in the Minimum Living Standards Security Act, legislated in 2000, which replaces (essentially incorporates) the earlier programme and includes provisions for food, clothing, housing, education, and health care, subsidized through cash and kind transfers for households who do not meet basic standards, with benefits linked to participation in labour programmes such as public works and job training.

Source: Blouin et al., 2007

SOCIAL PROTECTION : ACTION AREA 8.1

Establish and strengthen universal comprehensive social protection policies that support a level of income sufficient for healthy living for all.

more acceptable. Including the middle classes by means of universal programmes can enhance willingness of large parts of the population to pay the taxes needed to sustain universal and generous policies (Lundberg et al., 2007). Budgets for social protection tend to be larger, and perhaps more sustainable, in countries with universal protection systems. And in these countries, there tends to be less poverty and smaller income inequity than in countries with systems that target the poor (Korpi & Palme, 1998). Universal social protection systems can be tax based, contribution based, or a combination of the two.

Children

Universal social protection systems should protect all people across the lifecourse – as children, in working life, and in old age. Women and children are often the most unprotected of the population. Women do most of the world's work and have a reproductive role, but in most countries they work until they give birth, without access to maternity leave or benefits. Addressing child poverty clearly requires strong social protection measures, embedded within a broader set of policies that protect and promote a healthy standard of living and social inclusion of caregivers, including labour protection/rights, minimum income, childcare, and allowing flexible working hours. Box 8.2 describes the United Kingdom's child poverty strategy, which combines some of these elements.

Working age

The Commission emphasizes that everybody should be protected against the financial consequences of inability to work and loss of work, in a way that supports people to live healthy and flourishing lives. This means that governments, with employers, set up unemployment, sickness, and disability benefit schemes. It also means attending to the needs of people with disabilities and fighting discrimination of employers against people with disabilities. Furthermore, it includes treatment of physical and mental health problems, including addiction, that hamper finding and/or keeping a job, and providing lifelong opportunities for education and training to keep people up to speed with the changing requirements of the job market (see Chapter 7: *Fair Employment and Decent Work*). Social protection measures for those out of paid work can take different forms. In the EU, for example, a significant proportion of social provisions consist of benefits that are designed to replace or supplement earnings that individuals cannot find in the labour market for temporary or more durable reasons. Income replacement schemes usually take the form of three distinct kinds of provision: unemployment benefits (based upon previous earnings), unemployment assistance, and guaranteed minimum schemes. Some countries, such as India and South Africa, have set up employment guarantee schemes (see Chapter 7: *Fair Employment and Decent Work*).

Old age

Universal social pensions are an important element of a social protection system. They can substantially improve living standards for older people. Social pensions can raise the social status of older people within households, promote social inclusion and empowerment, and improve access to services. Moreover, they can contribute to gender equity, as women tend to live longer and often have less material resources or access to contributory pensions. Especially in low-income countries, social pension systems can also improve the well-being of other household members including children: the extra money that comes into the household can help improve, for example, school enrolment and nutrition (McKinnon, 2007). Thus, a social pension can help to break the intergenerational poverty cycle. Already several low- and middle-income countries have set up social pension schemes (Box 8.3).

BOX 8.2: NATIONAL STRATEGY TO ERADICATE CHILD POVERTY IN THE UNITED KINGDOM OF GREAT BRITAIN AND NORTHERN IRELAND

The national strategy to eradicate child poverty introduced in the United Kingdom in 1997 includes four elements: financial support for families, employment-related opportunities and support, tackling material deprivation through promoting financial inclusion and improving housing, and investing in public services. The strategy combines universal and targeted approaches. In the 18 years before the New Labour government took power, the number of children living in relative poverty in the United Kingdom had tripled to reach 34% or 4.3 million – the third highest rate in the industrialized world. To date, the percentage reduction in child poverty resulting from the strategy appears to have been modest, although important in absolute terms.

Source: SEKN, 2007

Developing, implementing, and evaluating pilot projects

Addressing health equity through a social determinants framework is a long-term investment. Low- and middle-income countries cannot be expected to implement a fully comprehensive suite of universal social protection policies overnight. It is, however, feasible gradually to develop these systems by developing and implementing pilot projects. Many low- and middle-income countries are starting to experiment with social protection programmes. These include social pension schemes and cash transfer programmes. The latter are being set up in Latin America, in particular (Fernald, Gertler & Neufeld, 2008), but also in several African countries (Bhorat, 2003; Schubert, 2005; UNICEF, 2007b). Process and impact evaluation tends to be rare, but is critical to the success of scaling up pilot projects to the national level (McKinnon, 2007). An example of a well-evaluated (targeted) cash transfer programme is Oportunidades in Mexico, which used randomly assigned treatment and control groups (Box 8.6).

Successful pilot projects can be progressively rolled-out to the national level, for example, starting with the most deprived regions. Sustainable development and implementation of social protection schemes are best achieved through piggybacking onto existing institutional structures (McKinnon, 2007).

In Lesotho, for example, pensions are disbursed using the countrywide post office network (Save the Children UK, HelpAge International & Institute of Development Studies, 2005).

Scaling up social protection programmes to the national level of course has implications for fiscal and institutional capacity and infrastructure. The lack of capacity and infrastructure in many low-income countries severely restricts programmes aiming to extend social protection (SEKN, 2007). Donors and international organizations, including the ILO, have an important role to play in building capacity for social protection in these countries. Building up universal social protection systems will require changes in the global economy and national economic policies, allowing all countries to reach the level of development at which this is feasible and sustainable in the long term (see Chapters 11 and 15: *Fair Financing; Good Global Governance*).

Once systems are implemented, uptake is important. Civil society organizations can play an important role in helping people become aware of and access their social security entitlements (HelpAge International, 2006a) (Box 8.4). They can also play an important role in getting and keeping social security high on the policy agenda, and in monitoring progress on government commitments regarding social protection (HelpAge International, 2006a).

BOX 8.3: UNIVERSAL SOCIAL PENSION – BOLIVIA

In Bolivia, 59% of older people live on less than a US$ 1/day. One annual payment of Bs 1800 (US$ 217) is available to all resident Bolivian citizens over the age of 65. Recipients collect the one-off annual payments in cash from affiliated banks, which are usually in urban areas. The pension makes up 1.3% of GDP. Half of recipients said that this social pension was their only source of income. It is generally spent on household expenses, but also on basic medication. In addition, the pension provides older people with capital that they can choose to invest in income-generating activities or for younger generations. Not only does this have a financial value, but it also has a social value, increasing their status within the family.

In 2004, 77% of those eligible were claiming the entitlement. However, pension coverage is particularly low among women. Unfortunately, they are also in greatest need. One problem is that identification documents are needed to register, and 16% of older people who are eligible for the pension scheme do not have identity documents, so cannot prove their eligibility. Many older people in rural communities have never had a birth certificate. HelpAge International, an NGO, supports socio-legal centres in La Paz and El Alto that help older people obtain a birth certificate from the government registry office so that they can receive their pension.

Reproduced, with minor editorial amendments, with permission of HelpAge International, from HelpAge International (2006b).

BOX 8.4: PROMOTING ACCOUNTABILITY TO OLDER PEOPLE AND UPTAKE OF PENSIONS – BANGLADESH

"In Bangladesh, an NGO, the Resource Integration Centre, worked with older people in 80 villages to form associations, which elected monitoring groups on older people's entitlements – the old age allowance, widow's allowance and access to health services. They found that significantly fewer people were receiving entitlements than were eligible – less than 1

in 10 in one area. The older people's associations held regular meetings with local government to help people claim pension entitlements; as a result, pension uptake increased five-fold, and banks improved their procedures for serving older people."

Reproduced, with permission of HelpAge International, from HelpAge International (2006a).

The generosity of social protection systems

Health and health equity are influenced not just by the degree of universalism, but also by the degree of generosity of social protection policies (Lundberg et al., 2007). Governments are advised to build up the generosity of social protection systems towards a level that is sufficient for healthy living. At the same time, minimum wages should also be sufficient for healthy living (see Chapter 7: *Fair Employment and Decent Work*), such that social protection policies and work policies are complementary.

Methods exist for calculating the minimum cost for healthy living. One methodology, proposed by Morris et al. (2007) (Box 8.5), builds a budget standard based on a basket of commodities deemed essential for healthy living. While the amount of money required for healthy living will be context dependent, such a methodology, or similar, could be adapted in all countries and used to inform minimum-wage and social welfare-benefit levels.

Low-income countries generally have limited financial resources to fund social protection programmes, and limited capacity to raise such funds given that a large part of their economy is informal and/or based on subsistence agriculture. The resources available may be further reduced by trade liberalization and tax competition (GKN, 2007). Resource constraints will often limit the generosity of social protection systems in low-income countries. Indeed, in practice the benefit level of existing universal schemes in low- and middle-income countries is often (very) limited (see Table 8.1). While insufficient and needing progressive strengthening, even a small amount of money on a regular basis can make an important difference in terms of well-being in poor countries (McKinnon, 2007; HelpAge International, 2006a). Low- and middle-income countries can progressively increase generosity to a level sufficient for healthy living, gradually protecting against a more comprehensive set of risks, where necessary with the help of donors.

Targeting

The Commission recommends that:

8.2 **Governments, where necessary with help from donors and civil society organizations, and where appropriate in collaboration with employers, use targeting only as back up for those who slip through the net of universal systems.**

While in many countries there may be a tendency to target social protection programmes to the most deprived, there are strong arguments for setting up universal protection systems, even in poor countries. Universal approaches to social protection tend to be more efficient than approaches that target the poor. Targeting is often costly and administratively difficult (HelpAge International, 2006a; McKinnon, 2007); universal systems require less administrative and institutional capacity and infrastructure. This is critical in settings where such capacity and infrastructure are the more binding constraints (provided donors contribute to or even cover the financial costs). In most poor countries, leakage to the rich costs less than the costs of means testing (World Bank, 1997). Moreover, targeting often does not produce the desired results. For example, it may leave out those who are just above the poverty line (McKinnon, 2007). Problems also include low uptake among eligible groups and inefficiencies due to the complex administrative systems required to monitor compliance, leading to irregular/erroneous payments and increased fraud (HelpAge International, 2006a; SEKN, 2007). Moreover, historical experience suggests that the form that social protection systems take, universal or targeted, tends to depend on what a system looks like from the outset: countries that start with targeted systems tend to continue along the same line (Pierson, 2000; Pierson, 2001; Korpi, 2001). For these reasons, it is advisable to create universal protection systems from the outset.

Despite these important drawbacks, means-tested or targeted cash transfers can have a significant positive impact on poverty reduction, living standards, and health and educational outcomes. Oportunidades, the conditional cash transfer programme in Mexico, for example, uses a combination of geographic and household-level targeting, and has shown important health effects (Box 8.6). Often, selective programmes based on means testing will continue to exist as complements to universal programmes (Lundberg et al., 2007). It is advised that targeting is only used as a back up for those who slip through the net of universal systems (Lundberg et al., 2007; SEKN, 2007).

BOX 8.5: MINIMUM INCOME FOR HEALTHY LIVING

An assessment was made of the cost of living among single people aged 65 without significant disabilities living independently in England. Based on consensual evidence, a basket of commodities considered necessary for healthy day-to-day living was priced including food and physical activity, housing, transport, medical care and hygiene, and costs relating to psychosocial relations/social inclusion (such as costs for telephone, newspapers, and small gifts to grandchildren and others). The total cost was considered indicative of the minimum disposable income that is now essential for health. The minimum cost of healthy living for this population group was assessed at £131.00/week (England April 2007 prices). This is substantially higher than the state pension for a single person in April 2007 of £87.30, and the Pension Credit Guarantee of £119.05 (which is means tested).

Source: Morris et al., 2007

Within universal social protection systems, conditionalities are sometimes used to stimulate specific behaviours such as use of health-care or education services. Again, an example is Oportunidades. Such cash transfer schemes are being pursued in many countries, including Brazil and Colombia, and in the high-income city New York (Office of the Mayor, 2007). Similarly, unemployment, disability, and sickness benefits, for example, can be conditional on enrolling in schemes that help find work. These conditionalities depend on the availability of jobs, according to people's capabilities, that provide long-term security with an income that is at least sufficient for healthy living (see Chapter 7: *Fair Employment and Decent Work*). While such programmes can have important positive (health) effects, the evidence for the added value of conditionalities per se is inconclusive (SEKN, 2007). A cash transfer programme in Ecuador showed positive effects on the physical, social-emotional, and cognitive development of children, even without conditionalities (Paxson & Schady, 2007).

Extending social protection systems to excluded groups

The Commission recommends that:

8.3. Governments, where necessary with help from donors and civil society organizations, and where appropriate in collaboration with employers, ensure that social protection systems extend to include those who are in precarious work, including informal work and household or care work (see Rec 7.4, 11.1, 13.3).

For all countries, rich and poor, it is important that social protection systems also protect people normally excluded from such systems: those in precarious work, including informal work and household or care work (WGEKN, 2007). This is particularly important for women, as family responsibilities often preclude them from accruing adequate benefits under contributory social protection schemes. Social protection systems, including pension schemes, should be set up so that they promote gender equity. A gender perspective must be incorporated into the design and reform of pension systems in order not to perpetuate gender inequities through social protection policies (WGEKN, 2007).

Including all through tax- and aid-based security systems

In many low- and middle-income countries, the majority of the population works in the informal sector and is therefore generally excluded from contributory social security schemes. In these countries, tax-based social protection programmes are of growing interest (HelpAge International, 2007; McKinnon, 2007). A number of low- and middle-income countries have, for example, set up universal or means-tested social pension systems (HelpAge International, 2006a) (see Table 8.1). It costs these countries 0.03-2% of GDP, depending on the size of the transfer and the size of the eligible population (HelpAge International, 2006a). Some are nationally financed, but for others donor support is needed (through general budget support and/or protected social protection sector programmes) (HelpAge International, 2006a). A combination of higher priority of social protection in public budgets and increased official development assistance can make rolling out social protection systems feasible in all countries (Mizunoya et al., 2006; Pal et al., 2005). Long-term and predictable funding mechanisms are needed and unpredictability of donor funding can be an important obstacle to the creation of social pension systems in many poor countries (HelpAge International, 2006a) (see Chapter 11: *Fair Financing*). Governments are advised to embed social security policies in poverty reduction strategies to ensure necessary donor funding (HelpAge International, 2006a). Existing schemes in countries such as Bolivia, Lesotho, Namibia, and Nepal show that creating a basic social protection system is administratively and practically feasible in low-

---

BOX 8.6: OPORTUNIDADES – CONDITIONAL CASH TRANSFER

An example of a conditional programme used to stimulate specific behaviour is Oportunidades (formerly Progressa), the conditional cash transfer programme in Mexico. The programme involves cash transfers to families provided that children aged 0-60 months are immunized and attend well-baby clinics where their nutritional status is monitored. These children are given nutritional supplements and their parents are given health education. Pregnant women receive prenatal care, lactating women receive postpartum care, other family members receive physical check-ups once per year (where they also receive health education), and adult family members participate in regular meetings where health, hygiene, and nutritional issues are discussed. An evaluation found that the programme had important health effects. Children born during the 2-year intervention period experienced 25% less illness in the first 6 months of life than control children, and children aged 0-35 months during the intervention experienced 39.5% less illness than their counterparts in the control group. Children in the programme were also one quarter as likely to be anaemic, and grew on average 1 cm more. Finally, the effects of the programme appear to be cumulative, increasing the longer the children stayed in the programme.

Source: ECDKN, 2007b

SOCIAL PROTECTION : ACTION AREA 8.2

Extend social protection systems to those normally excluded.

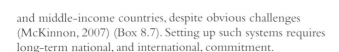
and middle-income countries, despite obvious challenges (McKinnon, 2007) (Box 8.7). Setting up such systems requires long-term national, and international, commitment.

The amount that pensioners receive from such schemes varies widely between countries, from US$ 2/month in Bangladesh and Nepal to US$ 140/month in Brazil. Few countries provide a pension above the absolute poverty line of US$ 1/day; all countries that do are middle- rather than low-income countries (Table 8.1). Protection systems and their generosity can be more rapidly increased with such external support (ILO, 2007b).

Including all through contributory social security systems

Tax-based financing is not the only way to set up universal social security systems in countries with a large informal sector. Box 8.8 describes an innovative initiative in India to set up a contributory social security system. The proposed system is based on contributions by employers by way of tax on their enterprise, by workers above the poverty line, and by the government.

Universal social protection systems are an important component of policies that seek to enable healthy living for all across the lifecourse – in rich and poor countries alike. Administrative and institutional capacity remains a critical barrier in many poor countries. Nevertheless, poor countries can progressively expand such systems by starting pilot projects and by gradually increasing the system's generosity, where necessary with help from donors.

BOX 8.7: UNIVERSAL SOCIAL PENSION SYSTEM IN LESOTHO

Since 2004, Lesotho has had a universal social pension scheme for all residents aged 70+ years. It is financed out of domestic resources and costs 1.43% of GDP. The benefit level is approximately the same as the national poverty line (about US$ 21/month). Monthly disbursement happens through the post office network that exists both in rural and urban areas (McKinnon, 2007). The age criterion of 70+, which reduces the cost of the programme, means that only a limited number of people benefit. The Government of Lesotho plans to lower the age limit to 65+, which would allow more people to benefit from the system.

Source: Save the Children UK, HelpAge International & Institute of Development Studies, 2005

BOX 8.8: SETTING UP A CONTRIBUTORY SOCIAL SECURITY SYSTEM IN INDIA

Of the workforce in India, 93% is informal. These workers have no security of work and income, nor statutory social security. The Self-Employed Women's Association (SEWA), a union of 1 million women workers in India, has been spearheading a national campaign for basic social security for informal workers. It developed a draft bill giving all informal workers the right to social security including, as a minimum, insurance, pension, and maternity benefits. Several national unions have joined this campaign. The national government set up a commission to develop laws and policies for informal workers. The commission developed a law that envisages basic coverage – health insurance, life and accident insurance, maternity benefits, and pension – for the 380 million workers in the informal economy. When fully implemented, these benefits will cost less than 0.5% of Indian GDP. Contributions from the government, employers as a group (by way of a tax on their enterprises), and workers above the poverty line will finance the social security coverage suggested by the commission. Workers below the poverty line will not need to provide any contributions. At the time of writing, the bill is being reviewed and is expected to be presented to Parliament in its next session.

Table 8.1: Social pensions in low- and middle-income countries

Country	Age eligibility (years)	Universal (U) or means tested (M)	Amount paid monthly (US$/ local currency)	% of population 60+ years	% of people 60+ receiving a social pension	Cost as % of GDP	Low- (L) or middle-income (M) country
Argentina	70+	M	US$ 88 273 pesos	14%	6%	0.23%	M
Bangladesh	57+	M	US$ 2 165 taka	6%	16%★	0.03%	L
Bolivia★★	65+	U	US$ 18 150 bolivianos	7%	69%	1.3%	M
Botswana	65+	U	US$ 27 166 pula	5%	85%	0.4%	M
Brazil (Beneficio de Prestacao Continuada)	67+	M	US$ 140 300 reais	9%	5%	0.2%	M
Brazil (Previdencia Rural)	60+ men 55+ women	M	US$ 140 300 reais	9%	27%★★★	0.7%	M
Chile	65+	M	US$ 75 40 556 pesos	12%	51%	0.38%	M
Costa Rica	65+	M	US$ 26 13 800 colones	8%	20%	0.18%	M
India	65+	M	US$ 4 250 rupees	8%	13%	0.01%	L
Lesotho	70+	U★★★★	US$ 21 150 loti	8%	53%	1.43%	L
Mauritius	60+	U	US$ 60 1978 rupees	10%	100%	2%	M
Moldova	62+ men 57+ women	M	US$5 63 lei	14%	12%	0.08%	L
Namibia	60+	M	US$ 28 200 dollars	5%	87%	0.8%	M
Nepal	75+	U	US$ 2 150 rupees	6%	12%	unknown	L
South Africa	65+ men 58+ women	M	US$ 109 780 rand	7%	60%	1.4%	M
Tajikistan	63+ men 58+ women	M	US$ 4 12 somoni	5%	unknown	unknown	L
Thailand	60+	M	US$ 8 300 baht	11%	16%	0.00582%	M
Uruguay	70+	M	US$ 100 2499 pesos	17%	10%	0.62%	M
Viet Nam	60+	M	US$ 6 100 000 dong	7%	2%	0.022%	L
Viet Nam	90+	U	US$ 6 100 000 dong	7%	0.5%	0.0005%	L

★Percentage of people aged 57+ years receiving a social pension; ★★paid annually; ★★★includes women 55+; ★★★★universal with a few exceptions, primarily people who are already receiving a substantial government pension (about 4% of those who would otherwise be eligible).

Reproduced, with permission of HelpAge International, from Help Age International (nd).

CHAPTER 9
Universal health care

"No one should be denied access to life-saving or health-promoting interventions for unfair reasons, including those with economic or social causes"

Margaret Chan, WHO Director-General (Chan, 2008)

THE RELATIONSHIP BETWEEN HEALTH CARE AND HEALTH EQUITY

Health-care systems[8] are a vital determinant of health. Yet, with the exception of rich industrialized countries, they are frequently chronically underresourced, and they are pervasively inequitable. Over half a million women die each year during pregnancy or delivery or shortly thereafter, virtually all in low- and middle-income countries (WHO, 2005b). Lack of access to and utilization of adequate maternity care is a key factor in this appalling statistic. In many countries, both poor and rich, costs of health care can lead to disastrous impoverishment. Every 30 seconds in the United States, someone files for bankruptcy following a serious health problem (National Coalition on Health Care, 2008). The health-care system needs to be designed and financed to ensure equitable, universal coverage, with adequate human resources. Health systems should be based on the PHC model, combining locally organized action on the social determinants of health as well as a strengthened primary level of care, and focusing at least as much on prevention and promotion as on treatment. Under these conditions, health care can offer much more than treatment for disease when it occurs. It can provide integrated, locally relevant, high-quality programmes and services promoting equitable health and well-being for all. And it can provide a common platform of security and social cohesion across societies and communities.

Inequitable distribution of health care

Health care is inequitably distributed around the world. The pattern of inequity in utilization is pronounced in low- and middle-income countries, but inequity is prevalent in high-income settings too. In the United States, minorities are more likely to be diagnosed with late-stage breast cancer and colorectal cancer than whites. Patients in lower socioeconomic strata are less likely to receive recommended diabetic services and more likely to be hospitalized for diabetes and its complications (Agency for Health Care Research and Quality, 2003). Inequities in health care are related to a host of socioeconomic and cultural factors, including income, ethnicity, gender, and rural/urban residency. As a fundamental contributor to welfare in every country, this is unacceptable.

Figure 9.1: Health-adjusted life expectancy (HALE) and private spending as a % of total health spending in 2000.

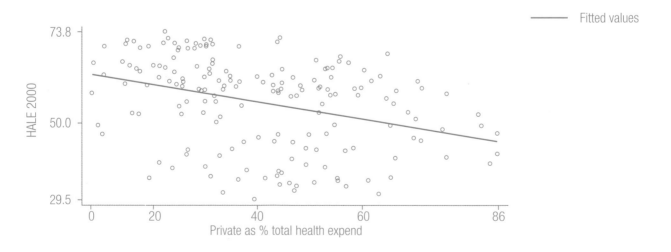

Reprinted, with permission of Palgrave Macmillan, from Koivusalo & Mackintosh (2005).

---

[8] Defined as the health system, "including preventive, curative and palliative interventions, whether directed to individuals or to populations" (WHR, 2000).

The health-care system – more than treatment of disease

Health care absorbs around 10% of global GDP, most spent in high-income countries compared with middle- and low-income countries. As employers, health-care systems provide work for around 59 million people (GKN, 2007). Health-care systems offer benefits that go beyond treating illness – especially where they are integrated with other services such as ECD programmes (ECDKN, 2007a). They can protect against sickness, generating a sense of life security, and can promote health equity through attention to the needs of socially disadvantaged and marginalized groups (HSKN, 2007). Health-care systems contribute most to improving health and health equity where the institutions and services are organized around the principle of universal coverage (extending the same scope of quality services to the whole population, according to needs and preferences, regardless of ability to pay), and where the system as a whole is organized around Primary Health Care (including both the PHC model of locally organized action across the social determinants of health, and the primary level of entry to care with upward referral).

Health-sector reform

However, broad global currents of macroeconomic policy change have strongly influenced health-sector reforms in recent decades in ways that can undermine such benefits. These reforms include encouragement of user fees, performance-related pay, separation of the provider and purchaser functions, determination of a package that privileges cost-effective medical interventions at the expense of priority interventions to address social determinants, and a stronger role for private sector agents. These have been driven strongly by a combination of international agencies, commercial actors, and medical groups whose power they enhance (Bond & Dor, 2003; Homedes & Ugalde, 2005; Lister, 2007). The result has been on the one hand an increasing commercialization of health care, and on the other, a medical and technical focus in analysis and action that have undermined the development of comprehensive primary health-care systems that could address the inequity in social determinants of health (Rifkin & Walt, 1986; Ravindran & de Pinho, 2005).

Opening the health sector to trade, reform processes have split purchasers and providers and have seen increasing segmentation and fragmentation in health-care systems. Higher private sector spending (relative to all health expenditure) is associated with worse health-adjusted life expectancy (Fig. 9.1), while higher public and social insurance spending on health (relative to GDP) is associated with better health-adjusted life expectancy (Koivusalo & Mackintosh, 2005). Moreover, public spending on health is significantly more strongly associated with lower under-5 mortality levels among the poor compared to the rich (Houweling et al., 2005). The Commission considers health care a common good, not a market commodity.

Underlying these reforms is a shift from commitment to universal coverage to an emphasis on the individual management of risk. Rather than acting protectively, health care under such reforms can actively exclude and impoverish. Upwards of 100 million people are pushed into poverty yearly through the catastrophic household health costs that result from payments for access to services (Xu et al., 2007).

Runaway commodification of health and commercialization of health care are linked to increasing medicalization of human and societal conditions, and the stark and growing divide of over- and under-consumption of health-care services between the rich and the poor worldwide. The sustainability of health-care systems is a concern for countries at all levels of socioeconomic development. Acknowledging the problem of sustainability in the context of a call for equitable health care is a vital first step in more rational policy-making, as is strengthening public participation in the design and delivery of health-care systems. The inverse care law (Tudor-Hart, 1971), in which the poor consistently gain less from health services than the better off, is visible in every country across the globe. A social determinants of health approach to health-care systems offers an alternative – one that unlocks the opportunities for greater efficiency and equity.

BOX 9.1: THAILAND – ACHIEVING UNIVERSAL HEALTH CARE

By early 2002, Thailand had achieved universal health-care coverage, incorporating a comprehensive package of curative services in outpatients, inpatients, accident and emergency, high-cost care, drugs provision reflecting the WHO Essential Drug Lists, and personal preventive and promotion services, with minimal exclusion (e.g. aesthetic surgery, renal replacement therapy for end-stage renal disease). The Universal Coverage scheme – primarily focusing on the financing side – was characterized by clear policy goals, defined participation, strong institutional capacity, and very rapid implementation (12 months). The agenda for universal coverage was set by the Prime Minister after electoral victory in 2001; policy

formulation was led by civil servants supported by policy reformers and researchers generating policy options through research-policy linkages. Based on previous experience of diverse health-care coverage schemes, the new universal coverage policy:

rejected a fee-for-service model;

adopted a capitation fee (paid to health-care provider from tax funds) as the payment method;

focused universal coverage on better use of primary care, with proper referral processes.

Source: HSKN, 2007

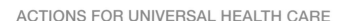
ACTIONS FOR UNIVERSAL HEALTH CARE

The Commission recommends that:

9.1   National governments, with civil society and donors, build health-care services on the principle of universal coverage of quality services, focusing on Primary Health Care (see Rec 5.2; 7.5; 8.1; 10.4; 13.6; 14.3; 15.2; 16.8).

Universal Primary Health Care

Virtually all high-income countries organize their health-care systems around the principle of universal coverage (combining mechanisms for health financing and service provision). But commitment to universal care is not limited to high-income countries. Thailand, for example, has shown leadership and success (Box 9.1).

Primary Health Care (combining the PHC model of action on the social determinants of health and an emphasis on the primary level of care, with effective upwards referral) implies comprehensive, integrated, and appropriate care, emphasizing disease prevention and health promotion. Evidence supporting the effectiveness of PHC approaches runs across the spectrum from high- to middle- and low-income settings (Box 9.2).

In Costa Rica, strengthened primary care (with improved access and the institution of multidisciplinary health teams) resulted in a reduction in the national infant mortality rate from 60 per 1000 live births in 1970 to 19 per 1000 in 1985. For every 5 years after the reform, child mortality was reduced by 13% and adult mortality by 4%, independent of improvements in other health determinants (PAHO, 2007; Starfield, 2006; Starfield et al., 2005). Evidence of the success of primary level services is also available from Africa (Democratic Republic of the Congo formerly Zaire, Liberia, Niger), Asia (China, India (the state of Kerala), Sri Lanka), and Latin America (Brazil, Cuba) (De Maeseneer et al., 2007; Doherty & Govender, 2004; Halstead et al., 1985; Macinko et al., 2006; Starfield et al., 2005; Levine, 2004).

Primary Health Care – community engagement and empowerment

The PHC model emphasizes community participation and social empowerment, even in the face of local power imbalance, resource constraints, and limited support from higher levels of the health system (Baez & Barron, 2006; Goetz & Gaventa, 2001; Lopez et al., 2007; Vega-Romero & Torres-Tovar, 2007). Social empowerment strategies can increase social awareness of health and health-care systems, strengthening

UNIVERSAL HEALTH CARE : ACTION AREA 9.1

Build health-care systems based on principles of equity, disease prevention, and health promotion.

BOX 9.2: PRIMARY HEALTH CARE, PRIMARY LEVEL CARE, AND POPULATION HEALTH

Evidence, mainly from high-income countries, shows that health-care systems that are organized around the primary care level have better health outcomes (Starfield et al., 2005).

Population health is better in geographic areas with more primary care physicians.

Individuals who receive care from primary care physicians are healthier.

There is an association between the special features of primary level care (e.g. preventive care) and improved health in the individuals who receive these services.

This last point suggests that it may not only be improved access to curative care that renders primary level care effective, but also its embodiment of the principles of disease prevention and health promotion.

Source: HSKN, 2007

BOX 9.3: EXAMPLES OF SOCIAL EMPOWERMENT STRATEGIES

Social empowerment strategies include the following:

increasing citizens' access to information and resources and raising the visibility of previously ignored health issues (the Panchayat Waves community radio programme in India; the participatory research and advocacy campaign on breast cancer in the United Kingdom; the Community Working Group on Health in Zimbabwe);

developing the consciousness, self-identity, and cohesion that underlie social action (South African study of micro-finance training and intimate partner violence for poor rural women);

involving population groups in priority-setting for planning (local theatre in the United Kingdom to identify alternative policy solutions through local Health Improvement Plans).

Source: HSKN, 2007

health literacy and mobilizing health actions (Goetz & Gaventa, 2001; Loewenson, 2003; Vega-Romero & Torres-Tovar, 2007) (Box 9.3).

Bangladesh's Urban PHC Project (Box 9.4) shows how public awareness of health needs, and partnership between local government and civil society, supports effective design and management of health care for marginalized urban groups.

Governments can take action to promote accountability of health-care systems to citizens (Murthy, 2007) (Box 9.5).

Evidence across the PHC literature supports the importance of including intended beneficiary groups in all aspects of policy and programme development, implementation, and evaluation. Advocacy – spearheaded by civil society – is required to raise attention and sustain support for services that address the health needs of poor women. Sex-specific needs in health conditions that affect both women and men must be considered, so that treatment can be accessed by both women and men without bias (WGEKN, 2007; Thorson et al., 2007; Bates et al., 2004; Huxley, 2007).

With a demographic shift in many regions towards older populations, health-care systems must focus on supporting healthy ageing. Global LEB is expected to continue to increase in both the developed and developing worlds so that the percentage of the population over age 65 years is predicted to increase from 7.4% in 2005 to between 13.7% and 19.1% in 2050 (Musgrove, 2006). Most growth is expected to occur in less-developed countries. Evidence suggests that disability,

usually due to chronic disease, is an important public health problem from age 45 years onwards. Major causes of age-related disability are neuropsychiatric disorders (the growing prevalence of conditions such as Alzheimer's disease), sight and hearing impairment, osteoporosis, arthritis, diabetes, and injury. Protective action on determinants of healthy ageing form the wider social context in which health-care services must be adapted (NAS Panel on Aging, 2006).

Prevention and promotion

Health care can do much more than treat disease when it happens. Research shows how a significant proportion of the global burden of both communicable and non-communicable disease could be reduced through improved preventive action (Lopez et al., 2006). Medical and health practitioners have powerful influence in the way society thinks about and provides health. They, alongside other advocates from across the fields of political, economic, social, and cultural action and activism, can bear witness to the ethical imperative, just as much as the efficiency value, of acting on the social causes of exposure and vulnerability to risk of poor health, and of action further upstream still (PPHCKN, 2007c; see also WHO's *Everybody's Business: Strengthening Health Systems to Improve Health Outcomes*). The PPHCKN is producing work across its departments showing how programmes can be better designed, delivered, and monitored to recognize health inequities and act on the social determinants of health. Options for action on mental health (Table 9.1) provides an example.

BOX 9.4: URBAN PRIMARY HEALTH CARE – BANGLADESH

The Urban PHC Project in Bangladesh is a partnership between municipal governments and civil society that aims to provide health services for populations living in informal settlements. City Corporations are working with 14 NGOs that set up health centres with funding from the ADB, UNDP, DFID, CIDA, and EU. The poorest women and children living in these settlements are offered subsidized good-quality primary health-care services and constitute 75% of all beneficiaries. The ultra-poor receive services free of cost. Coverage of primary care services increased from 400 000 people in 2001 to 5 million in 2004 served by 124 primary care facilities.

Source: KNUS, 2007

BOX 9.5: GOVERNMENT ACTION FOR PUBLIC ACCOUNTABILITY IN HEALTH CARE

Government actions that increase public accountability in health care include the following:

legislation on the right to health, and on rights of citizens to information and to participate in public policy and budgeting (see Chapter 10: *Health Equity in All Policies, Systems, and Programmes*);

legislation on the right of citizens to participate in hospital management and health-service delivery, and in quality assessments of provider clinics and providers; establishment of mechanisms for self-regulation by health professionals, and for protecting patient rights;

strengthening gender equity accountability of health-care systems through ombudsmen centres on sexual and reproductive health and rights and national- and state-level committees to monitor sexual and reproductive health programmes.

Source: HSKN, 2007

Table 9.1: Mental health – determinants and interventions

Differentials	Determinant	Intervention
Differential health-care access	Lack of available services	Improving availability of mental health services through integration into general health care
	Unacceptable services	Ensuring that mental health staff are culturally and linguistically acceptable
	Economic barriers to care	Providing financially accessible services
Differential consequences	Financial consequences of impact of depression on productivity	Support to caregivers to protect households from financial consequences of depression; rehabilitation programmes
	Social consequences of depression	Antistigma campaigns; promotion of supportive family and social networks
	Financial consequences of depression treatment	Reduce cost
	Lifestyle consequences of depression	Mental health promotion, including avoidance of substance abuse
Differential vulnerability	Early developmental risks	Promote ECD programmes
	Early developmental risks, maternal mental illness, weak mother–child bonding	Mother–infant interventions, including breastfeeding
	Developmental risks for adolescence	Depression prevention programmes targeting adolescents
	Development risks for older adults	Education and stress-management programmes; peer support mechanisms
	Inaccessibility to credit and savings facilities	Improve access to credit and savings facilities for poor
Differential exposure	Violence/crime	Violence/crime prevention programmes
	Social fragmentation	Promoting programmes building family cohesion and wider social cohesion
	Natural disasters	Trauma and stress support programmes
	Injury prevention	Targeting conditions of multiple deprivation
	Inadequate housing	Housing improvement interventions
	Poor neighbourhoods	Relocation programmes
	Unemployment	Employment programmes, skills training
Socioeconomic context and position	Lack of government policy and legislation; human rights framework	Strengthening mental health policy; legislation and service infrastructure
	Substance abuse	Alcohol and drugs policies
	Stigma	Mental health promotion programmes
	Unemployment	Economic policies to promote stability and financial security, and provide adequate funding for a range of public sector services (health, social services, housing)
	Financial insecurity	Welfare policies that provide a financial safety net
	Work stress	Protective labour policies (e.g. restrictions on excessive shift work, worker rights protection, job security)
	Lack of education	Mandating basic education, incentives, financial support

Source: PPHCKN, 2007d

Using targeted⁹ health care to build universal coverage

Coverage is not simply a matter of availability of drugs and services. It implies adequate, quality services reaching, and being utilized by, all those who need them. The Tanahashi model (Fig. 9.2) demonstrates five levels or steps that individuals, groups, or populations in need must pass through to obtain effective services or interventions, and how the proportion of people able to access care diminishes at each stage. Traditional disease programmes focus on effective and contact coverage. The PPHCKN is identifying entry points to overcome barriers, improving national programmes at each step (see Chapter 15: *Good Global Governance*).

In low-income countries, where public funding is limited and public spending commonly pro-rich, some argue that universal coverage is unlikely to be achieved in the short term and, as a policy goal, distracts attention from the critical need to experiment with other ways of extending health-care coverage to poorer groups (Gwatkin et al., 2004). While

it is important that all countries build a universal health-care system, ensuring that services preferentially benefit disadvantaged groups and regions can be an important strategy in the short term. Geographical or group-specific targeting and universal access are not contradictory policy approaches. Brazil and the Bolivarian Republic of Venezuela (Box 9.6) provide examples of the way large-scale national targeted health-care programmes can work towards universalism – establishing and enlarging right of access, promoting utilization, and channelling benefits, initially, towards the most disadvantaged groups in the population.

Yet care should be taken with targeting. Experience shows that it is difficult to expand small-scale projects designed preferentially to benefit the poor into national-scale action to address inequity (Ranson et al., 2003; Simmons & Shiffman, 2006).

Figure 9.2: Effective services for universal coverage.

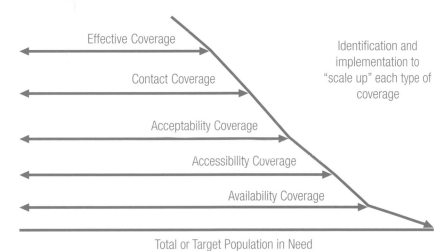

Reprinted, with permission of the publisher, from Tanahashi (1978).

---

9 'Targeted' refers to the range of social – including health-care – policy options whose central objective is to channel scarce health-care resources – in the immediate or medium term – preferentially towards poor and disadvantaged groups and regions.

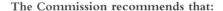
The Commission recommends that:

9.2 National governments ensure public sector leadership in health-care systems financing, focusing on tax-/insurance-based funding, ensuring universal coverage of health care regardless of ability to pay, and minimizing out-of-pocket health spending (see Rec 10.4; 11.1; 11.2).

Health-care financing – tax and insurance

Universal coverage requires that everyone within a country can use the same range of (good quality) services according to needs and preferences, regardless of income level, social status, or residency, and that people are empowered to use these services. It extends the same scope of benefits to the whole population (though the range of benefits varies between contexts), and it incorporates policy objectives of equity in payments, financial protection (Box 9.7), and equity of access to acceptable services.

There are a number of different models of health-care system financing, from general taxation, through mandatory universal insurance, to voluntary and community-based insurance schemes, and direct, out-of-pocket payment. Of these, the Commission advocates pre-payment methods of financing through general taxation (Box 9.8) and/or mandatory universal insurance for health equity (HSKN, 2007).

In Asia, public spending on health was redistributive in 10 of 11 countries, while four others achieved a pro-poor, or even, distribution of health benefits (O'Donnell et al., 2007; O'Donnell et al., 2005). In five of seven Latin American countries, public spending on health was either proportionally distributed across rich and poor groups or weighted to the poor (PAHO, 2001). Even in Africa, where concern has been expressed about inequity of public health-care expenditure, spending was found to be redistributive in all of the 30 countries studied (Chu et al., 2004). Health-care spending reached those in the lowest income categories (Kida & Mackintosh, 2005).

BOX 9.6: BRAZIL – THE FAMILY HEALTH PROGRAMME (PSF)

Established in the 1990s, PSF involves the provision of free universal access to primary care as the gateway to a publicly funded unified health-care system. Under the system, Family Health Teams (ESF) were set up covering a population of between 3000 and 4000 people each, and consisting of a general practitioner, a nurse, a nurse assistant, and a 'community agent' selected from the local population. Some ESFs also had Oral Health Teams. Initially, PSF focused on poor areas, but from 1998 onwards, the approach was adopted by the Federal Government as a strategy for transforming the existing national model of health assistance, and financial incentives were given to municipalities to encourage them to adopt the programme.

By 2006, 82 million people (46% of the population) were covered; coverage significantly increased in poor regions in the north and northeast; coverage was higher in cities with poorer populations.

Between 1988 and 2006, the programme created 330 000 new jobs.

Between 1998 and 2003, among cities with low Human Development Index, those with high PSF coverage saw the infant mortality rate decrease by 19%, while those with low PSF coverage saw it rise.

BOLIVARIAN REPUBLIC OF VENEZUELA - 'BARRIO ADENTRO

Barrio Adentro aims to transform the health-care system and has been a catalyst for initiatives aimed at wider social, political, cultural, and economic development. The programme began with the establishment of free primary care centres in informal settlements in Caracas but expanded into a national initiative providing primary health care to more than 70% of the population by 2006. In the early period of development, Barrio Adentro staff identified illiteracy and malnutrition as key priorities for public health and in response the government announced additional 'social missions' to enhance rights to land, education, housing, and cultural resources, and to promote recognition for indigenous people.

By 2006, 19.6 million people (73% of the population) were covered.

Between 2003 and 2005, there was an accelerated decline in the infant mortality rate and prevalent childhood diseases, with increased identification and follow-up of chronic illnesses.

Source: SEKN, 2007

UNIVERSAL HEALTH CARE : ACTION AREA 9.2

Ensure that health-care system financing is equitable.

The potential for redistributive health-care systems to offer health equity gains is further suggested by evidence from low- and middle-income countries that public health-care spending has a greater impact on mortality among the poor than the non-poor (Bidani & Ravallion, 1997; Gupta, Verhoeven & Tiongson, 2003; Wagstaff, 2003). So even where the poor receive less of the public spending subsidy than the rich, they may still secure relatively greater health gains than richer groups (O'Donnell et al., 2005; Wagstaff et al., 1999). This might be partly explained by the finding that health-care use among the poor is significantly more strongly related to public spending on health than health-care use among the rich (Houweling, 2005). Clearly, the emphasis on progressive tax-based health care depends on capacity to achieve adequate levels of domestic revenue (and/or adequate international aid) (see Chapter 11: *Fair Financing*).

Where taxation capacity and/or available sources of tax are weak, an alternative form of pre-payment is a national, mandatory health insurance scheme. However, especially in low-income settings, such financing can be heavily reliant on external funding, in the initial instance at least, and this raises questions about long-term sustainability. The Ghana example (Box 9.9) has shown signs of dependence, but also shows how bold moves towards universal pre-payment are possible.

Smaller-scale insurance schemes may be useful as a way of increasing health services among very poor communities and households, but the small size of the risk pool, and the potential for fragmentation among multiple schemes, can have a negative impact on health equity. Strengthened risk sharing is associated with better average LEB and more equitable child survival rates (HSKN, 2007). The Thai case study (Box 9.10, Fig. 9.3) shows how financial coverage was extended to lower-income groups through the tax-funded Universal Coverage scheme, initially complementing other health insurance schemes, but building through the national insurance agency the potential to pool funds across schemes.

BOX 9.7: EQUITY AND PROTECTION

The essence of financing arrangements for universal coverage is to ensure protection against the financial costs of ill-health for everyone. In the context of low- and middle-income countries, financing universal coverage essentially means substantially reducing the often very high amounts paid out of pocket for health care, and substantially increasing the share of health financing that comes from tax funding and/or contributory health insurance. The implications of

such changes for who pays and who benefits will depend on the financing source(s), the scope of risk pooling arrangements, the approach to purchasing, and the determinants of use of services, including the influence of any mechanisms designed to target benefits to specific groups.

Source: HSKN, 2007

BOX 9.8: PROGRESSIVE HEALTH-CARE FUNDING – EVIDENCE FROM MIDDLE-INCOME AREAS

Areas where general tax funding makes up a greater share (e.g. Hong Kong SAR, Sri Lanka, Thailand) appear to have a more progressive pattern of health

financing than those dependent more on mandatory social health insurance financing (e.g. Korea).

Source: HSKN, 2007

BOX 9.9: MANDATORY HEALTH INSURANCE IN GHANA

While a growing number of African countries are considering or are in the early phases of introducing mandatory health insurance, the Ghanaian government has made the boldest moves in this direction of any African country to date. The government has made an explicit commitment to achieving universal coverage under the National Health Insurance (NHI), but recognizes that coverage will have to be gradually extended and the aim is to achieve enrolment levels of about 60% of residents in Ghana within 10 years of starting mandatory health

insurance. Ghana's NHI explicitly includes both those in the formal and informal sectors from the outset, building on a long Ghanaian tradition of community-based health insurance schemes. Secondly, although there are different sources of funding for the formal and informal sectors, they will belong to one unified scheme. It should be noted that there are signs of severe financial stress in the Ghana health insurance programme, deriving from its reliance on external funding support.

Source: HSKN, 2007

Despite recent interest in social health insurance (Box 9.11), progressive tax-based funding offers particular advantages (Mills, 2007; Wagstaff, 2007). Examples of tax-based systems include Canada, Sweden, and the United Kingdom. In some situations, such as falling employment, it may be difficult to extend mandatory insurance; and even within insurance systems, tax funding must be used fully or partially to subsidize the costs of care provided to groups who are hard to reach through insurance, such as the informally employed or self-employed.

Community-based insurance schemes played an important role in the evolution of universal coverage in Europe and Japan (Ogawa et al., 2003), as well as in Thailand, and are currently important in China and some African (Carrin et al., 2005) and transitional countries (Balabanova, 2007). Although such schemes may offer financial protection benefits to some among the poor, cross-national evidence suggests that limited coverage, frequent exclusion of the very poorest, and weak capacity can limit the impact they have on equity and undermine their sustainability (Lagarde & Palmer, 2006; Mills, 2007). There is evidence that micro-insurance schemes for health suffer from similar problems and that, while they may offer immediate opportunities to extend coverage to those normally unable to achieve more formal insurance cover, they should be carefully regulated and monitored (Siegel et al., 2001). Separate insurance programmes may also face difficulties in achieving high coverage of the target population (Mills, 2007). Community-based and micro health insurance arrangements should only be implemented with caution, therefore, and efforts must be made to safeguard access for socially disadvantaged groups.

BOX 9.10: THAILAND – TAX-FINANCED UNIVERSAL HEALTH CARE

In the process of health-care system reforms in Thailand, a universal coverage model was built out of pre-existing health insurance schemes, including the Civil Service Medical Benefits Scheme (CSMBS) and the Social Security Scheme (SSS). Direct taxation was chosen as the funding mechanism for pragmatic reasons – the desire for speedy implementation. It has since been assessed as an equitable funding model in comparison with social insurance or other contributory schemes. Evidence from the Health and Welfare Survey conducted by the National Statistical Office indicates that, compared with the CSMBS and SSS, the Universal Coverage scheme extended benefits much more towards the poor. Where 52% of beneficiaries under the CSMBS belonged to the richest quintile, 50% of the Universal Coverage scheme beneficiaries belong to the poorest two quintiles. The scheme has resulted in a reduced incidence of catastrophic health expenditure from 5.4% to 2.8-3.3%.

Source: HSKN, 2007

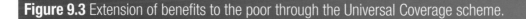

Figure 9.3 Extension of benefits to the poor through the Universal Coverage scheme.

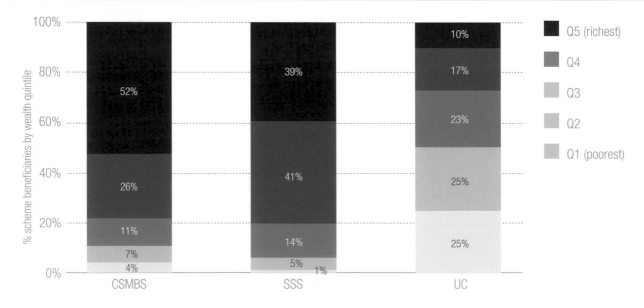

CSMBS = Civil Service Medical Benefits Scheme; SSS = Social Security Scheme; UC = Universal Coverage Scheme; Q = wealth quintile.
Source: HSKN, 2007

There are circumstances, in rich and poor country contexts, in which health-care users pay fees directly for services. In instances where such direct fee paying does not exacerbate inequity, it can be a component of health-care financing. However, where user fees adversely impact social inequity, or equity of health-care access, utilization, and/or benefit, they should be removed. Systematic reviews of available evidence clearly show that introduction of user fees in low- and middle-income countries has led to falling utilization levels (Lagarde & Palmer, 2006; Palmer et al., 2004) (Box 9.12). Out-of-pocket payments generate utilization inequities and impoverish women and lower-income and socially marginalized groups (Box 9.13).

The Commission recommends that:

9.3 National governments and donors increase investment in medical and health personnel, balancing health-worker density in rural and urban areas (see Rec 6.4; 16.5).

There is often geographical imbalance in the distribution of health workers within countries, which affects health-care service equity. More equitable distribution of the health workforce is likely to require national measures to improve overall human resource availability, as well as differential implementation between geographical areas to address the particular needs of underserved areas.

BOX 9.11: SOCIAL HEALTH INSURANCE

The concept of social health insurance is deeply ingrained in the fabric of health-care systems in Western Europe. It provides the organizing principle and a preponderance of the funding in seven countries – Austria, Belgium, France, Germany, Luxembourg, the Netherlands, and Switzerland. Since 1995, it has also become the legal basis for organizing health services in Israel. Previously, social health insurance models played an important role in a number of other countries that subsequently changed to predominantly tax-funded arrangements in the second half of the twentieth century – Denmark (1973), Italy (1978), Portugal (1979), Greece (1983), and Spain (1986).

Moreover, there are segments of social health insurance-based health-care funding arrangements still operating in predominantly tax-funded countries such as Finland, Sweden, and the United Kingdom, as well as in Greece and Portugal. In addition, a substantial number of central and eastern European countries have introduced adapted social health insurance models – among them, Hungary (1989), Lithuania (1991), the Czech Republic (1992), Estonia (1992), Latvia (1994), Slovakia (1994), and Poland (1999).

Amended, with permission of the publisher, from Saltman et al. (2004).

BOX 9.12: UGANDA – USER FEES IMPOSITION AND ABOLITION

Uganda introduced user fees on a universal basis in 1993. Although revenue generation was relatively low (generally less than 5% of expenditure), it was an important source of funds for supplementing health worker salaries, maintaining facilities, and purchasing additional drugs. However, there was a dramatic decline in the utilization of health-care services and there were growing concerns about the impact on the poor. User fees at public sector facilities were abolished in March 2001, with the exception of private wards. Utilization of health services increased immediately and dramatically. The poor particularly benefited from the removal of fees. Utilization of

health services (percentage who when sick sought professional care) increased from 58% to 70% in the case of the poorest quintile and from 80% to 85% for those in the richest quintile. National immunization coverage increased from 41% in 1999/2000 to 84% in 2002/03. This could not have been achieved without significant government financial support. Moreover, attention is required to other expenses such as drugs and transport costs, and the elimination of unofficial payments (Balabanova, 2007; O'Donnell et al., 2007).

Source: HSKN, 2007

The 2006 World Health Report (WHO, 2006) concludes that the actions with the most potential to improve personnel availability relate to salaries and payment mechanisms, combined with availability of materials and equipment needed and flexibility and autonomy to manage work. Experience in eastern and southern Africa also suggests that non-financial incentives (e.g. training, welfare provision, career paths, support, and supervision) may play a significant role in motivating health workers' choice of whether to work and stay at particular levels of service, and may have a more sustained effect in situations of high inflation and economic instability (Caffery & Frelick, 2006; Dambisya et al., 2005) (Box 9.14).

Human resources, both formal and informal, are an integral part of health-care systems. A majority of the health workforce is female, and the contributions of women to formal and informal health-care systems are significant but undervalued and unrecognized. This is partly due to the unavailability of sex disaggregated data on the care economy (WGEKN, 2007).

Women providing informal or auxiliary health services should be strongly supported in the health-care system, and closely tied in with higher levels of care service.

Across the health-care system, health-care workers offer a powerful lobby to lead the way in better integrating health care and the social determinants of health. Community health workers, while by no means the 'magic bullet' for health-care systems, offer a number of potential benefits in sustaining and developing health human resources. In most cases, community health workers are associated with lower costs in terms of training finance and time; they provide significant value to local health services provision, with minimal risk of brain-drain out-migration; depending on recruitment, they are often more willing to be posted in (or indeed are recruited from) rural areas; and they are often more conversant with the norms, traditions, and health needs of the communities they serve (Canadian Health Services Research Foundation, 2007).

BOX 9.13: OUT-OF-POCKET SPENDING AND HEALTH EQUITY

Out-of-pocket payment by patients at the point of service delivery negatively influences access to care.

In Asia, health-care payments pushed 2.7% of the total population of 11 low- to middle-income countries below the very low poverty threshold of US$ 1/day.

A cross-country study in sub-Saharan Africa found that, "the poorer the quintile, the higher the rate of use of private facilities for [acute respiratory infection (ARI)], the lower the rate of treatment for ARI, the higher the percentage of children that lack immunization entirely, and the worse the child mortality rate."

In the United States, the average employee contribution to company-provided health insurance has increased more than 143% since 2000. Average out-of-pocket costs for deductibles, co-payments for medications, and co-insurance for physician and hospital visits rose 115% during the same period.

The average out-of-pocket medical debt for those who filed for bankruptcy in the United States was US$ 12 000; 68% of those who filed for bankruptcy had health insurance, and 50% of all bankruptcy filings were partly the result of medical expenses (http://www.nchc.org/facts/cost.shtml).

Source: HSKN, 2007

BOX 9.14: REVERSING THE INTERNAL BRAIN DRAIN IN THAILAND

The internal brain drain in Thailand was reversed by providing:

combined financial and non-financial incentives for working in rural areas that included: changing physicians' status from civil servants to contracted public employees; housing; and recognition;

support through a wider programme of sustained rural development.

The differential availability of doctors between the rural northeast and Bangkok fell from 21 in 1979 to 8.6 in 1986.

Source: HSKN, 2007

UNIVERSAL HEALTH CARE : ACTION AREA 9.3

Build and strengthen the health workforce, and expand capabilities to act on the social determinants of health.

Aid for the health workforce

Increases in aid and debt relief should contribute to the strengthening of health-care systems, including contributing to recurrent costs such as human resource recruitment and training. This is not, however, always the case. Countries applying for debt relief under the Highly Indebted Poor Countries (HIPC) initiative must complete a PRSP – a national development plan – as part of the qualifying process. Each PRSP (acting as a gateway more broadly for the flow of aid to a given recipient) is moderated by means of a shorter timeframe plan for controlling expenditure – the Medium-Term Expenditure Framework (MTEF). Although not explicitly placing a cap on recurrent costs such as recruitment and salaries for much-needed health-care staff, the MTEF has been found to discourage such expenditure, leading to underinvestment in the human capacity critical for health-care systems (Box 9.15).

Global health initiatives (GHI) – such as the Global Fund for AIDS, Tuberculosis and Malaria, the Global Alliance for Vaccines and Immunisation, Stop TB, Roll Back Malaria, and the Multi-Country AIDS Programme – have brought significant new resources to international development and health. There is, however, a danger that large new funding lines, running parallel to national budgeting, distort national priorities for allocation of expenditure and action (Box 9.16). At the same time, GHI – often offering higher salaries than those available in the public sector – may cream off health human resources from the national health system, exacerbating personnel scarcity.

The Commission recommends that:

9.4   International agencies, donors and national governments address the health human resources brain-drain, focusing on investment in increased health human resources and training, and bilateral agreements to regulate gains and losses.

Adequate numbers of appropriately skilled health workers at the local level are fundamental to extending coverage, improving the quality of care, and developing successful partnerships with the community and other sectors (Kurowski et al., 2007). In many parts of the world, however, low wages coupled with lack of infrastructure and poor working conditions lead to emigration of valuable and experienced human resources (GKN, 2007). Some high-income countries actively recruit doctors and nurses in Africa and Asia. International action can help to redress this (Box 9.17).

BOX 9.15: DEBT RELIEF, POVERTY REDUCTION, AND PAYING FOR HEALTH WORKERS

Part of the approval process for many PRSPs (conditional in the agreement and provision of debt relief under the HPIC programme) is the completion of an MTEF. MTEFs are set in negotiations between ministries of finance and the IMF, which prioritize very low inflation and avoiding fiscal deficits rather than addressing poverty or health needs. This process limits the size of the total budget and, within the budget, non-discretionary expenditures such as debt repayments tend to be prioritized, limiting sectoral budgets. One study of four African countries found that health ministries had difficulty influencing this budget-setting process. Although the IMF stipulates that ceilings are not placed on recurrent costs such as the health sector wage bill, there is evidence that in practice the MTEF process has had a suppressant effect on adequate budget allocations to investment in the health workforce.

Source: GKN, 2007

BOX 9.16: GLOBAL HEALTH INITIATIVES

While GHIs have brought enormous new levels of funding to health-care systems within low- and middle-income countries (US$ 8.9 billion in 2006 for HIV/AIDS alone), there is a concern that their vertically managed programmes have potential to undermine the population health orientation of health-care systems and exacerbate health inequity. As the GHIs provide an estimated 90% of total development assistance for health (DAH) services, they have become major actors in global health policy. All GHIs need to plan for, finance, and address the impact on health systems, in particular addressing any potential drain on local and national health human resources.

Source: HSKN, 2007

Health-care systems are an important social determinant of health. Strengthened focus on the primary level of care, and wider action to build a broader Primary Health Care orientation within the health-care system, including community engagement in the assessment of needs, is vital. Within countries, increased financial allocations to health care are needed in almost every conceivable setting – most pressingly in low-income countries. More than this, though, equitable modes of financing, removing any costs at the point of service that deter use or degrade equity of access and benefit, are key. This means public sector, pre-payment methods, with smaller-scale schemes used only as subsidiary strategies. An adequate supply of health workers requires not only investment in recruitment and training – including improved training in the social determinants of health as a core part of medical and health curricula – but also action to stop the haemorrhage of health workers migrating out of low- and some middle-income countries.

BOX 9.17: POLICY OPTIONS TO STOP THE HEALTH HUMAN RESOURCES BRAIN DRAIN

A number of policy options exist to address – and stop – the brain drain of health human resources from poorer countries. These include:

return of migrant programmes (costly and largely unsuccessful);

restricted emigration (weak, resulting often only in delaying migration) or immigration (modestly successful, although criticized for singling out health workers over other migrants);

bi/multilateral agreements to manage flow between source and destination countries (somewhat successful);

strengthening domestic health human resources in source countries (strongly supported in the literature, but questionable from the perspective of source countries in the context of global markets);

restitution (including two-way health human resources flows, and increased contribution from high-income receiving countries to health and health-training systems in low-income source countries).

Preference tends towards bilateral agreements and restitution as promising policy areas.

Source: GKN, 2007

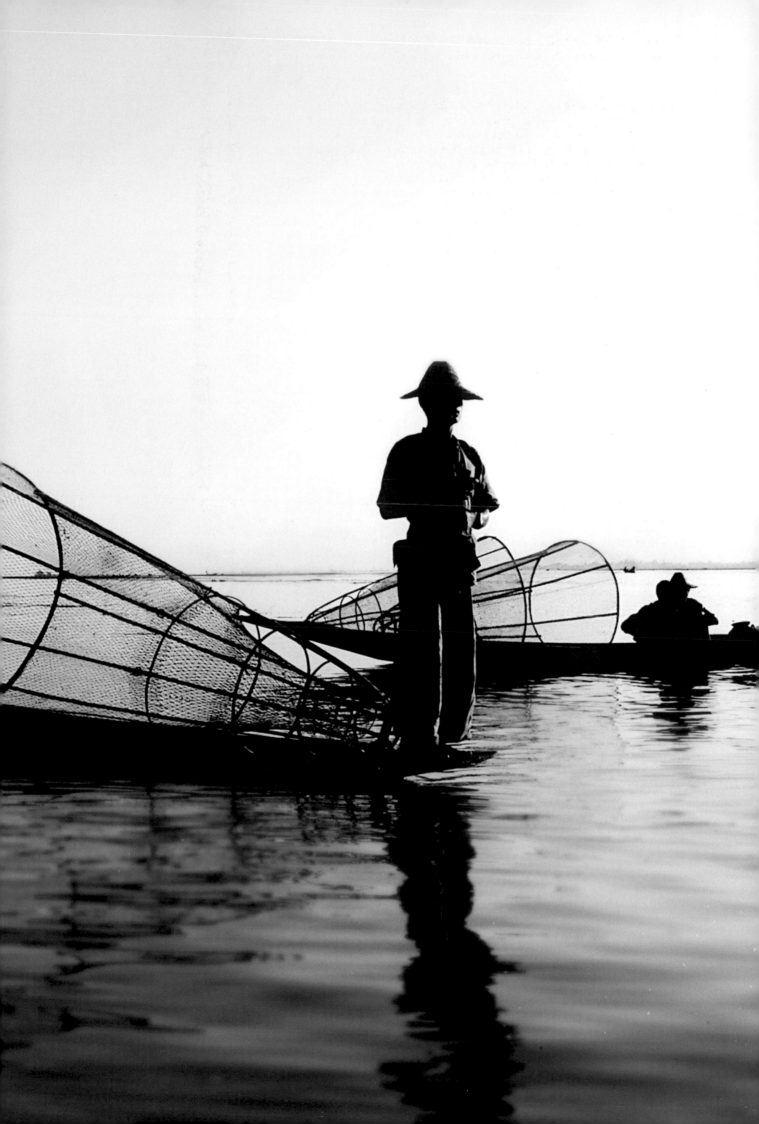

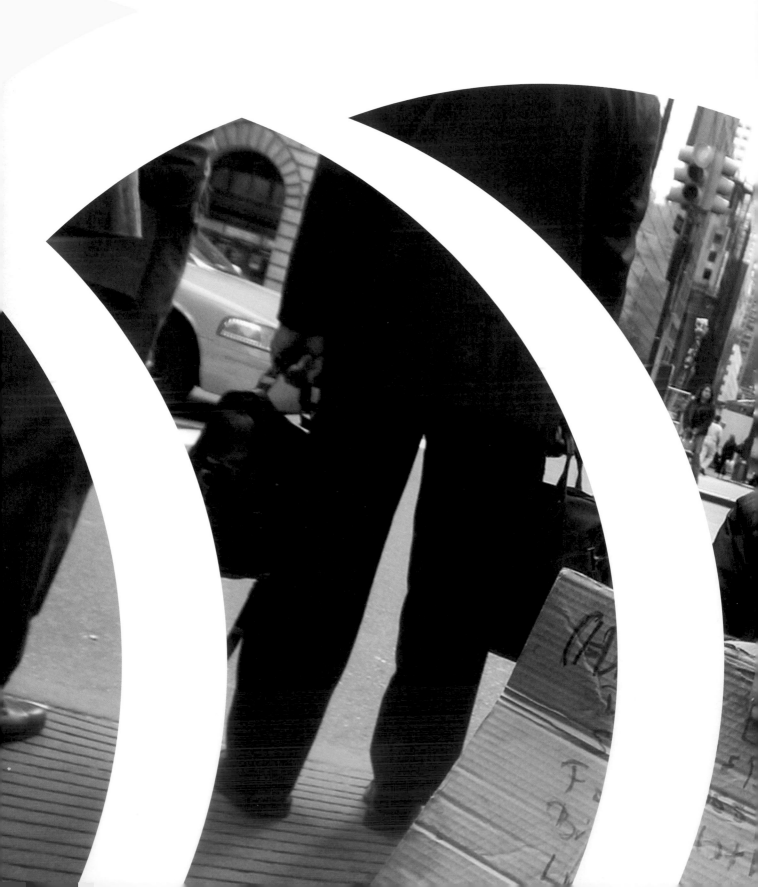

TACKLE THE INEQUITABLE DISTRIBUTION
OF POWER, MONEY, AND RESOURCES

The second of the Commission's three principles of action is:

Tackle the inequitable distribution of power, money, and resources – the structural drivers of the conditions of daily life – globally, nationally, and locally.

That some people live with much and others with little; that some enjoy long comfortable lives, while others live short, and often brutal, ones – and that these differences can be seen globally as well as within countries – is not a condition of nature. Nor is it randomly assigned. Inequity in the conditions of daily lives is shaped by deeper social structures and processes; the inequity is systematic, produced by policies that tolerate or actually enforce unfair distribution of and access to power, wealth, and other necessary social resources.

The chapters that follow map out some of the underlying, more structural aspects of society that influence health equity – social norms and political choices feeding into processes of policy formation, and thus leading to the inequitable conditions of growing, living, and working described in Part 3. Across all of these, the collective value of health equity, the vital role of public action, and thus the centrality of empowered public sector leadership emerges compellingly.

We are under no illusions, though, regarding the reality of government around the world today. It is not always benign, not always committed to social justice. In many instances, even where commitment is strong, capacity (be it institutional, financial, technical, or human) is weak or underdeveloped. And where commitment and capacity are strong, the wider global context can, increasingly, act as a brake as much as an accelerator on the creation of the conditions necessary for good and equitable health. Building political will and institutional capacity is central to all the Commission's recommendations. And that building process is not government's alone. Rather, it is through the democratic processes of civil society participation and public policy-making, supported at the regional and global levels, backed by the research on what works for health equity, and with the collaboration of private actors, that real action for health equity is possible.

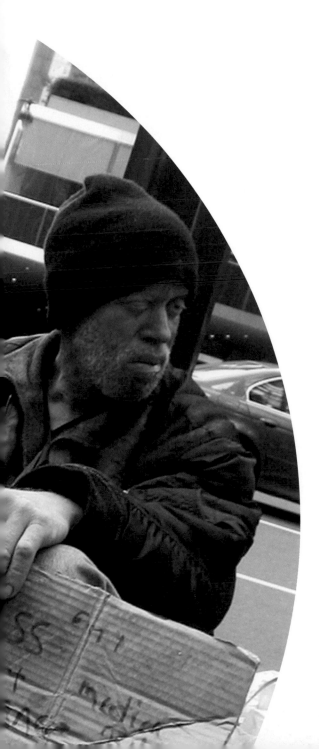

CHAPTER 10
Health equity in all policies, systems, and programmes

"If health is present in every dimension of life, it also implies that risk is everywhere. This has significant consequences for how we frame health policies and where we assign responsibilities for health in society."

Illona Kickbusch (2007)

HEALTH EQUITY: GREATER THAN THE HEALTH SECTOR

Every aspect of government and the economy has the potential to affect health and health equity – finance, education, housing, employment, transport, and health, just to name six (Marmot, 2007). While health may not be the main aim of policies in these sectors, they have strong bearing on health and health equity. A policy agenda that aims to address the social determinants of health and that is pro-equity therefore demands a relationship between health and other sectors (Vega & Irwin, 2004) at global, national, and local levels.

Policy coherence

Different government policies, depending on their nature, can either improve or worsen health and health equity. Urban planning, for example, that produces sprawling neighbourhoods with little affordable housing, few local amenities, and irregular unaffordable public transport does little to promote good health for all (NHF, 2007).

Policy coherence is crucial – this means that different government departments' policies complement rather than contradict each other in relation to the production of health and health equity. For example, trade policy that actively encourages the unfettered production, trade, and consumption of foods high in fats and sugars to the detriment of fruit and vegetable production is contradictory to health policy, which recommends relatively little consumption of high-fat, high-sugar foods and increased consumption of fruit and vegetables (Elinder, 2005). Working towards coherent policy involves a process through which policies in all government departments are checked for the extent to which they are consistent with the goal of health equity.

A critical starting point for a social determinants approach to health and health equity is, of course, within the health sector itself. Resourced and organized well, it can offer benefits that go beyond treating illness (see Chapter 9: *Universal Health Care*). It can promote health equity through specific attention to the circumstances and needs of socially disadvantaged and marginalized groups (HSKN, 2007) and provide leadership in promoting coherent policies across government (PPHCKN, 2007c).

Recognizing the role of and barriers to intersectoral action for health

ISA for health – coordinated policy and action among health and non-health sectors – can be a key strategy to achieve policy coherence and for addressing, more generally, the social determinants of health and health equity (PHAC, 2007). The 1978 International Conference on Primary Health Care in Alma Ata (WHO & UNICEF, 1978), the first International Conference on Health Promotion in Ottawa in 1986 (WHO, 1986), the 1997 WHO Global Conference on Intersectoral Action for Health and, more recently, the 2005 Bangkok Health Promotion conference (WHO, 2005d) and the 2006 EU's Finnish presidency theme of Health in All Policies (Stahl et al., 2006) each recognized that political, economic, social, cultural, environmental, behavioural, and biological factors can all favour health or be harmful to it, and acknowledged and legitimized the expansion of the territory of health and proposed policy actions in all sectors of society.

While the global evidence base and strategic call for integrated action on societal-level factors has been mounting, it is still not systematically translated into policy approaches and even less so into integrated pro-equity policy. Not all countries are resourced to embrace such a policy response to health equity. For many low- and middle-income countries, limited investment over time in infrastructure and human resources as a result of the structural adjustment policies of the 1980s and 1990s has reduced state capacity, exacerbated by the unprecedented double burden of infectious and chronic diseases (Epping-Jordan et al., 2005). Others have argued that the rhetoric of practicality and fiscal limitation has supported a continuing silo focus on 'disease-centred' approaches, making little impression on the burden of disease in low- and middle-income countries (Magnussen et al., 2004). There is also the recognition that ISA for health has a fundamental tension with the structural framework within which government operates (Vincent, 1999). And of course not only are there competing mandates between government departments, there may be, and often are, competing interests and ideologies and territorial protection (Logie, 2006).

Although progress may be slow, public health systems are being transformed from discrete interventions that address specific diseases to broad social, cultural, and economic reforms that tackle the root causes of ill health (Baum, 2008; Gostin et al., 2004; Locke, 2004). Coherent policy-making and ISA have been used globally to address a wide range of health and socioeconomic public policy challenges, including action on specific determinants of health and specific populations, communities, diseases, and health behaviours (CW, 2007). The global obesity epidemic is a good example of a socially patterned health outcome that is a consequence of changes in a constellation of social factors. The interconnected nature of the causes of obesity has generated ISA often comprising coherent sectoral responses and community-level action (Box 10.1).

To a lesser extent, broad policy frameworks that explicitly address health equity – for example, Finland, Sweden, and the United Kingdom (Stahl et al., 2006) – have outlined ISA as a key strategy (PHAC, 2007).

Beyond government

Health can be a rallying point for different sectors and actors – whether it is a local community designing a health plan for themselves (Dar es Salaam, United Republic of Tanzania's Healthy City Programme), enabling citizens to vote for priorities in local resource allocations for health (participatory budgeting in Porto Alegre, Brazil), decreasing dengue incidence (Marikina Healthy Cities Programme, Philippines), or involving the entire community in designing shared spaces that encourage walking and cycling (Healthy by Design, Victoria, Australia) (Mercado et al., 2007). Involving key people and institutions and reaching beyond government to involve civil society are vital steps towards integrated action for health equity.

The argument for a coherent approach to health equity through action on the social determinants in all socioeconomic and sociocultural contexts is unequivocal. There is, however, no 'one size fits all' approach, but rather principles that can be adapted to action in a range of contexts. In some contexts, action within a single sector will have enormous impact on health equity. In other cases, integrated action across sectors will be vital.

BUILDING A COHERENT APPROACH TO HEALTH EQUITY

Coherent action is needed within and between sectors at all levels of governance, from global through to local. The recommendations in this chapter draw on the learning from the country work stream of the Commission (CW, 2007; PHAC, 2007; PHAC & WHO, 2008b) and concentrate particularly on national government with some reference to global input from WHO and the role of civil society at the national and local levels. See Chapter 15 (*Good Global Governance*) for more details on ISA and policy coherence at the international level and Chapter 12 (*Market Responsibility*) for coherence of contributions from the private sector.

Health equity as a marker of societal progress

The Commission recommends that:

10.1. **Parliament and equivalent oversight bodies adopt a goal of improving health equity through action on the social determinants of health as a measure of government performance (see Rec 13.2; 15.1).**

Making health equity a marker of the progress of society requires its adoption and leadership at the highest political level within a nation. Parliament, or other governing body, is a key institution for promoting health equity through its representative, legislative, and oversight roles (Mususka & Chingombe, 2007). As the experience from the United Kingdom demonstrates, political leadership at the cabinet level is pivotal. During the 1980s and 1990s, the evidence assembled in the Black Report made little impact on government policy. Since 1997, with a fresh look at health inequities in the Acheson Report, there has been political will and the United Kingdom government has made social justice a priority of its socioeconomic policy, with a cross-government strategy to reduce health inequities (see Box 10.3).

The health sector is a defender of health, advocate of health equity, and negotiator for broader societal objectives. It is important therefore that ministers of health, supported by the ministry, are strongly equipped to play such a stewardship role within government, as was the case in the United Kingdom. Improving the understanding among all political actors of the social determinants of health can help to prepare the political ground (see Chapter 16: *Social Determinants of Health: Monitoring, Research, and Training*). Similarly, the strategic presentation of information on the health equity situation,

---

BOX 10.1: INTERSECTORAL ACTION ON OBESITY

Obesity is becoming a real public health challenge in transitioning countries, as it already is in high-income nations. Obesity prevention and amelioration of existing levels require approaches that ensure an ecologically sustainable, adequate, and nutritious food supply; material security; a built habitat that lends itself to easy uptake of healthier food options and participation in both organized and unorganized physical activity; and a family, educational, and work environment that positively reinforces healthy living and empowers all individuals to make healthy choices. Very little of this action sits within the capabilities or responsibilities of the health sector. Positive advances have been made between health and non-health sectors – for example, healthy urban living designed by urban planners and health professionals working together, and bans on advertisements for foods high in fats, sugars, and salt during television programmes aimed at children. However, a significant challenge remains: to engage with the multiple sectors outside health in areas such as trade, agriculture, employment, and education, areas in which action must take place if we are to redress the global obesity epidemic.

Source: Friel, Chopra & Satcher, 2007

HEALTH EQUITY IN ALL SYSTEMS : ACTION AREA 10.1

Place responsibility for action on health and health equity at the highest level of government, and ensure its coherent consideration across all policies.

demonstrating the costs of health inequity, highlighting synergies between sectors, and highlighting opportunities for intervention, are vital actions that encourage political uptake and can be spearheaded by ministers of health.

Policy coherence – mechanisms to support health equity in all policies

In addition to strong political support and leadership, reaching the goal of health equity through cross-government policy coherence requires the creation or strengthening of processes and structures within government and other agencies. It requires transparent information links across government departments, information, and analytical resources (Picciotto et al., 2004).

The Commission recommends that:

10.2. National government establish a whole-of-government mechanism that is accountable to parliament, chaired at the highest political level possible (see Rec 11.1; 11.2; 11.5; 12.2; 13.2; 16.6).

A whole-of-government mechanism concerned with health and health equity can take various forms. For example, a number of Southern African Development Community countries have set up parliamentary portfolio committees to track the activities of government sectors such as health, education, mining, agriculture, and transport. A number of the reform programmes in East and Southern Africa have been accompanied by specialist professional support and specific budgets for the work of the portfolio committees. The example

of the Zambian parliamentary Portfolio Committee on Health, Community Development, and Social Welfare illustrates a comprehensive approach to tackling HIV/AIDs that actively involved various sectors (Box 10.2).

Identifying win–win policy solutions

Central to the effectiveness of a whole-of-government mechanism is the assembly of support-of-government and administrative actors with broad mandates and a clear articulation of the benefits for each sector. It is helpful to identify priorities within different sectors and establish agreed short- and long-term health equity goals and objectives that integrate health equity policy elements into the agendas of each sector (CW, 2007). Finding policy solutions that both meet the needs of the different sectors and lead towards a shared vision will help to create political and administrative buy-in. The Health in All Policies Initiative in the state of South Australia provides an example of work undertaken recently in a high-income country to build on an existing state Strategic Plan and develop the skills and mechanisms for a whole-of-government approach to health and health equity (see **http://www.dh.sa.gov.au/pehs/publications/ public-health-bulletin.htm**).

Adapting to the context

Depending on the level of support provided by political contexts, different policy and sectoral approaches to action on the social determinants of health are more or less feasible (PHAC, 2007). For example, in contexts where equity is high

---

BOX 10.2: ZAMBIA PORTFOLIO COMMITTEE ON HEALTH, COMMUNITY DEVELOPMENT, AND SOCIAL WELFARE

The Zambian Portfolio Committee on Health, Community Development, and Social Welfare undertook an analysis of the HIV and AIDS situation in 1999, in collaboration with both the government and NGO stakeholders. Concerned with the rising HIV/AIDS statistics, the Committee undertook a performance review of government policy on HIV/AIDS in 2000. The Committee also undertook a comparative study visit to Senegal on HIV and AIDS. Arising from this, the Committee made recommendations that would see greater participation of Members of Parliament (MPs) in health matters that relate to HIV/AIDS. The recommendations contained in the Committee's report to Parliament in November 2002 included, among others, the following ISAs:

Government should consider facilitating the establishment of reproductive health activities encompassing HIV/AIDS/sexually transmitted infection (STI) prevention and control in all constituencies.

In order to sensitize the labour force, trade unions, in conjunction with the Zambia Federation of Employers and Chamber of Commerce and Industry, should incorporate HIV/AIDS prevention and control activities in their programmes at work places.

In order to sensitize school children to the danger of HIV/AIDS, government should consider introducing sex education encompassing HIV/AIDS into the school syllabus.

Government should regulate social activities that are suspected of promoting the spread of HIV, such as the sale of alcohol and opening and closing times of bars and nightclubs.

The government, NGOs, and community-based organizations should work together to set up telephone hotlines and to provide free information and counselling to the public.

The Government and all stakeholders should, as a matter of urgency, approach international drug companies and funding agencies to negotiate for a significant reduction in the cost of antiretroviral drugs to improve accessibility among those in need.

MPs and other decision-makers should strengthen their knowledge about the HIV/AIDS situation in Zambia, including awareness of the main opportunities and challenges faced by the country.

Source: Musuka & Chingombe, 2007

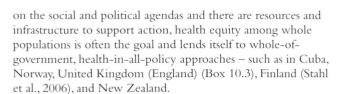
on the social and political agendas and there are resources and infrastructure to support action, health equity among whole populations is often the goal and lends itself to whole-of-government, health-in-all-policy approaches – such as in Cuba, Norway, United Kingdom (England) (Box 10.3), Finland (Stahl et al., 2006), and New Zealand.

In other contexts, ISA may not be feasible. In these instances, attention to the nature of policy and action within sectors, working towards coherent policies, will help reach the goal of improved health and health equity. As the Sri Lanka example illustrates (Box 10.4), despite the Sri Lankan Prime Minister's recognition of and commitment to ISA, existing structures and

capacities were not able to support it. What did result, however, was coherent and effective action within the different sectors, which in turn helped to ensure the adoption of primary health care as the main approach to health.

It is important to continue supporting innovative government management models and incentive structures that can encourage intersectoral cooperation such as work on priority objectives between health and one other ministry. For example, in Mozambique, the Ministry of Health worked with the Ministry of Public Works to develop water and sanitation interventions to reduce infant mortality. In Brazil, there has been collaboration between the Ministry of Health and the

---

BOX 10.3: CROSS-GOVERNMENT ACTION ON HEALTH INEQUITIES, THE UNITED KINGDOM

The Acheson report on health inequities exposed the limitations of individual agendas within social justice and health inequities and the importance of joined-up action. In 2002, as part of the formal government-wide spending negotiations, the Department of Health and the Treasury led discussions between 18 departments to inform a delivery plan for the targets and identify the contribution required from each part of government. The Treasury's financial and political authority was instrumental and brought departments to the table to engage in a cross-cutting goal. It facilitated agreement between departments to combine expertise and resources behind government priorities.

The 2003 Programme for Action identified 82 funded commitments, owned by 12 government departments, which in the following 3 years would lay a foundation for achieving the 2010 targets and provide a sustainable impact on the wider determinants of health. The Programme for Action provided a strategic framework to direct all actions towards a single goal. This prescribed coordination at both national and

local levels of government and strong performance management systems to drive delivery. An open process of regular audit, reporting, and review provides understanding of the target trajectory and the ability to refine the approach. Status reports were published in 2005 and 2008.

The target has put pressure on the government to coordinate activities. This has required good communication between departments and Treasury leadership. National frameworks now mandate health inequities as a top priority for health planners and local government, while central guidance and support has targeted underperforming areas and promoted best practice. The current Secretary of State for Health has made health inequities his priority, challenging the National Health Service, which has its 60th anniversary in 2008, to live up to its founding principles of universality and fairness.

Source: Hayward, 2007

BOX 10.4: SRI LANKA – A COHERENT SECTORAL APPROACH TO HEALTH

Sri Lanka underwent a rapid health transition during the period 1950-1975 that prolonged life and reduced mortality and fertility. The improvement in health occurred simultaneously with improvement in other states of well-being. Each sector simultaneously pursued its goals to improve the conditions for which it was responsible. Intersectoral processes did not lead to clearly articulated programmes of ISA for health in which the sectors other than health identified their contribution to health and consciously coordinated their activities to produce a desired health outcome. This failure is attributed to the existing structures of decision, the lack of capacity to identify intersectoral links and become proactive on them, and the prevailing administrative culture.

The Sri Lankan case demonstrates processes that for the most part act independently of each other but act simultaneously to improve well-being as a whole with health as an integral component. These processes required (1) an overall social development strategy, (2) a political process that evolves a high degree of consensus for such a strategy, (3) as far as possible equal weight and commitment to be given to each of the key indicators, and (4) shared responsibility for the programme at the highest level of government.

Source: PHAC & WHO, 2008

Action within the health sector

Ultimately, to address the social determinants of health and health equity requires action across the whole of government and other key stakeholders. However, the health sector itself is a good place to start building support and structures that encourage action on the social determinants of health and health equity. And the minister of health, supported by the executive branch of government, must provide strong stewardship for ISA for health and health equity, committing time and financial resources to the development of relevant skills and capacity among the health workforce and providing reward structures for intersectoral working.

The Commission recommends that:

10.4. The health sector expands its policy and programmes in health promotion, disease prevention, and health care to include a social determinants of health approach, with leadership from the minister of health (see Rec 9.1).

Skills and capacity

Taking a social determinants approach within the ministry of health will require not only political will but adequate finances and personnel within the ministry. It is likely to require broadening the skills and knowledge mix of programme staff due to:

- the necessity to diversify and target the set of interventions to cater for the specific needs and circumstances of different population groups;

- the expanding range of up-stream interventions required to influence the social determinants before they manifest in differential vulnerabilities and health outcomes;

- requirements for policy and public dialogue, cross-programme and -sector coordination, and understanding and management of complex social, economic, and political change processes.

Closer links between a diversity of complementary disciplines such as public health, health promotion, urban planning, education, and social sciences will help expand the conceptual and practical ways of working together in a social determinants of health framework. Development is needed of formal and vocational training that includes the spectrum of social determinants of health (see Chapter 16: *Social Determinants of Health: Monitoring, Research, and Training*). The example from Cuba illustrates how ISA was progressively built up in the country, incorporating skills development as a central backbone to ISA for health (Box 10.9).

Financial support for action on the social determinants of health

Critical to the successful application of a social determinants of health framework within the ministry of health's policy and programmatic focus is resource allocation at a level that makes a demonstrable difference (see Chapter 11: *Fair Financing*). Learning from different countries' methods of raising money for health promotion activities (IUHPE, 2007), hypothecated taxation from, for example, tobacco could create a sustainable source of money for action that utilizes a social determinants of health framework. Dedicating a certain percentage of national health insurance funds to action on social determinants of health is another way to ensure resource allocation. Supporting such resource generation and allocation requires incentive structures within the ministry of health, including financing and departmental awards to increase accountability on social determinants of health and health equity issues, ensuring that health sector programmes monitor equity impacts.

Institutional strengthening

Institutionalizing, implementing, and managing health equity in all policies, systems, and programmes requires, among other things recommended elsewhere in this report, technical capacity and knowledge of the social determinants of health. These are skills that are rarely taught in public health, management, and policy institutions. In particular, the workforces in the ministry of health in many countries lack training in areas that are important for addressing the social determinants of health such as social epidemiology, intersectoral planning and policy-making, and monitoring/evaluation related to the health sector and ISA. Ministries of health in few countries have experience in developing economic and political arguments for tackling the social

---

BOX 10.9: CUBA – TOOLS TO MONITOR AND EVALUATE THE EFFECTIVENESS OF INTERSECTORAL ACTION

The development of the Cuban public health system has gone through three phases, with an evolving emphasis on intersectoral collaboration. A focus on curative medicine and coverage extension in the 1960s gave way to a greater emphasis on prevention, regulation, and risk groups in the 1970s and 1980s, with a growing use of intersectoral planning commissions and the development of polyclinics that provided holistic approaches to treatment. In the 1990s, the focus expanded to embrace family and community health, with an even greater focus on ISA through the creation of local health councils and the enshrinement of ISA as one of the central principles of public health delivery. Training programmes were developed and implemented to strengthen intersectoral collaboration skills among public health professionals and decision-makers. A team from the National Health School has carried out a systematic evaluation of intersectoral activities using a standardized questionnaire and methodology that addressed a number of key intersectoral dimensions, including level of knowledge about ISA among players in the health sector and other sectors, and presence of ISA in the strategic objectives of municipalities and municipal health councils.

Source: WHO & PHAC, 2007

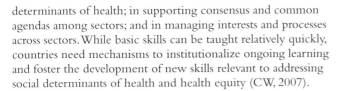
determinants of health; in supporting consensus and common agendas among sectors; and in managing interests and processes across sectors. While basic skills can be taught relatively quickly, countries need mechanisms to institutionalize ongoing learning and foster the development of new skills relevant to addressing social determinants of health and health equity (CW, 2007).

The Commission recommends that:

10.5. WHO support the development of knowledge and capabilities of national ministries of health to work within a social determinants of health framework, and to provide a stewardship role in supporting a social determinants approach across government (see Rec 15.3; 16.8).

WHO is the UN specialised agency mandated to lead on health and health equity globally. It has been central to the work of the Commission and will be critical to the sustainability of action on the social determinants of health and health equity. Part of WHO's responsibility includes providing technical capacity and knowledge building on the social determinants of health within Member States. The country work stream of the Commission led by WHO aimed to promote, demonstrate, and bridge knowledge to policy and implementation in order to address socially determined health inequities. WHO identified a core group of interested governments in all regions of the world to work with in order to build the basis for change in the future, and to identify new ways that WHO can support work on social determinants of health and health equity in the context of national policy-making and planning. It is critical that WHO build on the country work, supporting existing partner countries and encouraging action on the social determinants of health and health equity in new countries (see Part 6).

Chapter 16 (*Social Determinants of Health: Monitoring, Research, and Training*) outlines various recommendations specific to WHO. It is critical to ISA that WHO share the evidence and learning from the Commission across countries and use this to support ministries of health to play a stewardship role in:

1. making the argument for such an approach and increasing the visibility of social determinants of health and health equity issues;

2. creating national and local institutional structures to take forward the social determinants of health and health equity agenda;

3. developing a national action plan in relation to this;

4. developing the appropriate workforce competencies through short- and long-term training programmes.

WHO has already moved to transform some of its organizational structures in order to better support ministries of health in their efforts to develop and implement national policy on social determinants of health and health equity. In addition to regional focal points to coordinate social determinants of health work, Regional Offices have initiated work to strengthen the evidence base, advocate social determinants of health policies and programmes, foster partnerships between countries, and support ISA. Coherence between the strategic actions of WHO regional and national offices is necessary to promote coherence between different government departments within Member States.

The Commission established the PPHCKN based within WHO headquarters (see Chapter 9: *Universal Health Care*). This network focused on WHO programmes and health conditions, with the aim of expanding the definitions and practices of what constitutes public health actions and interventions to include the social determinants and how public health programmes are organized. Key learning from this network highlights the need to articulate and provide evidence of the relationship between socioeconomic status and health outcomes; to advocate social and economic change; to enhance the evidence base for social determinants of health and inequity in health; and to strongly advocate the need for and benefits of social interventions to prevent increased prevalence of HIV, tobacco use, malnutrition, diabetes, alcoholism, risky sex, indoor air pollution, and transgenerational effects of under-5 mortality. WHO must now transfer to ministries of health in

---

BOX 10.10: ACTIVE INVOLVEMENT OF THE AFFECTED COMMUNITY – SEX WORKERS IN KOLKATA

In the early 1990s, the All India Institute of Hygiene and Public Health (AIIHPH) initiated a conventional STI treatment and prevention programme in a red-light district in north Kolkata. The Sonagachi HIV/AIDS International Project (SHIP) was implemented through an intersectoral partnership of WHO, AIIHPH, the British Council, and a number of ministries and local NGOs. Sex workers in the area were poor and marginalized. The project quickly moved beyond traditional treatment and education modalities to focus on the empowerment of the sex workers. Key interventions during the first five years included vaccination and treatment services for the sex workers' children, literacy classes for the women, political activism and advocacy, micro-credit schemes, and cultural programmes. The sex workers created

their own membership organization, the Durbar Mahila Samanwaya Committee (DMSC), that successfully negotiated for better treatment by madams, landlords, and local authorities. In 1999, the DMSC took over management of SHIP, and has since expanded to include 40 red-light districts across West Bengal. It has an active membership of 2000 sex workers and has established a financial cooperative. The strong occupational health focus and the emphasis on giving sex workers more control over their bodies and living and working conditions has resulted in low rates of HIV infection and STIs in Sonagachi relative to the rest of the country.

Source: WHO & PHAC, 2007

Member States and other global institutions the learning from this innovative introduction of a social determinants of health framework to health outcome-focused programmes.

The health sector as a catalyst beyond government

A central element of ISA is increased social participation in policy processes (see Chapter 14: *Political Empowerment – Inclusion and Voice*). Ministries of health can act as a catalyst to involve key people and institutions and reach beyond government to involve those affected by policies (Box 10.10).

While highest-level government oversight is needed to push and coordinate ISA and to ensure sustainability, local-level government and community ownership is a prerequisite to sustained results. Government-NGO collaboration can increase the reach of action and win early results (Box 10.11). There are many existing intersectoral programmes and frameworks, such as Healthy Cities, Municipalities, Villages and Islands, that take a social determinants approach to health and health equity, that may be explored for their applicability in different contexts.

The private sector has a major responsibility both in the production of health inequity and in solving the problem of inequity. Effective engagement of the private sector for health equity is critical and discussed in more detail in Chapters 7, 12, and 15 (*Fair Employment and Decent Work; Market Responsibility; Good Global Governance*). An example of the global recognition of the role the private sector plays in health is the WHO Diet and Physical Activity Strategy, which specifically requested companies to be more engaged in tackling diet- and activity-related ill-health. A review of the practices of 25 of the world's largest food companies by Lang and colleagues (2006) identified that only four had any policies on food advertising and only six had policies specifically relating to children.

Making health equity a shared value across sectors is politically challenging but is needed globally. The recommendations outlined in this chapter illustrate the need for commitment at the highest level of government to health and health equity through a social determinants framework. Attention within the health and non-health sectors to ensure that the nature of their policies do not have negative consequences for health and health equity is critical. And integrated action, both within government and with the voluntary and private sectors, is an important element of a concerted approach to health equity.

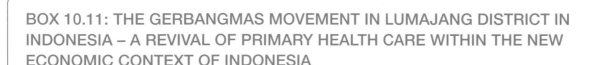
BOX 10.11: THE GERBANGMAS MOVEMENT IN LUMAJANG DISTRICT IN INDONESIA – A REVIVAL OF PRIMARY HEALTH CARE WITHIN THE NEW ECONOMIC CONTEXT OF INDONESIA

Following the principles of primary health care as expressed in the Alma Ata Declaration, in 1986 Indonesia launched the integrated health posts (Posyandus). While these achieved impressive coverage, with 254 154 Posyandus operating in 2004, the quality and general performance is varied and has deteriorated considerably. One contributing reason has been drop-out of the health volunteers associated with economic and ideological transition, reducing voluntarism, and collectivism.

To redress the situation, the District Health Office initiated and spearheaded a mechanism to coordinate multisectoral interventions to rejuvenate community health development. It mobilized support from the highest political authority in the district and enrolled an NGO as partner. In January 2005, the elected head of Lumajang district launched GERBANGMAS as a strategy of community empowerment and the local government defined three functions of the Posyandus: community education, community empowerment, and community service.

The multisectoral village GERBANGMAS teams are provided with a general budget allocation from the local government, which is matched by the community and used for activities as well as to provide incentives for health workers. To guide investment and development, 21 indicators have been defined. Only about one third of these are traditional health indicators, such as use of family planning. The rest address determinants of health, including poverty reduction, literacy, waste management, housing, and mobilization of youth and the elderly. One proof of the functioning of the village team is that 12 sectoral bodies, including fisheries, public works, labour and transmigration, agriculture, and religious offices, provide budget support through the village team. All indicators have improved, both the health-specific and the upstream determinants of health.

Source: PPHCKN, 2007c

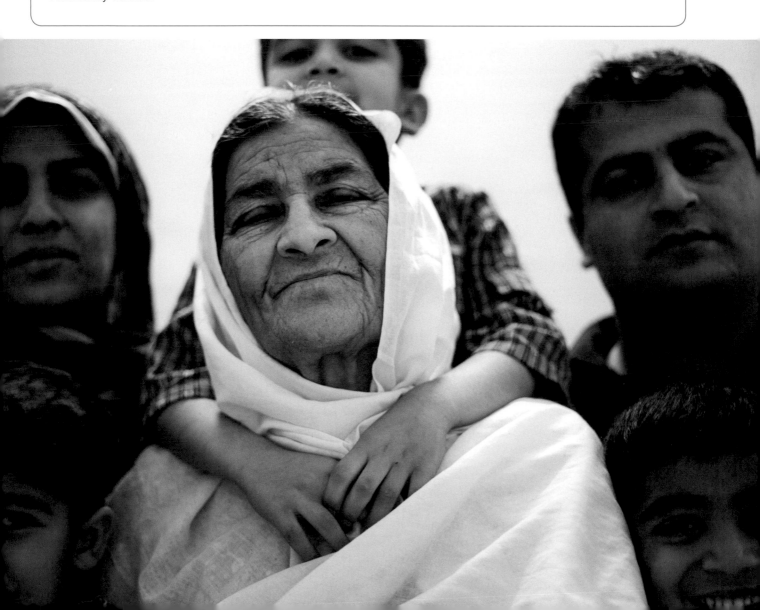

CHAPTER 11
Fair financing

"Equity is complementary to the pursuit of long-term prosperity. Greater equity is doubly good for poverty reduction. It tends to favour sustained overall development, and it delivers increased opportunities to the poorest groups in a society." Francois Bourguignon (2006)

THE RELATIONSHIP BETWEEN FAIR FINANCING AND HEALTH EQUITY

For countries at all levels of economic development, increasing or re-allocating public finance to fund action across the social determinants of health – from child development and education, through living and working conditions, to health care – is fundamental to improved welfare and health equity. Within countries, adequate financial resources, progressively obtained, proportionately invested across the social determinants of health, and allocated equitably across population groups and regions, are fundamental. Given the drastic limits on domestic financing in low-income countries, official financial flows in the form of aid and debt relief are critical to addressing dramatic global health inequities. In 1970, rich countries pledged to give 0.7% of their GDP in official development assistance (ODA). Thirty-five years later, they were managing an average of 0.33%. The annual global requirement for health-related aid – that is, DAH, defined as aid allocated to activities with health as their main purpose – is estimated at US$ 27 billion in 2007, simply to finance basic life-saving health services. In 2005, the total external debt owed by developing countries was US$ 2.7 trillion, with a servicing bill of US$ 513 billion in that year. We should, as Sachs suggests, "recognise the iron laws of extreme poverty ... A typical sub-Saharan African country has an annual income of perhaps $350 per person per year ... The government might be able to mobilise 15 per cent of the $350 in taxes from the domestic economy. That produces a little over $50 per person per year in total government revenues (and in many countries much less). This tiny sum must be divided among all government functions: executive, legislative, and judicial offices; police; defence; education and so on" (Sachs, 2007).

The importance of public finance

Health equity relies on an adequate supply of and access to material resources and services; safe, health-promoting living and working conditions; and learning, working, and recreational opportunities. Supply of and access to these, in turn, requires public investment and adequate levels of public financing, and/or regulation of markets where private provision can be an effective and efficient means of equitable access. All of this implies the need for more and fairer forms of public financing. The emphasis on public financing is related to the importance of public goods in building action on the social determinants of health, and the importance of public investment in order to reach all socioeconomic groups. Traditionally, governments are expected to play an active role in providing public goods. Left solely to the market, such goods are undersupplied (GKN, 2007). Even where goods and services can be efficiently and equitably provided through the private sector, it is vital to ensure the effective authority and capacity of the government to manage market regulation (see Chapter 12: *Market Responsibility*). Coherent national action on social determinants of health and health equity requires the adoption – *and financing* – of 'health in all policies' (Stahl et al., 2006; see Chapter 10: *Health Equity in All Policies, Systems, and Programmes*).

In any country, economic inequality – including inequity in public financing – needs to be addressed to make progress towards health equity. Universal public services and infrastructure played a vital role in the historical development of today's rich countries (Szreter, 2004). Yet there is still considerable inequity in the financing of public services within countries. Whether the issue is health care, transportation infrastructure, or social protection, those social groups and regions with the highest need often receive proportionately the least public investment. The prevalence of an urban bias in public investment is reflected in worse health outcomes and lower service use in rural areas, especially in low- and middle-income countries.

BOX 11.1: GLOBAL ECONOMIC GROWTH AND PRO-POOR DISTRIBUTION

Recently, it has been calculated that, "each $1 of poverty reduction ... requires $166 of additional global production and consumption, with all its associated environmental impacts which adversely affect the poorest most. Coupled with the constraints on global growth associated with climate change, and the disproportionately adverse net impact of climate change on the poor, this casts serious doubt on the dominant view that global growth should be the primary means of poverty reduction. Rather than growth, policies and the global economic system should focus directly on achieving social and environmental objectives."

The Commission does not underestimate the critical value of economic growth. But it does point to the serious potential environmental consequences, and minor impact on poverty, of growth models that are inattentive to the distribution of the benefits of growth.

Reprinted, with permission of the publisher, from Woodward & Simms (2006b).

Economic growth and distribution

The view that economic growth alone can solve the global poverty problem has been widely challenged – not least by Szreter (2004), Sachs (2005), and UN-HABITAT (2006). Instead, both more equitable within-country distribution of resources and increased international financial transfers are necessary to reduce poverty and improve health, not only under the ethical imperative to alleviate avoidable suffering, but equally at the pace expressly desired by governments through the MDGs (KNUS, 2007). Studies in Latin America strongly suggest that even a little redistribution of income through progressive taxation and targeted social programmes can go further in terms of poverty reduction than many years of solid economic growth, because of the extremely unequal distribution of income and wealth in most countries in the region (Paes de Barros et al., 2002; de Ferranti et al., 2004; Woodward & Simms, 2006b) (Box 11.1).

Domestic revenues

Critical weaknesses – in particular for developing countries – exist in the current domestic and international arena of public financing. Low-income countries often have weak income tax institutions and mechanisms and a majority of the workforce operating in the informal sector. These countries are relatively more reliant on import tariffs for public revenue. Trade liberalization has seriously reduced the availability of such tariff revenues since the 1970s (GKN, 2007) (Fig. 11.1).

Many countries have not been able to replace these losses with other sources of public revenues or taxation. As a consequence, a majority of low-income countries have seen a net decline in overall public revenues (however, for many low income countries, this trend has been arrested or reversed since 1998). Middle-income countries have fared slightly better, but in general trade liberalization has translated into a reduced capacity of national governments to support public expenditures in health, education, and other sectors (Baunsgaard & Keen, 2005; Glenday, 2006). High-income countries, with already well-established taxation systems and existing public infrastructures, have been able to move away from tariff revenues with minimal loss in fiscal capacity. But increasing intensity of global tax competition (real or perceived) has also had negative effects on national fiscal capacity, even in high-income countries (Tanzi, 2001; Tanzi, 2002; Tanzi, 2004; Tanzi, 2005).

Aid and debt relief

Strengthening adequate domestic public financing for action on health equity and the social determinants of health will be a medium- to long-term process. In the shorter term, many resource-poor countries will continue to rely on external financing through aid and debt relief. Solid evidence now exists that aid financing can contribute both to general economic growth in recipient countries (McGillivray et al., 2005) and more directly to improved health (Mishra & Newhouse, 2007). However, the total flow of aid remains chronically low relative to the scale of need and, in the case of the majority of donors, far below the 0.7% of GDP commitment made by OECD countries in 1969. Donors continue to appear ambivalent about the value of aid, with persistent failure to meet the 0.7% of GDP commitment and a consistent shortfall between funds committed and those actually disbursed. In 2005, only 70% of aid committed was actually delivered. A considerable portion of aid remains tied to donor country trade and security interests, while there is evidence that donor allocations follow their own geostrategic interests as much as – if not more than – global conditions of need (Box 11.2).

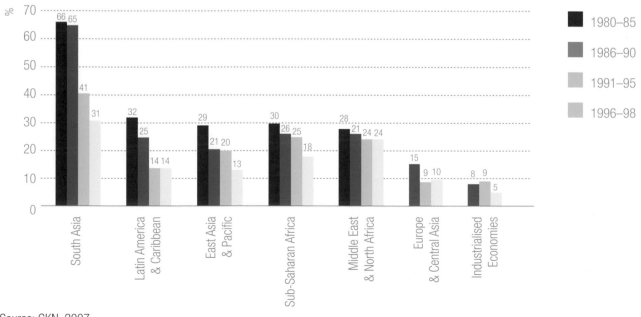

Figure 11.1 Proportion of tariffs in total revenue by region, 1980–1998.

Legend:
- 1980–85
- 1986–90
- 1991–95
- 1996–98

South Asia: 66, 65, 41, 31
Latin America & Caribbean: 32, 25, 14, 14
East Asia & Pacific: 29, 21, 20, 13
Sub-Saharan Africa: 30, 26, 25, 18
Middle East & North Africa: 28, 21, 24, 24
Europe & Central Asia: 15, 9, 10
Industrialised Economies: 8, 9, 5

Source: GKN, 2007

There is also evidence of what might be called a trust deficit between donors and recipients, leading to multiple and onerous conditions placed on aid that heighten transaction costs on often weak recipient country bureaucracies and constrain recipients' freedom to determine developmental and financing priorities. The net effect is periodic, effectively punitive, reversals in aid flows that create volatility (Fig. 11.2, Box 11.3), which has been shown to harm health (Bokhari, Gottret & Gai, 2005).

Development assistance for health

The part of total global aid allocated to action on health (DAH) tends to be confined largely to financing action within the health sector. Much aid for health remains locked within

a range of narrowly defined health interventions, privileging treatment over investment in prevention. The large (US$ 15 billion) allocation of finance for action on HIV/AIDS under the Presidential Emergency Plan for AIDS Relief (PEPFAR) is a good example of this (Fig. 11.3, Box 11.4).

Meanwhile, the considerable weight of remaining debt, some of it unquestionably 'odious', continues to draw public resources away from developmental investments. Debt crises among developing countries were the result of rising prices of oil; poor needs assessments and loan designs (both on creditor and debtor sides) and high rates of loan diversion; worsening loan repayment conditions; and both falling prices and falling

---

BOX 11.2: GLOBAL AID AND GLOBAL NEED

Over 60% of the total increase in ODA between 2001 and 2004 went to Afghanistan, the Democratic Republic of Congo, and Iraq – in spite of the fact that the three countries account for less than 3% of the

developing world's poor. Much of the ODA increase in 2005 can be accounted for by debt relief to Iraq and Nigeria.

Figure 11.2 Official development assistance disbursements for health in selected countries.

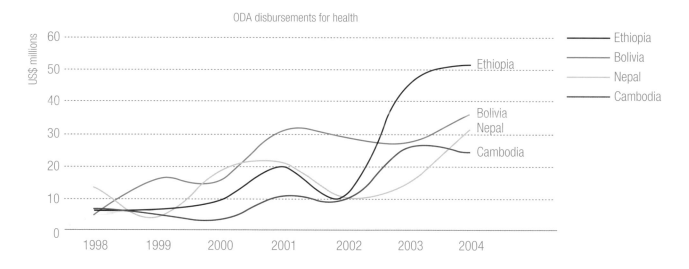

Reprinted, with permission of the author, from World Bank (2006a).

BOX 11.3: AID VOLATILITY

Even though aid to health has been increasing, aid volatility not only reduces the capacity of recipient governments to plan expenditure, but it is also directly and negatively associated with health outcomes. Econometric analysis of child mortality across 75 developing countries between 1995 and 2000 found

that, "both low levels [of aid] and high volatility of donor funding for health explained the relatively slow progress of some countries in reducing under-five mortality".

Source: Bokhari, Gottret & Gai, 2005

developed-country demand for the exports of indebted countries. The hardest-hit countries, the HIPCs, have seen a massive increase in debt over the past four decades, while their per capita incomes have stagnated. Debt is negatively associated with social sector spending, in particular adversely affecting public investment in non-wage goods such as infrastructure (GKN, 2007).

Debt relief, while promising, remains limited largely to HIPC qualifying countries, leaving other resource-poor countries unjustifiably without relief on repayments. It is, in any case, a slow process with – again as with aid – onerous conditions that limit national capacity to invest in needed social sector spending (Box 11.5). Figures for the 35 of the 40 HIPCs located in sub-Saharan Africa underline the basic problem – while these countries have received US$ 294 billion in loans and paid back US$ 268 billion between 1970 and 2002, they were still left with a debt stock of US$ 210 billion circa 2004 (UNCTAD, 2004).

Besides aid and debt relief, conditions for growth and improved domestic public finance capacity can be supported by the international community through several avenues – for example, clearer global agreements and more efficient global action to extend security to countries at risk of conflict;

expanded action to monitor production of and trade in natural resources; increased international legislative standards for rich country business relations with low- and middle-income trading partners; and support for the development of preferential trade agreements that allow for protection to countries attempting to build the capacity to engage on viably competitive terms in the global marketplace (Collier, 2006).

ACTIONS FOR FAIR FINANCING

The Commission recommends that:

11.1 Donors, multilateral agencies, and Member States build and strengthen national capacity for progressive taxation (see Rec 8.1; 8.3; 9.2; 10.2).

Progressive taxation

Strengthening domestic revenues for equitable public finance requires stronger progressive taxation. This implies strengthening tax systems and capacities, particularly building institutional capacity in low-income settings (Box 11.6). Taxation should focus on direct – such as income or property taxes – over indirect forms – such as trade or sales taxes[10]. Tax regimes in East Asia between 1970 and 1999 showed a strong and persistent emphasis on direct tax, with less emphasis on

Figure 11.3 Changes in spending allocation under the President's Emergency Plan for AIDS Relief, 2004–2006.

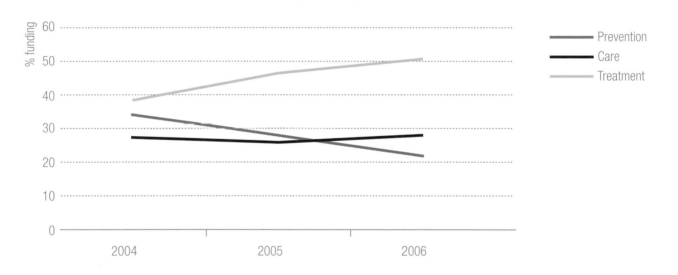

Source: USAID, 2006

FAIR FINANCING : ACTION AREA 11.1

Strengthen public finance for action on the social determinants of health.

---

10 In relation to taxation and transnational corporations, measures to reduce capital flight and tax avoidance via transfer pricing are probably at least as important as the reduction of tax incentives for investing in export processing zones (GKN, 2007).

other types, while tax regimes in sub-Saharan Africa showed a heavy reliance on indirect – sales and trade – taxes (Fig. 11.4). Notwithstanding other contributing factors, East Asia saw strong growth and improvements in health throughout the period, while sub-Saharan Africa experienced large-scale stagnation and, in some cases, decline.

Many countries, with relatively weak tax systems and high rates of informal labour complicating tax efforts, have relied on indirect tax revenues, such as trade tariffs, as income for public spending. High- and middle-income countries should not demand further tariff reductions in bilateral, regional, and world trade negotiations with low-income countries still reliant on tariffs for public revenue. And low-income countries should be extremely careful in agreeing to reduce tariffs prior to creating or improving alternative revenue streams. Dedicated aid and technical support should be made available to strengthen capacity for direct taxation in the longer term. Multilateral efforts are required not only to reduce the adverse impact of trade and financial market liberalization on national fiscal resources, but also to strengthen a globally enforceable framework to reduce international tax avoidance and capital flight (Box 11.7).

Measures to combat the use of offshore financial centres to avoid national tax regimes would provide resources for development at least comparable to those made available through new taxes. One estimate is that the use of offshore financial centres for tax avoidance costs developing countries US$ 50 billion per year in lost revenues (Oxfam Great Britain, 2000). The value of (personal) assets held in offshore accounts has been put at between US$ 8 and US$ 11.5 trillion, not including real estate (Tax Justice Network, 2005). The losses due to this tax avoidance amount to at least US$ 160 billion annually – that is, about the estimated value of the additional development assistance required to reach the MDGs (UN Millennium Project, 2005). Curbing tax avoidance would increase the fiscal capacity of governments in rich and poor countries alike. It would also reduce economic inequities, since most of the opportunities in question are available only to the wealthy.

The Commission recommends that:

11.2 New national and global public finance mechanisms be developed, including special health taxes and global tax options (see Rec 9.2; 10.2).

There are further options for strengthening public finance, used in low-, middle-, and high-income countries but perhaps particularly relevant in terms of immediate capacity to leverage additional finance in low-income settings. New health taxes have been introduced or are being considered in several countries: Ghana's value added tax levy of 2.5%; Zimbabwe's 3% personal and income tax levy for HIV/AIDS; and tobacco and alcohol taxes in Thailand (HSKN, 2007). Tax collection efficiency has improved in South Africa; in Bolivia tax reform increased revenue sixfold in the 1980s (Wagstaff, 2007).

Tax in a globalized world

The increasingly globalized nature of economic practices, including offshore tax havens, provides a strong argument in favour of the development of a system of global taxation – not least in recognition of interdependent interests and the increasing importance of global public goods for population health. A tax on airline tickets, with revenues specifically targeted for purchase of drugs to treat HIV/AIDS, tuberculosis, and malaria and to support public health systems in poor countries, has already been implemented by several countries (Farley, 2006; Ministries of the Economy, 2006). A tax on foreign currency transactions to reduce financial instability (the Tobin Tax) was originally proposed by economist James Tobin. This – and similar tax proposals – was subsequently identified as one among many potential sources of revenue for financing health systems in low- and middle-income countries, moving closer to the mainstream of development policy thought (Gottret & Schieber, 2006). One estimate is that such a tax at a very low rate (0.02%) would raise US$ 17-35 billion per year, with higher estimates available in the literature (Nissanke, 2003).

BOX 11.4: AID AND HIV/AIDS

A breakdown of PEPFAR allocations between 2004 and 2006 not only shows a preference for investment in treatment over prevention, but a significant shift in funding away from preventive action, from over one third in 2004 to less than one quarter two years later. PEPFAR is one of the most significant single lines of international health funding in the last 20 years. It is important money, but it highlights a worrying discontinuity between donor rhetoric and the reality of donor practice, which continues to privilege medical and curative intervention, particularly where that meets the requirements of a domestic policy agenda.

FAIR FINANCING : ACTION AREA 11.2

Increase international finance for health equity, and coordinate increased finance through a social determinants of health action framework.

An alternative proposal to the Tobin Tax is the Currency Transaction Development Levy, designed as a 'solidarity levy' specifically to generate new global public finance for development (Hillman et al., 2006). The Currency Transaction Development Levy could be implemented unilaterally by countries or currency unions. It is estimated that it could raise US$ 2.07 billion annually if implemented by the United Kingdom, US$ 170 million if implemented by Norway, and US$ 4.3 billion if implemented throughout the Euro zone

(Hillman et al., 2006). Although cautious about the merits of a currency transaction tax, the UN High-level Panel on Financing for Development (Zedillo et al., 2001) stressed the need for new sources of development financing, and proposed the establishment of an International Tax Organization to limit tax competition and evasion. Whatever may be the merits of any single proposal, taxing financial transactions to raise revenue for development is now widely regarded as both feasible and appropriate. As in the case of debt cancellation, if

BOX 11.5: DEBT RELIEF AND SOCIAL SPENDING

Nepal spends more on debt than education. It has only one teacher to every 180 children. Debt relief is likely to be delayed by conditions set by creditors. Chad spent US$ 66 million on debt service in 2006. It is one of the many countries charging some kind of fee for school. Only one third of girls in Chad go to school. Globally, another US$ 17 billion per year is needed to provide education for all girls and boys. In 2005, developing countries altogether spent 30 times this amount on servicing debt. The World Bank and IMF say that Kenya's debt is 'sustainable' and it is therefore not eligible for debt relief. Kenya's last two budgets allocated US$ 350 million more to paying

debts than to education. Over 1 million Kenyan children do not go to primary school. Repeated studies have shown the positive impact of debt relief on social services, most of them agreeing that education is the biggest winner. After receiving debt relief, Malawi, and Uganda, and United Republic of Tanzania all abolished primary school fees. This helped over 1 million more children into school in each country. Debt relief paid for training of 4000 teachers each year in Malawi, and salaries for 5000 community teachers in Mali.

Source: Jubilee Debt Campaign, 2007

BOX 11.6: STRENGTHENING NATIONAL AND INTERNATIONAL TAX

Develop efficient and just tax systems. A basic requirement for strengthening public revenues is a broad based tax system. Taxation should be based on ability to pay, and rich individuals, large landowners, and private companies should be taxed accordingly. Governments should use fiscal policies actively to reduce disparities in income and wealth distribution.

Strengthen tax authorities and financial administrations. In many countries, the tax administration still needs to be developed, or at least strengthened. This involves a legal framework as well as necessary staff and technical infrastructure.

Effective taxation of transnational corporations. An essential element of an efficient tax system includes the effective taxation of transnational corporations. Tax holidays or tax incentives for transnational investors in EPZs [export processing zones] are counterproductive in this regard.

Binding regulations on transparency of payment flows. Taxes and royalties from foreign investments in the oil, natural gas, and mining sectors are of great importance to resource-rich countries ... but are often not disclosed by governments or by the companies involved. Therefore, all publicly-traded companies

should be required to disclose information about taxes, royalties, fees, and other transactions with governments and public sector entities in all of the countries in which they operate.

Combating corruption and bribery. More decisive rules and procedures are necessary both in affected countries and at the international level. The UN Convention Against Corruption, which came into force in December 2005, should be ratified as soon as possible and implemented.

Strengthened international tax cooperation. Pivotal to the success of national tax reforms is improved cooperation between governments on the international level. A better-coordinated [international] tax policy would benefit the majority of countries (with the exception of some of the more aggressive tax havens). As yet, there is no intergovernmental global forum to deal with questions of taxation. For years, there have been calls for the creation of an International Tax Organization to close this global governance gap. It should be established under the auspices of the UN.

Reprinted, with permission of the publisher, from Martens (2007).

any such new revenue-raising initiatives are to be effective, they must be genuinely additional to existing development finance, rather than merely substituting for current revenue streams.

The Commission recommends that:

11.3 Donor countries honour existing commitments by increasing aid to 0.7% of GDP; expand the Multilateral Debt Relief Initiative; and coordinate aid use through a social determinants of health framework (see Rec 13.6; 15.2).

Critiques of aid's relation to economic growth in recipient countries contributed to a downturn, prominently in the 1990s, in ODA (Friedman, 1958; Bauer, 1981; Boone, 1996; Easterly, 2006; Quartey, 2005; Rajan & Subramanian, 2005; Schneider, 2005; Svensson, 2000). New empirical analysis – partly the result of improving data – shows a more positive relation between ODA and growth (GKN 2007). Meta-analyses report consistently positive associations across dozens of individual empirical studies (Clemens et al., 2004; McGillivray et al., 2005). Collier and Dollar (2000) estimate that aid sustainably lifts around 30 million people per annum out of absolute poverty. While the Commission endorses the contribution of aid to economic growth, the emphasis should be on its contribution to meeting basic health-related needs.

Development assistance for health

DAH, in reality aid primarily devoted within the health sector, has increased substantially in recent years (Fig. 11.5). However, total DAH remains too low to cover the need for health services. The Commission on Macroeconomics and Health estimated that aid for health needs to rise to around US$ 34 per capita per annum by 2007, rising again to US$ 38 per capita by 2015 (recently re-estimated to be closer to US$ 40 per person), in order to "deliver basic treatment and care" (CMH, 2001).

The total volume of DAH must increase. But beyond aid allocated as finance to basic health-related interventions, the Commission urges donor and recipient countries to adopt a more comprehensive social determinants of health framework to advance the volume of aid as a whole, the coordination of contributions, and the alignment of aid spending with the wider development plans of recipient countries, following the Paris Declaration on Aid Effectiveness in 2005.

A social determinants of health framework for aid

Aid coordination and alignment can be improved through increasing the emphasis on globally pooled funds, multilaterally managed and transparently governed. Recipients' eligibility and donor allocations would be determined according to agreed needs and developmental objectives (broadly following

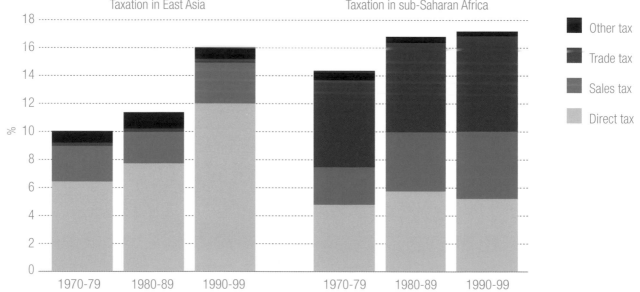

Figure 11.4 Taxation in East Asia (left) and sub-Saharan Africa (right), 1970–79, 1980–89, and 1990–99.

Reprinted, with permission of the publisher, from Cobham (2005).

FAIR FINANCING : ACTION AREA 11.3

Fairly allocate government resources for action on the social determinants of health.

the major elements of the social determinants of health framework), with multi-year stability of donor inputs and recipient receipts. The establishment of a new multilateral institution dedicated to an expanded, reliable, more coherent system of global aid may seem unrealistic. However, the example provided by the International Finance Facility for Immunization (Box 11.8), and the ongoing processes of UN reform, suggest that such innovations are not only viable, but necessary (see Chapter 15: *Good Global Governance*).

In the more immediate term, the proportion of aid that is tied – for example, to donor trade interests – should be reduced,

and the proportion provided as general budget support should be substantially increased (Box 11.9). Donors have recognized for some time the cross-sectoral nature of health and the imperative to act not just on the immediate causes of poor health and health inequity but on the wider determinants. Beyond the rhetoric, however, donor practices in aid in general and in health in particular remain heavily sector-specific and technocratic (Sachs, 2004). The advantage of general budget support aid is that it provides a 'purer' form of aid support to the whole of the recipient government. The proviso to a recommendation to increase general budget support

Figure 11.5 Development assistance for health 1973–2004: 5-year moving average, commitments.

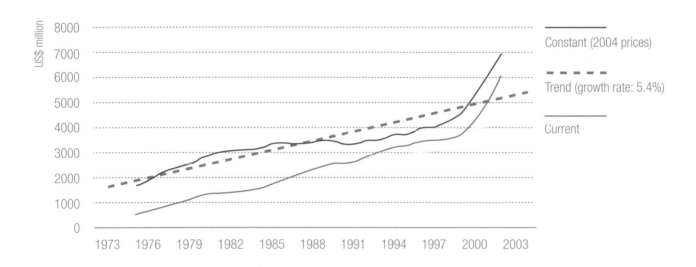

Reprinted, with permission of the author, from DAC (2005).

BOX 11.7: TAX COMPETITION AND 'FISCAL TERMITES'

Globalization has limited the ability of governments to collect taxes by increasing the opportunity of corporations and wealthy individuals to minimize their tax liabilities by shifting assets, transactions, and even themselves from high- to low-tax jurisdictions. The former Chief of the IMF's Fiscal Affairs Department has identified a number of 'fiscal termites' that diminish the fiscal capacity of governments in rich and poor countries alike. These include the hypermobility of financial capital and of high-income individuals with highly marketable skills as, "high tax rates on financial capital on highly mobile individuals provide strong incentives to taxpayers to move the capital to foreign jurisdictions that tax it lightly or to take up residence in low tax countries". A termite not identified

here, but one of increasing concern, arises from the growing importance of intra-firm trade among components of transnational corporations – according to one estimate, one third of total world trade in the late 1990s. This creates multiple opportunities for corporations to reduce their tax liabilities through transfer pricing (setting the price for goods and services between actors within an organization, allowing for artificially low turnover reporting in higher-tax environments). One recent estimate is that such mispricing accounted for financial outflows of over US$ 31 billion from Africa to the United States between 1996 and 2005.

Source: GKN, 2007

– to reduce the risk of such aid leaking away from health-related activities – is that the money is tied to specific social determinants of health action plans, and that recipients honour their accountability to such plans.

The PRSP constitutes perhaps *the* major organizing framework for development spending under the IMF's Poverty Reduction and Growth Facility. The PRSP is supposed to promote within-country consensus on development needs and coherence in development planning. As such, it presents a real opportunity to strengthen aid coordination and alignment through a framework of sectoral investments very similar to the social determinants of health framework.

However, criteria for PRSP process and performance – in particular, heavy emphasis on macroeconomic controls –

appear to have had an adverse impact on national policy space and public spending on, for example, education and health care, even when development assistance funds for these have been available (Ambrose, 2006; Ooms & Schrecker, 2005). While the IMF does not explicitly set limits on health spending, its overall policies and targets – partly articulated through the PRSP's MTEF – limit the resources available for health care and health personnel, and health ministries have difficulty influencing the budget-setting process (Wood, 2006).

From a social determinants of health point of view, the Poverty Reduction Strategy Process has been something of a missed opportunity. PRSPs hold great promise for more accountable cross-sectoral working, yet governments, led principally by finance ministries, are not seizing the opportunity, nor

---

BOX 11.8: THE INTERNATIONAL FINANCE FACILITY FOR IMMUNIZATION

The International Finance Facility for Immunization Company (IFFIm) is a new multilateral development financing institution, supported by sovereign donors (currently the governments of France, Italy, Norway, South Africa, Spain, Sweden, and the United Kingdom). President Lula of Brazil has also pledged the support of Brazil. The World Bank is the Treasury Manager for IFFIm. IFFIm's financial base consists of legally binding payment obligations from sovereign donors. It is intended that IFFIm borrow operating funds in the international capital markets over the next 10 years, up to a prudently limited proportion of the sovereign obligations making up its financial base (gearing ratio).

IFFIm's central aim is to help save more children's lives and to do so faster, in order to support the achievement of the MDGs. The Facility was designed

to accelerate the availability of funds to be used for health and immunization programmes in 70 of the poorest countries around the world. By investing most resources initially – 'frontloading' – the funding programme is designed to increase significantly the flow of aid, and to ensure reliable and predictable funding flows for immunization programmes and health system development during the years up to and including 2015. An anticipated IFFIm investment of US$ 4 billion is expected to help prevent 5 million child deaths between 2006 and 2015 and more than 5 million future adult deaths by protecting more than 500 million children in campaigns against measles, tetanus, and yellow fever.

Amended, with permission, from
http://www.iff-immunisation.org/

BOX 11.9: ENHANCING THE COHERENCE OF AID – SHIFTING TO GENERAL BUDGET SUPPORT

Traditional forms of international aid have flowed predominantly outside the formal budget processes of recipient countries. This means of delivery has been criticized for its negative impact on recipient government capacity to plan expenditure. Policy conditions and spending restrictions have further restricted the national policy space of recipient countries in taking action on the social determinants of health – in particular, for example, where aid is not allowed to flow to core institutional costs such as the public sector wage bill. A key mechanism to finance and strengthen recipient countries' capacity

to plan cross-sectoral developmental action is the shift among donors to general budget support. Under general budget support, aid flows through government budgetary processes, enhancing recipient governments' control over the development and enactment of policies that the aid is designed to finance. General budget support currently comprises a relatively small component of overall aid, but there are indications that it will increase.

Source: GKN, 2007

are international agencies providing them with adequate incentives, support, and opportunities to do so. Many PRSPs remain devoid of attention to major determinants of health, such as employment. Properly used, through more inclusive and responsive national stakeholder consultations, the PRSP provides a potentially powerful tool for organized action by aid recipient governments and civil society partners on poverty reduction, using a social determinants of health framework (Box 11.10).

Debt relief

Debt cancellation for HIPCs has made possible increases in public spending on such basic needs as health care and education in several recipient countries (World Bank Independent Evaluation Group, 2006). However, its 'success' has been uneven, and an urgent need exists for more debt relief, deployed more effectively in support of social determinants of health.

A first mechanism for augmented relief is redefining the level of sustainable debt service of low- and middle-income countries such that it is consistent with achieving basic health-related needs. The Millennium Project recommended that debt sustainability should be redefined as the level of debt consistent with achieving the MDGs, which for many HIPCs will require 100% debt cancellation and for middle-income countries, more debt relief than has been on offer (UN Millennium Project, 2005). A second mechanism is a separate debt relief initiative for heavily indebted middle-income economies, housed either at the World Bank or IMF. This would help middle-income countries to avoid a future debt crisis and to protect social expenditures in the face of a high debt burden (Dervis & Birdsall, 2006). A third option is a *feasible net revenue approach* to debt forgiveness, based on a per capita minimum income of US$ 3/day at purchasing power parity (Edward, 2006). Using this approach, Mandel finds that 31-43% of all outstanding developing country debt – affecting 93 to 107 nations – needs to be cancelled if poverty is to be reduced and the MDGs met (Mandel, 2006). Extended debt relief should be conditional on clear commitments by recipient governments to measurable increase in social sector spending, allowing for regular evaluation of performance by civil society actors. The benefits of debt relief will only be apparent if they are truly additional to revenue already raised from development assistance (Bird & Milne, 2003; Arslanalp & Henry, 2006).

The Commission recommends that:

11.4 International finance institutions ensure transparent terms and conditions for international borrowing and lending, to help avoid future unsustainable debt.

Future debt responsibility

The international community should recognize that, given the large capital requirements of poor countries, borrowing on international markets will be inevitable in the future. There is evidence that indebted countries in receipt of relief have seen their total stock of debt start to rise again after 2000 (Fig. 11.6).

Future international credit arrangements need to expand the focus from narrow indicators of economic sustainability towards an agreement on the need for 'debt responsibility'. The concept of debt responsibility has economic, social, and political aspects. Broader measures of economic vulnerability must be used when assessing the likelihood of a country encountering debt problems – these might include the country's dependence on primary commodities and the frequency of natural disasters or the size of the HIV/AIDS epidemic. But the concept of debt responsibility goes further than this. More transparency is needed in the process of incurring debt itself: government borrowers and lenders should be subject to legislative scrutiny, with public participation in important economic decisions. The strong creditor control over the HIPC process has re-invigorated calls for a more balanced approach to debt cancellation. The UN Conference on Trade and Development (UNCTAD) (2006) and debt campaigners have called for reforms to the international financial architecture to ensure an orderly bankruptcy procedure and independent arbitration between creditors and debtors. It is worth recalling, in relation both to aid increase and debt reduction, that recipients of increasing resources must be accountable to demonstrable improvements in social spending for social determinants of health action, and verifiable positive trends in health equity.

BOX 11.10: STRENGTHENING THE POVERTY REDUCTION STRATEGY PAPER

Strengthening the PRSP requires:

more explicit emphasis on the PRSP as a process of national cross-sectoral coherence in decision-making and ISA;

more support from donors and national governments for funding cross-sectoral work on the social determinants of health;

more international focus on increasing ISA in the health field, led by WHO;

more support to health ministries attempting to engage with finance ministries and the IMF on the size of the health budget;

assured access to flexibilities in expenditure planning (MTEF) for key recurrent costs (such as health human resources).

Source: GKN, 2007

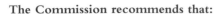
The Commission recommends that:

11.5 National and local governments and civil society establish a cross-government mechanism to allocate budget to action on social determinants of health (see Rec 10.2).

Fair allocation

Many governments recognize the need to increase public sector spending across a coherent set of policies and interventions that act on health. For health to be considered in all aspects of policy-making, it needs to be budgeted for in the plans and actions of individual ministries and departments (Box 11.11; see Chapter 10: *Health Equity in All Policies, Systems, and Programmes*).

The Commission recommends that:

11.6 Public resources be equitably allocated and monitored between regions and social groups, for example, using an equity gauge (see Rec 5.2; 14.3; 16.2).

In addition to financing coherent cross-sectoral policies for poverty reduction and the social determinants of health, there is a need to ensure that such financing is allocated fairly across national regions, to address geographical inequity. An approach to this is the equity gauge (Box 11.12). The development and testing of a model equity gauge – with potential to be generalized to address wider social determinants of health – for dissemination and use among Member States might be taken up as a collaborative endeavour led by WHO and the World Bank, working with civil society actors such as the Global Equity Gauge Alliance (GEGA) (see Chapter 16: *Social Determinants of Health: Monitoring, Research, and Training*).

Adequate public finance, equitably sourced and coherently spent, is vital to progress on health equity. In the long term, capacity to tax and commitment to progressive taxation are key to fair financing within countries. In the more immediate future, higher levels of better-coordinated aid and debt relief, applied to poverty reduction through a social determinants of health framework, are a matter both of life and death and of global justice.

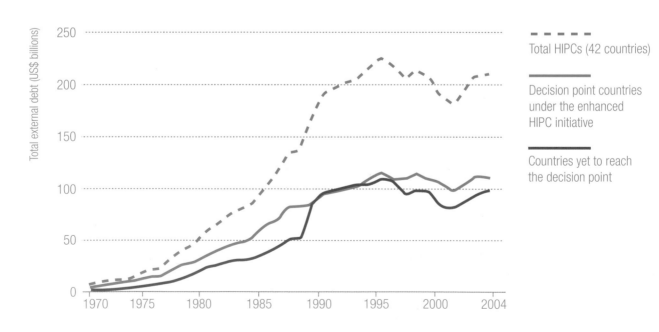

Figure 11.6 Total external debt of Highly Indebted Poor Countries, 1970–2004 (billions of dollars).

Reprinted, with the permission of the authors, from UNCTAD (2006).

BOX 11.11: FINANCING ACTION ACROSS THE SOCIAL DETERMINANTS OF HEALTH

The lack of financial mechanisms to support ISA has been identified as a common barrier to ISA. However, a number of models highlight financial tools and mechanisms that may hold promise, and which may be applied nationally and internationally:

Financial allocations exclusively for ISA, with clear criteria on what does or does not constitute ISA. This can be combined with regulations that provide legal instruments to enforce ISA in certain situations.

ISA as a **condition of funding** (see Chapter 10: *Health in All Policies, Systems, and Programmes*).

Cost-sharing or resource pooling involves financial contributions by a range of government and NGOs for a specific population or issue that aligns with the organizations' mandates. This can include in-kind resource contributions (e.g. people, information, expertise, physical space, and technology) by sectors or organizations that have limited financial resources.

Source: **http://www.phac-aspc.gc.ca/publicat/2007/cro-sec/index_e.html**

BOX 11.12: FAIRLY APPORTIONING FINANCE – THE EQUITY GAUGE APPROACH

To ensure geographic coverage, including underserved areas, and to sustain comprehensive service availability in all countries, it is important to implement mechanisms that allocate available tax funding between populations and areas relative to need – for example, allocating budgets between geographic areas on the basis of formulae that weight population numbers according to need rather than on the basis of historical expenditure patterns. Experience shows the real potential of such mechanisms even in low-income contexts, despite informational and political challenges. Where a patchwork of financing sources exists (including, for example, international funding and community-based health insurance revenue), the resource allocation mechanism should take account of all funding sources to ensure an overall distribution that is equitable.

An equity gauge is an active approach to addressing inequities in health that not only *monitors* inequities, but also incorporates concrete *actions* to bring about *sustained reductions* in unfair disparities in health and health care. In this sense, an equity gauge functions more like a thermostat than a thermometer, not just measuring – or gauging – equity and inequity, but also triggering actions to reduce inequities. An equity gauge seeks to reduce unfair disparities in health through three broad spheres of action, referred to as the pillars and each essential to an effective equity gauge: (a) assessment and monitoring, to analyse, understand, measure, and document inequities; (b) advocacy, to promote changes in policy, programmes, and planning; and (c) community empowerment, to support the role of the poor and marginalized as active participants in change rather than passive recipients of aid or help.

Source: HSKN, 2007

CHAPTER 12
Market responsibility

"Imagine a trading regime in which trade rules are determined so as to maximize development potential, particularly of the poorest nations in the world. Instead of asking 'how do we maximize trade and market access?' negotiators would ask 'how do we enable countries to grow out of poverty?'"

Dani Rodrik (2001)

THE RELATIONSHIP BETWEEN THE MARKET AND HEALTH EQUITY

Markets can bring health benefits in the form of new technologies, goods and services, and improved standard of living. But the marketplace can also generate negative conditions for health. Commercialization of vital social goods such as education and health care, and the increased availability of and access to health-damaging commodities, can and do produce health inequity. A key objective of economic policy should be the creation of an environment that generates livelihoods that promote health equity for all people. This implies a set of commitments to equitable distribution of resources; effective national and supranational regulation of those products, activities, and conditions that damage health or lead to health inequities; and enforceable social rights. Markets are important. But renewed government leadership is urgently needed to balance public and private sector interests – as is a global economic system which supports that leadership.

Global market integration

Key features of globalization in the past three decades have been the integration of most of the world's countries into the global marketplace and the spread of market relations into increasingly more areas of social life within those countries. This process has been facilitated by such measures as liberalization of trade regimes and deregulation in selected domestic markets. Consequences, in countries rich and poor alike, have included the emergence of genuinely global labour markets (although not labour mobility), extensive privatization, and a commensurate scaling back of the state. These processes have intensified the commodification and commercialization of vital social determinants of health including water, health care, and electrical power. They have also increased the availability of health-damaging products such as processed foods high in fats, sugars, and salt, and tobacco and alcohol. The public sector's role in regulating the market to achieve collective objectives such as health equity has, in many cases, been severely diminished.

Evidence suggests that globalization's enlarged and deepened markets are inherently 'disequalizing' (Birdsall, 2006). They reward more efficiently countries that already have productive assets – financial, land, physical, institutional, and human capital – over those primarily low- and middle-income countries that lack them. Globalization also favours already-rich countries, and groups within countries, because they have greater resources and power to influence the design of the rules. Thus

markets and their effects require moderation in favour of those whom they put at relative disadvantage, not only with regard to stronger public sector leadership within countries, but in terms of major improvements in global governance of, for example, international financial markets (see Chapter 15: *Good Global Governance*). The banking crisis arising in 2008 out of 'subprime' mortgages bears witness to the disproportionate risks borne by some social groups, notably the poor, and the need for stronger regulation.

Even globalization's vaunted 'winners', such as China, achieved much of their growth without adhering to anything approximating free market policies. Most of China's poverty reduction and improvements in population health occurred before integration into the global market. Between 1952 and 1982, infant mortality fell from 200 to 34 per 1000 live births and LEB increased from about 35 to 68 years (Blumenthal & Hsiao, 2005). Indeed, it is since China deregulated its domestic markets and accelerated export-oriented industrial development that both income inequality and inequity in access to health care have increased dramatically (Akin et al., 2004; Akin et al., 2005; French, 2006; Dummer & Cook, 2007; Meng, 2007). Today there are large health differences between China's coastal regions and the interior provinces. More broadly, the period of market integration has seen income inequality, within and between countries, rise sharply.

Trade and investment – inequitable global negotiations

Structural inequities in the global institutional architecture maintain unfairness in trade-related processes and outcomes. Trade and investment agreements have often been characterized (a) by asymmetrical participation among signatory countries, especially low-income countries with relatively weak trade-negotiating capacity, and (b) by inequalities in bargaining power that arise from differences in population size and national wealth. Such agreements are often entered into without adequate assessment of the full scale of the social risks – including risk of increasing inequality and health inequity – that they entail. This is partly because government departments or ministries and civil society organizations with mandates and expertise relevant to public health seldom participate in trade negotiations. Global institutions and processes, such as the Codex Alimentarius Commission (Box 12.1), show how health and health equity perspectives have been underrepresented in critical areas of international economic negotiations.

Bilateral investment agreements constitute another example of international trade-related arrangements that underestimate or actively exclude health issues. Aside from the fact that bilateral, and regional, agreements can undermine or adversely impact the health conditions of multilateral agreements (see TRIPS below), evidence suggests that frameworks such as bilateral investment agreements are disproportionately concerned with facilitating foreign direct investment and are comparatively inattentive to health.

Transnational corporate influence

Transnational corporations that organize production across multiple national borders have flourished as trade liberalization has broadened and deepened. The revenues of Wal-Mart, BP, Exxon Mobil, and Royal Dutch/Shell Group all rank above the GDP of countries such as Indonesia, Norway, Saudi Arabia, and South Africa (EMCONET, 2007). The combination of binding trade agreements that open domestic markets to global competition and increasing corporate power and capital mobility have arguably diminished individual countries' capacities to ensure that economic activity contributes to health equity, or at least does not undermine it. This is not to suggest that private sector actors (individuals or corporations) are innately bad. Rather, it is to state that many have grown immensely powerful in economics and in political influence, and that their power must be accountable to the public good as well as dedicated to private economic ends.

Protecting public provision and regulating private supply

Public sector leadership relative to the private sector should be strengthened in two respects: protecting equitable access to goods and services critical to well-being and health (such as water), and controlling availability of goods and services that are harmful. The question of which goods and services require protected status or regulatory control will vary from one country context to another, but examples can be given:

Water

An estimated 1.2 billion people worldwide, almost all of them in low- and middle-income countries, lack access to improved water supplies (UNESCO, 2006a). Ensuring people's access to water and sanitation is essential to life, and a clear responsibility of the state. Globalization has spurred new insight into provision of water and sanitation services, especially where government capacity is weak. That said, the role of the public sector – not least a historical track record in the equitable management of water provision – remains central. The examples given (Box 12.2) show the potential adverse impacts of water privatization. There is a much larger evidence base (Loftus & McDonald, 2001; Jaglin, 2002; Budds & McGranahan, 2003; McDonald & Smith, 2004; Galiani et al., 2005; Mehta & Madsen, 2005; Debbane, 2007; Aiyer, 2007) suggesting that wholesale privatization of water should be discouraged.

Health care

Health sector reform has focused on a narrow conception of technical and economic efficiency, privileging 'cost-effective' medical intervention, and increasing commercialization – in spite of significant evidence of cost-ineffectiveness. Available evidence indicates that commercialization in health services, including health insurance, creates inequities in access (Barrientos & Lloyd-Sherlock, 2000; Bennett & Gilson, 2001; Cruz-Saco, 2002; Barrientos & Peter Lloyd-Sherlock, 2003; Hutton, 2004) and in health outcomes (Koivusalo & Mackintosh, 2005), whether such commercialization is led

---

BOX 12.1: REPRESENTATION WITHIN THE CODEX ALIMENTARIUS COMMISSION

The Codex Alimentarius Commission is an important body that has been jointly formed by FAO and WHO to, "develop food standards, guidelines and related texts such as codes of practice under the Joint FAO/WHO Food Standards Programme. The main purposes of this Programme are protecting health of the consumers and ensuring fair trade practices in the food trade, and promoting coordination of all food standards work undertaken by international governmental and non-governmental organizations". The Codex has assumed much greater power since the establishment of the WTO. Codex standards are used by the WTO as benchmarks in the event of trade disputes. It is important that FAO and WHO ensure the impartiality of this body. Current arrangements suggest biased participation and inequitable representation, resulting in an imbalance between the goals of trade and consumer protection. A review in 1993 found 26 representatives from public interest groups compared with 662 from industry.

Source: Friel et al., 2007

BOX 12.2: WATER PRIVATIZATION IN ARGENTINA AND BOLIVIA

Since 1993, the French company Suez-Lyonnaise has been the major partner in the privatized utility company supplying water to Buenos Aires' 10 million inhabitants, one of the largest water concessions in the world. Utility prices were raised by more than 20% after privatization. Poorer families – if connected to the supply at all – could no longer afford to pay their water bills.

In September 1999, the international water-led consortium Aguas del Tunari was awarded a 40-year concession for the water and sanitation system of Cochabamba, the third largest city in Bolivia. Water tariffs increased by up to 200% in order to cover the costs of a massive engineering scheme.

Sources: Loftus & McDonald, 2001; http://www.foe.co.uk/resource/briefings/gats_stealing_water.pdf

by domestic or foreign actors. Almost all health systems are 'mixed', involving both private and public initiatives. The Commission recognizes this. A key issue is, therefore, how much and how well government is able to oversee the function of its mixed system, plan fair provision, and regulate private sector input. In middle-income countries, higher levels of commercialization are systematically associated with worse and more unequal health-care access and health outcomes (HSKN, 2007). In low-income settings, unregulated fee-for-service commercialization is particularly damaging to health outcomes. In terms of health equity, publicly financed health care, regardless of ability to pay, is the preferred policy option. (See Chapters 9 and 11: *Universal Health Care; Fair Financing*).

Labour

Work – both its availability and the conditions in which it is undertaken – is critical to people's social functioning and equitable health. Global market integration and liberalization have had a heavy impact on labour and working conditions. The emergence of a 'new international division of labour' is exemplified by the relocation of labour-intensive production (e.g. in the textile and garment industries) to sites in the developing world selected on the basis of low wages and minimal protection for workers, often located in EPZs (Fröbel et al., 1980). Even in the richest economies there are segments of the labour force where conditions are very poor. Legislation and formal regulatory frameworks promoting healthy work, and protecting workforces, are often poorly developed or enforced, both internationally and nationally. Labour standards are not a component of global trade agreements and although they are included in some bilateral or regional agreements, they are often ambiguous or lack enforcement provisions. (See Chapter 7: *Fair Employment and Decent Work*).

Food, tobacco, and alcohol

Trade reforms, and the growing influence of foreign direct investment, can affect diet and the nutrition transition by removing barriers to entry for transnational food companies and supermarkets expanding into new markets. Trade liberalization – opening many more countries to the international market – combined with continuing food subsidies has increased the availability, affordability, and attractiveness of less healthful foodstuffs, and transnational food companies have flooded the global market with cheap-to-produce,

Figure 12.1 Fast food consumption (1995 and 1999) in selected countries.

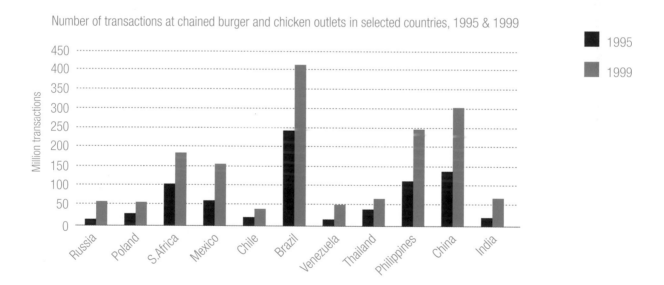

Number of transactions at chained burger and chicken outlets in selected countries, 1995 & 1999

Reprinted, with permission of the publisher, from Hawkes (2002).
Source: Euromonitor data in Hawkes (2002).

BOX 12.3: THE COSTS OF SMOKING

A study using 1998 data in China found that medical costs for premature tobacco deaths amounted to US$ 2.76 billion, or 6% of all Chinese medical costs.

In India in 2000, the Indian Council of Medical Research estimated the costs of three major tobacco-related diseases (cancer, heart disease, and chronic obstructive lung disease) at 270 billion rupees (US$ 5.8 billion), more than the direct contribution of the tobacco industry to Indian government revenue of 70 billion rupees (about US$ 1.5 billion).

Source: PPHCKN, 2007c

energy-dense, nutrient-empty foods (Fig. 12.1). (See Chapter 6: *Health Places Healthy People*).

Increased global market integration has also seen expanding production and consumption of health-damaging commodities such as tobacco and alcohol. Currently, more than 1.3 billion people smoke cigarettes worldwide – more than 1 billion men and about 250 million women – one in five of the world's population and one in three of all those over 15 years old. That figure is expected to rise to more than 1.7 billion by 2025 if the global prevalence rate of tobacco use remains unchanged (PPHCKN, 2007c). Box 12.3 outlines the costs of smoking.

There are nearly 2 million alcohol-related deaths per year, of the same order as HIV/AIDS at 2.9 million. Absolute levels of alcohol-related disease and disability are as high in the poorest countries of Africa and America as in Western Europe and North America. Alcohol-related disease is highest in the former Soviet Union and Central Asia, amounting to 13% of the total burden. In the Russian Federation itself it is even higher (PPHCKN, 2007b). A society without effective alcohol policies is likely to experience a sharp rise in alcohol problems during economic development. The transition in the former Soviet Union is a striking example. In the Russian Federation, the 'shock therapy' and economic liberalization in 1992 included a total deregulation of trade in alcoholic beverages. The subsequent mortality rise in the Russian Federation has been linked to a rise in binge drinking of alcohol (Leon et al., 1997; PPHCKN, 2007b).

ACTIONS FOR MARKET RESPONSIBILITY

The Commission recommends that:

12.1 WHO, in collaboration with other relevant multilateral agencies, supporting Member States, institutionalize health equity impact assessment, globally and nationally, of major global, regional, and bilateral economic agreements (see Rec 10.3; 16.7).

A key recommendation from the Commission is that caution be applied by participating countries in the consideration of new global, regional, and bilateral economic (trade and investment) policy commitments. Before such commitments are made, understanding the impact on health and health equity is vital. WHO should re-affirm its global health leadership by initiating a review of trade and investment agreements – working collaboratively with other multilateral agencies – with a view to institutionalizing health equity impact assessment as a standard part of all future agreements. WHO can also strengthen the capacity of Member States, their ministries of health, and civil society organizations to prepare positions for bilateral and multilateral trade negotiations.

To do this, WHO will need to augment its existing research and policy expertise, including economics, law, and the social sciences. Specific attention needs to be given to addressing trade-related negotiations on domestic regulation, subsidies, and government procurement – and those affecting globally organized production and financial markets – and trade in goods and services with direct effects on health. This may

---

BOX 12.4: WORLD HEALTH ORGANIZATION: DIAGNOSTIC TOOL AND COMPANION WORKBOOK IN TRADE AND HEALTH – A PRIORITY FOR 2008/2009

WHO is working with WTO, the World Bank, World Intellectual Property Organization, UNCTAD, international experts, and trade and health policy-makers from 10 countries to develop a diagnostic tool and companion workbook on trade and health. This new phase of work adopts a more systematic and broader perspective on the linkages between trade and health. The diagnostic tool examines five components of that relationship: 1) macroeconomics, trade, and health; 2) trade in health-related products, including medicines and intellectual property-related issues; 3) trade in products hazardous to health, such as tobacco products; 4) trade in health services – e-commerce, health tourism, foreign direct investment in health, cross-border movement of health professionals; and 5) trade in foodstuffs. The

diagnostic tool and its companion workbook, which document best practices, data sources, decision trees, and international norms and standards, will be ready for implementation in 2009. The implementation of the diagnostic tool will enable policy-makers to develop national policies and strategies related to trade and health and to identify their capacity-building needs in this area. In recent years, there has been a substantial increase in the amount of external resources provided to developing countries for capacity building in trade. 'Aid for trade' presents an opportunity to support countries to develop capacity on trade and health.

Source: WHO, **http://www.who.int/trade/resource/tradewp/en/index.html** and personal communication

---

MARKET RESPONSIBILITY : ACTION AREA 12.1

Institutionalize consideration of health and health equity impact in national and international economic agreements and policy-making.

require collaboration with other UN agencies, such as UNCTAD, ILO, FAO, UNESCO, and the UN Department of Economic and Social Affairs, to create a cross-sectoral and more extensive evidence base for understanding issues related to global economic governance, globalization, and social determinants of health. WHO is already engaging with other global institutions, and has made support for Member States in trade negotiation capacity a priority (Box 12.4). However, such support needs to be much more effectively focused on the issue of health *equity*.

Health equity impact assessment in economic agreements

Since the health equity implications of international agreements and their impact on national policies and programmes are not always fully evident, health equity impact assessment is key to coherent cross-government policies and programmes. It is essential that health equity assessment be applied to policies or major programmes outside the health sector, too (MEKN, 2007a) (see Chapter 16: *The Social Determinants of Health: Monitoring, Research, and Training*). Examples from Slovenia and Thailand, although focused on general health rather than health equity, demonstrate the feasibility and potential of such assessment processes (Boxes 12.5 and 12.6).

The institutionalization of health equity impact assessment is clearly still in its infancy – and presents real issues in terms of required technical skills and institutional capacity in many countries, especially those with low and middle incomes. However, the example of environmental impact assessment provides some basis for optimism. Notwithstanding serious recognized shortfalls in the methodology, conduct, and enforcement of environmental impact assessment, environmental impact has become – in the space of a generation – a widely acknowledged criterion in the processes of policy-making across the board.

Flexibility in agreements

Commitment to trade agreements should not constrain signatory countries, after signing, from acting to mitigate unforeseen adverse impacts on health and health equity.

There is a clear need for more flexibility in the way signatory status to international agreements can be modified over time. The General Agreement on Trade in Services (GATS) provides exceptions in cases of environmental or health hazard, but the provision is narrow and appears to require demonstration of actual harm, limiting national capacity to exercise precautionary measures (Box 12.7). Although flexibilities

---

BOX 12.5: HEALTH IMPACT ASSESSMENT IN THAILAND

Among low- and middle-income countries, only Indonesia, Sri Lanka and Thailand have some policy procedures or frameworks to support HIA. Thailand is the only country that has been successful at explicitly introducing HIA as part of its recent health sector reforms. HIA is now required as part of the new National Health Act 2002. National and regional HIAs have been focused on infrastructure or development projects, seeking to balance the health of local communities with other policy pressures.

For example, the HIA of Pak Mon Hydro Power Dam showed that the local villages had suffered due to a reduction in fishery resources, which had a negative impact on local income and socioeconomic status.

The HIA has led to the needs of the local villages being taken into account and mitigation measures initiated to improve rural livelihoods by changing the dam opening frequency to aid a return of the fishing industry. Thailand has also developed HIA at a national policy level, for example, looking at the health and economic effects of sustainable agriculture. The Thai example shows that it is possible in a short timescale to implement a strong and effective system of HIA of policy if there is government commitment, the presence of a policy framework, and sufficient resources.

Source: Lock, 2006

BOX 12.6: SLOVENIA – HEALTH IMPACT ASSESSMENT OF AGRICULTURE, FOOD, AND NUTRITION POLICIES

In December 2001, the Slovenian Ministry of Health and the WHO European Region proposed to undertake an HIA of agriculture, food, and nutrition policies, stimulated by Slovenia's application to join the EU and the influence that the Common Agricultural Policy legislation would have on national agricultural policy. The results of the HIA were presented to the Intergovernmental Committee on Health. Recommendations covered agricultural issues including the fruit and vegetable, grain, and

dairy sectors and rural development funding. An unforeseen outcome of the HIA was that the health and agricultural sectors began to support each other in the types of policies that they wanted implemented in Slovenia after EU accession. The EU negotiations were very successful and Slovenia was allocated more than other accession countries.

Source: MEKN, 2007a

are formally written into the Trade-related Aspects of Intellectual Property Rights (TRIPS) agreements, governments – particularly in many low- and middle-income countries with limited technical and institutional capacity – have in many cases derived only limited benefit from such flexibilities, and have in others been encouraged not to use them at all (Box 12.8).

At a more general level, international market-related trade agreements could include more strongly worded provisions by which countries with widely different needs and developmental strategies can opt out of their signatory status (for limited periods and under transparent conditions) where domestic conditions – including evidence of adverse impact on health and health equity – suggest the need (Box 12.9).

The Commission recommends that:

12.2 Government policy-setting bodies, with support from WHO, ensure and strengthen representation of public health in domestic and international economic policy negotiations (see Rec 10.2).

BOX 12.7: GENERAL AGREEMENT ON TRADE IN SERVICES

In principle, GATS only applies to sectors that governments voluntarily release to the market. However, Article 6.4 appears to imply that all service-sector regulations can be contested across the board. This contradicts assurances given by the WTO and governments supporting the agreement that GATS rules will only apply in those sectors that governments have offered up. Furthermore, the agreement contains a stringent article that prevents countries from altering commitments (part of the GATS rules) once they have been set.

Sources: http://www.foe.co.uk/resource/briefings/gats_stealing_water.pdf; Woodward, 2005; Adlung, 2005; Mehta & Madsen, 2005

BOX 12.8: WORLD TRADE ORGANIZATION AGREEMENT ON TRADE-RELATED ASPECTS OF INTELLECTUAL PROPERTY RIGHTS

GKN makes several recommendations on trade-related agreements in intellectual property rights (IPR) and TRIPS:

Avoid further concessions in bilateral or free trade agreements that increase the level of IPR protection for pharmaceuticals and, if such concessions have already been made, provide for compensatory measures to support access to drugs.

Maximize use of the flexibilities provided by TRIPS and explore the use of compulsory licences of patented essential medicines.

WHO should evaluate mechanisms other than patents, such as contests, public-interest research funding, and advance purchase agreements, to encourage development of drugs for diseases that disproportionately affect developing countries and assist member countries to implement such mechanisms.

These are supported by recommendations from the Commission on Intellectual Property Rights.

Sources: GKN, 2007; Commission on Intellectual Property Rights, 2002

BOX 12.9: SAFEGUARDING HEALTH AND HEALTH EQUITY IN AGREEMENTS

"The WTO has in place a 'safeguard' designed to protect countries from a surge in imports. The Agreement on Safeguards allows (temporary) increase in trade restrictions under a very narrow set of conditions, primarily demonstrable threat to a domestic industry ... A broader interpretation of safeguards would acknowledge that countries may legitimately wish to restrict trade or suspend existing WTO obligations – exercising 'opt-outs' – for reasons going beyond competitive threats to their industries ... Developmental priorities are among such reasons, as are distributional concerns or conflicts with domestic norms or social arrangements ... The current agreement could be recast as an 'Agreement on Developmental and Social Safeguards', which would permit the application of opt-outs under a broader range of circumstances."

Reproduced, with permission of the author, from Rodrik (2001).

Health is implicated across the breadth of WTO trade agreements. But throughout the field of trade negotiation processes, the voice of public health has too often been absent or muted. Supported by WHO, Member States can strengthen their capacity to represent health interests in the consideration of trade (Box 12.10).

The Commission recommends that:

12.3   National governments, in collaboration with relevant multilateral agencies, strengthen public sector leadership in the provision of essential health-related goods/services and the control of health-damaging commodities (see Rec 6.3; 7.3).

The areas covered below are illustrative examples, not an exhaustive list.

Water

It is vital to ensure – through regulation (nationally) and development assistance (internationally) – that equity in access remains central to all water policy. It must be recognized that a 'full-cost pricing' approach to extending vital services to the poor is indifferent to equity concerns. To the extent that cost recovery is required in such services, systematic cross-subsidies are needed to ensure all households have sufficient access to meet all basic needs independently of ability to pay (Box 12.11, Fig. 12.2).

BOX 12.10: HEALTH PARTICIPATION IN TRADE NEGOTIATIONS – GOVERNMENT, CIVIL SOCIETY, AND REGIONS

In Malaysia, the Ministry of Health was proactive in the decision to import generic antiretroviral drugs under the 'government use' provision of TRIPS, even in the face of strong opposition from within the national government cabinet. In Sri Lanka in 2003, activists and advocates challenged a TRIPS-related bill in the Supreme Court that would knowingly increase inequity, denying people equal access to equal health services. In national GATS negotiations, the Pakistani Ministry of Health made an offer on professional services in the health sector that excluded health services provided by public institutions. The objective of this exclusion was to ensure future regulatory flexibility to improve accessibility to health services through subsidies, universal service obligations, or other measures.

The Secretariat of the Common Market on Eastern and Southern Africa is coordinating comprehensive assessments of the state of trade in services (including health services) in this region, in preparation for economic partnership agreements with the EU and GATS negotiations. Low-income countries may not have the resources to create a distinct unit or committee to deal with trade and health, and regional collaboration may be the best way to ensure internal coherence.

Amended, with permission of the publisher, from Blouin (2007).

BOX 12.11: DESIGNING WATER TARIFFS FOR EQUITY

A central challenge in the market management of access to water and sanitation services is the design of a subsidized tariff. The slope and shape of the tariff curve determines whether the overall impact is progressive. Subsidies that cover a small basic amount do not ensure equitable access if the price

rises sharply once this amount has been consumed. This has been the unintended effect of Free Basic Water in Johannesburg and Durban, South Africa, where minimally adequate use is unaffordable for many households.

Source: GKN, 2007

MARKET RESPONSIBILITY : ACTION AREA 12.2

Reinforce the primary role of the state in the provision of basic services essential to health (such as water/sanitation) and the regulation of goods and services with a major impact on health (such as tobacco, alcohol, and food).

Health care

A core objective of all health–systems policy must be to ensure that everyone has access to competent, quality care independently of ability to pay (see Chapter 9: *Universal Health Care*). Theoretically, market regulation can shape the role and behaviour of the private sector within the health system. In practice, evidence that it can do so in ways that enhance health equity is lacking. Until governments have demonstrated their ability to effectively regulate private investment and provision in health services in ways that enhance health equity, they should avoid making any health services commitments in binding trade treaties that affect their capacities to exercise domestic regulatory control. It is not clear that any government, anywhere in the world, has met this test (HSKN, 2007; GKN, 2007). The example of health insurance is instructive. It is clear that health insurance can support health-care financing, but it must not, in so doing, undermine health equity (Box 12.12).

Labour

National governments, working in collaboration with employers and workers' organizations, should adopt and effectively implement the ILO's four core labour standards (see Chapter 7: *Fair Employment and Decent Work*). However, caution is required in processes of enforcing internationalized labour standards by way, for example, of 'social clauses' in trade agreements. These can be used by countries with greater resources for compliance to protect domestic industries through invoking sanctions on poor compliance, often in low- and middle-income countries. Rather than the WTO penalizing countries that fail in their obligations, it would be better to increase the power of those organizations (such as the UN Environment Programme, ILO, FAO, WHO) with the specialized knowledge to make good adjudications. The role of workers themselves in promoting and protecting decent working conditions (Box 12.13) can be critical.

Figure 12.2 Johannesburg water – convex tariff curve and ideal-type concave curve.

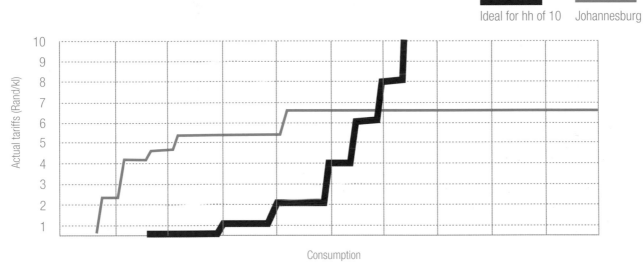

Ideal for hh of 10   Johannesburg

hh = households.
Reprinted, with permission of the author, from GKN (2007).

BOX 12.12: REGULATING HEALTH INSURANCE FOR EQUITY

Health insurance not only shelters people from large out-of-pocket payments, but also allows for pooling (i.e. spreading financial risks among the participants). However, it is unlikely that the expansion of private foreign insurance will have a large-scale positive impact on improving access to services. Given costs and marked evidence of market failure in private health insurance, this is arguably not a viable option for risk pooling at the national level in low- and middle-income countries. The evidence from Latin America shows that private insurers, be they foreign or domestic,

tend to serve the higher-income and lower-risk groups who can pay relatively high financial contributions to receive coverage. In Chile, for example, elderly people and women of fertile age face much higher premiums. One way to address this discrimination is to introduce regulations to limit such behaviour by insurers. A major caveat here, though, is that there is very little evidence of countries actually doing this.

Source: HSKN, 2007

In countries where many rely on agriculture for basic household living, governments should act to protect the livelihoods of farming communities exposed to cost and competition pressures through agricultural trade agreements (Box 12.14) (see Chapter 6: *Healthy Places Healthy People*). Recent evidence on trade reforms and food security suggest that a key policy lesson for developing countries is that, "trade reform can be damaging to food security in the short to medium term if it is introduced without a policy package designed to offset the negative effects of liberalization" (GKN, 2007). Where agricultural trade reform and liberalization is being pushed forward, a targeted subsidy for agricultural inputs is one measure highlighted to manage the initial negative impact.

Food

Governments will need to develop regulatory strategies to address the impact of globalized food production and trade on the nutritional quality of national and local diets. Food-related policy-making and trade agreements need to concentrate on the three key aspects of nutrition and health equity: availability, accessibility, and acceptability. The example of controls on consumption of soft drinks (Box 12.15) offers some broader insights into options for action.

BOX 12.13: TRANSFORMING EXPLOITATION IN THE GARMENT INDUSTRY – BANGLADESH

Under the Multi-fibre Arrangement (1974-2004, abolished under the WTO Uruguay Round Agreement), Bangladesh saw massive growth of its garment industry. Ready-made garments are now the leading national export – accounting for around three quarters of annual export receipts, the overwhelming majority of exports – and the industry employs an estimated 2.5 million workers. Garment-manufacturing employers sought women employees because they provided low-cost labour, were perceived to be docile, and had low occupational mobility. Previously there had been little attention to women's rights, with minimal avenues for women to exercise leadership. Women had few opportunities to access the formal labour market and there was highly discriminatory investment in girls' education and health compared to boys'. The garment industry has begun to change women's position. Approximately 80% of employees in the garment industry are women and women's employment in non-export industries is estimated to be 7%. Increased female employment is leading to increased attention to women workers' rights; increased activities aiming to organize women and cultivate female leaders; more workforce options for women with relatively higher and more regular wages; more support in households for girls' education due to the incentive of future income; greater ability among women to negotiate public spaces when commuting and working; increased empowerment of women as their economic role in households increases their

power; and increased preference for delayed marriage and childbirth.

But wages in the garment industry are low, there is high stress, and working conditions are poor and hazardous. Research conducted in Dhaka in 2006 reported women regularly working 80 hours per week for 5 pence an hour. The factories included in the research were supplying the United Kingdom stores Primark, Tesco, and Asda, which have all made a commitment to pay a minimum wage of £22 a month – calculated as a living wage in Bangladesh. Workers in the industry went on strike led by the National Garment Workers Federation and won a 50% rise in the minimum wage to £12 a month – progress, even if still well below a living wage. The case study of the Bangladesh garment industry powerfully illustrates the benefits that can accrue when major companies locate in low-income countries, but also points to the potentially profound social changes that this can trigger even when conditions fall far short of good labour practice. The contribution could be much greater if private sector companies took their 'corporate social responsibility' more seriously. As elsewhere, the emphasis here is that globalization can bring tremendous benefits but that, unregulated, it will certainly not benefit all, and will harm many. The implication is not to resist the globalization processes of market integration, but to make them better and fairer.

Source: SEKN, 2007

BOX 12.14: PROTECTING AGRICULTURAL LIVELIHOODS

Effective agricultural development – development that generates jobs and widely shared growth in income – depends on land distribution patterns, access to inputs such as capital and labour, environmental conditions, and access to markets. Strong agricultural development and equitable land distribution together provide a solid basis for economic growth and poverty reduction. Farmers' prosperity depends on their resource base and their market power. For low-income countries whose economies are still heavily dependent on agriculture, sequencing of reforms is critical. Raising agricultural productivity and creating non-agricultural employment should precede trade reforms such as the reduction of tariffs on crops grown by low-income households.

WTO's Agreement on Agriculture (Uruguay Round) discourages or prohibits national policies that seek to manage agricultural price or production. For the majority of developing countries, the demands of food security make it important to be able to provide production incentives, for example, stable domestic prices (almost impossible in an open global market). Recognizing the potential that new negotiations may limit further national policy space to promote

food security, FAO advocates special and differential treatment at the WTO, where developing countries would have greater flexibility in the application of the WTO rules:

Numbers of subsistence and resource-poor farmers. Where governments allocate most or all support to such farmers, they should be exempt from any further cuts to domestic support.

Economic vulnerability. Where countries are highly dependent on the export of just one or two crops, FAO recommends allowing high government spending levels to support productivity increases, improved standards, and phased programmes to buy out less efficient producers.

Physical vulnerability. Temporary special and differential treatment may be needed for countries whose producers suffer a disaster, such as an earthquake, flood, or war. In such cases, governments may need a period of unrestricted investment to build up herds or restore perennial crops.

Source: GKN, 2007

BOX 12.15: MARKET REGULATION AND NUTRITION – SOFT DRINKS

There are a number of examples of approaches to market regulation in the field of foods. Limiting availability can be an effective means of limiting consumption ... A first step is to consider limiting availability in places that specifically target children, schools being the notable example. In Brazil, laws have recently been passed in three municipalities to ban the sale of certain foods in school cafeterias, including soft drinks. In Oman, Saudi Arabia, and the United Arab Emirates, carbonated soft drinks are banned in schools. This policy is also being implemented in the United States. Price has a very real effect on consumption, although increasing prices raises issues of equity ... Packaging regulations are another possible option. In Mexico, there were limits on packaging until 1991. As a result, up to 75% of Coke sold was in the single serve glass bottle, limiting consumption.

Options for action:

Begin a dialogue about whether regulating or setting standards for the marketing of fatty, sugary, and salty processed foods would be appropriate and, if so, at what scale: local, national, or international. This dialogue should include the food industry alongside international, governmental, and NGOs.

Carry out an econometric analysis to gain greater understanding of the effects of global brands of processed foods on consumption patterns (as opposed to local or regional brands), and of the effects of marketing these products relative to other factors that influence food choice.

Amended, with permission of the publisher, from Hawkes (2002).

Tobacco and alcohol

The development of the WHO's FCTC is an excellent (if rare) example of coherent, global action to restrain market availability of a lethal commodity (Box 12.16). The Commission urges the 12 countries in Africa, 13 countries in the Americas, 12 countries in Europe, and 5 countries in the Middle East that are not part of the FCTC to ratify and enforce the FCTC. This includes G8 countries – Italy, Russian Federation, and the United States – as well as WHO's host country, Switzerland.

Strategies at the global and national levels need to be complemented by actions at the local policy level and behaviour-change interventions. An example of such a strategy includes local taxation policy – though the potential for exacerbating inequity through taxation that impacts regressively on the poorest needs to be taken into account – and a wider set of supply-and-demand measures (Box 12.17).

Learning from the FCTC, the Commission urges WHO to initiate a discussion with Member States on regulatory action for alcohol control (Boxes 12.18 and 12.19). The WHO European Region suffers the highest levels of alcohol-related disease and violence, with very large differences in alcohol-related mortality between countries. European policy discussion has been characterized by a conflict of view: is alcohol a commodity like any other, or should it be seen as a public health concern, whose trade could be regulated to protect people's health? The Commission urges governments in the WHO European Region and globally to work together to limit alcohol-related harm.

A responsible private sector

Private sector actors can behave in ways that undermine public interest, but they can also contribute powerfully to public good. There is some evidence of small moves towards greater social contribution, but it is of limited credibility. Corporate social responsibility has been promoted as a vehicle for improving the positive social impacts of private sector actors. To date, however, corporate social responsibility is often little more than cosmetic. One of its principal shortcomings is that, being voluntary, it lacks enforcement (Box 12.20), but also that little evaluation has been attempted. An exception to this problem is the Ethical Trading Initiative. An independent evaluation of the impact of the Ethical Trading Initiative Code of Labour Practice, for example, reported a number of areas of improvement (Barrientos & Smith, 2007). But voluntary initiatives will inevitably be limited in their impact. Corporate accountability may be a more meaningful approach.

BOX 12.16: THE FRAMEWORK CONVENTION ON TOBACCO CONTROL

Clear evidence exists that trade liberalization, when applied to tobacco, leads to adverse health consequences. World Bank research found that reduced tariffs in some parts of Asia resulted in a 10% increase in smoking rates above what it would have been without trade liberalization. Increases within certain population groups, such as teenage males (18.4% to 29.8% in 1 year) and teenage females (1.6% to 8.7%) in Republic of Korea was even starker. To prevent trade policy taking precedence over health protection, health organizations and WHO have urged the exclusion of tobacco from trade treaties. The FCTC notably acknowledges the link between trade and tobacco but contains no provisions to address it.

Sources: GKN, 2007; Gostin, 2007

BOX 12.17: STRATEGIES TO CONTROL TOBACCO – THAILAND

In its report on "Thailand – restrictions on importation of and internal taxes on cigarettes," the 1990 General Agreement on Tariffs and Trade (GATT) Panel decided that, "GATT-consistent measures could be taken to control both the supply of and demand for cigarettes, as long as they were applied to both domestic and imported cigarettes on a national-treatment basis". It was therefore concluded that the restriction of foreign imports of cigarettes was not necessary if other measures could be taken. The future harmonization of tobacco control policies, including price increases, ad valorem taxes, and advertising bans, could be introduced as long as the policies did not discriminate between foreign and domestic products. Thus, the Panel provided a general mechanism for tightening tobacco control without breaking WTO rules. Following the GATT Panel decision, Thailand maintained its advertising ban and has upheld other strict measures to control tobacco use. Thailand's strong legislation is a model of what countries can do when confronted with multinational tobacco companies and their advertising.

Source: Bettcher et al., 2000

BOX 12.18: EVIDENCE FOR ALCOHOL CONTROL

There is substantial evidence that an increase in alcohol prices reduces consumption and the level of alcohol-related problems. In most countries and especially in countries with low alcohol tax rates, tax-induced price increases on alcoholic beverages lead to increases in state tax revenues and decreases in state expenses related to alcohol-related harms. The effects of price increases, like the effects of other alcohol control measures, differ among countries depending on such factors as the prevailing alcohol culture and public support for stricter alcohol controls. However, the effects on alcohol-related harms are definite and the costs low, making it a cost-effective measure. In addition, stricter controls on the availability of alcohol, especially via a minimum legal purchasing age, government monopoly of retail sales, restrictions on sales times, and regulation of the number of distribution outlets, are effective interventions. Given the broad reach of all these measures, and the relatively low expense of implementing them, they are highly cost effective.

Source: http://www.euro.who.int/document/E82969.pdf

BOX 12.19: STRATEGIES TO CONTROL ALCOHOL

Worldwide, alcohol taxation – in the form of special excise duties, value added taxes, and sales taxes – has proven among the most popular and effective societal-level intervention to reduce the overall volume of drinking and, in turn, may particularly reduce alcohol-attributable chronic health problems. Taxation policies rely on the economic law of supply and demand: adding a tax increases the price of alcohol. The higher price then means that consumers can afford to buy less of their preferred alcoholic beverage. Taxation policies may be bolstered by the concentration of market power in government-controlled alcohol monopolies that control prices, production, imports, and sales. This approach has been prevalent in North America and parts of South America, Eastern Europe, and the Nordic countries. In the latter, careful tinkering with alcohol controls has produced remarkable success with changing patterns of consumption as well, for example by reducing the availability of forms of alcohol that tend to be consumed in binge drinking and by promoting lower-strength beverages, such as low-alcohol content beer.

Source: PPHCKN, 2007b

BOX 12.20: BUILDING CORPORATE SOCIAL RESPONSIBILITY – PUSH FROM BELOW

While it is fair to say that corporate social responsibility makes a positive contribution to the human rights of those working in transnational corporations, it is also fair to say that it only makes a difference to those few corporations targeted by consumers or who are already thinking ethically and responsibly. Other industries are not so well inclined. Such anomalies, and the somewhat piecemeal approach of the corporate social responsibility movement, should alert global citizens to the need for a more systematic approach.

Source: Kemp, 2001

Civil society action, especially by trade unions, including action by stakeholders and consumers, can increase pressure for greater social accountability by private sector organizations, including demanding greater formal regulatory action (Box 12.21).

The marketplace and private sector actors have, without doubt, great power in influencing social conditions, including many if not all the major social determinants of health. But that influence – globally, regionally, nationally, and locally – must be benign. From fair participation in the global institutions through which market policies are formulated, through trade and investment-related agreements, to the regulation of commercial activities and products, the role of the public sector, both to provide and to regulate, remains vital.

BOX 12.21: CIVIL SOCIETY – INFLUENCING SHAREHOLDERS

In recognition of the limits of voluntary initiatives, a number of international civil society organizations have formed a social movement focusing on corporate accountability and fair-trade and market-access issues for poor countries more generally (War on Want, Christian Aid, World Development Movement, Trade Justice Movement coalition, Third World Network, Oxfam, International Gender and Trade Network). One approach has been to target shareholders in an attempt to gain support for resolutions to be passed at Annual General Meetings. These would require

companies to appoint independent auditors to ensure that workers in supplier factories and farms are guaranteed decent working conditions, a living wage, job security, and the right to join a trade union of their choice. Given the emphasis on shareholder value, and the leverage of institutional shareholders, it should be noted that the effectiveness of this kind of civil society action is unproven.

Source: SEKN, 2007

CHAPTER 13
Gender equity

" [T]here is the need to look at women's issues in a holistic manner and to address them as part of overall societal and developmental concerns. It will not be possible to attain sustainable development without cementing the partnership of women and men in all aspects of life."

Gertrude Mongella (1995)

GENDER EQUITY AND HEALTH

Gender inequities are pervasive in all societies. Gender biases in power, resources, entitlements, norms, and values and in the organization of services are unfair. They are also ineffective and inefficient. Gender inequities damage the health of millions of girls and women (WGEKN, 2007). They influence health through, among other routes, discriminatory feeding patterns, violence against women, lack of access to resources and opportunities, and lack of decision-making power over one's own health. Furthermore, survival and development of all children, boys and girls, are strongly related to the position of women in society (Caldwell, 1986; Cleland & Van Ginneken, 1988). It has been estimated, for example, that women's lower status in South Asia is the strongest contributor to child malnutrition in that region (Smith & Haddad, 2000).

Gender relations of power are expressed through norms and values, and internalized through socialization. These are manifest in the extent to which: laws promote gender equity, women earn the same income as men for equivalent work, and women's economic contributions are included in national accounts. Moreover, gender biases tend to be reproduced in the way in which organizations are structured and programmes are run.

> Currently, an estimated 495 million women worldwide are illiterate (64% of all illiterate adults). (UNESCO, 2007a)

In daily life, gender relations of power often underpin unequal access to and control over material and non-material resources and unfair divisions of work, leisure, and possibilities of improving one's life. Girls in some countries are fed less and are more physically restricted (WGEKN, 2007). Gender inequities in education, particularly secondary education, remain large. Women have less land, wealth, and property in almost all societies, yet they have higher burdens of work in the 'economy of care' – ensuring the survival, reproduction, and security of people, including young and old. For many women, childcare responsibilities represent the single most important barrier to participation in the waged labour market (Barriento, Kabeer & Hossain, 2004). Yet even where women do increasingly enter the labour market, they continue to bear unequal burdens for childcare and unpaid work in the household (WGEKN, 2007). The deepening of such a double burden has implications for women's health, both their occupational health and the consequences of insufficient rest and leisure (WGEKN, 2007). Moreover, the feminization of

work forces has been simultaneous with increased casualization (WGEKN, 2007). In addition, women are typically employed in lower paid, less secure, and informal occupations (WGEKN, 2007). Even for equivalent work, women worldwide are paid 20-30% less then men (Fig. 13.1) (UNICEF, 2006).

An extreme, though common, manifestation of gender inequity is intimate partner violence. While widespread, and with serious consequences for health and well-being, intimate partner violence remains widely ignored in policies and services (WHO, 2005a).

Within the health sector, gender power relations translate into differential access to and control over health resources within and outside families; unequal divisions of labour and benefits in formal, informal, and home-based parts of the health-care system (see Chapter 9: *Universal Health Care*); and gender biases in the content and process of health research (see Chapter 16: *Social Determinants of Health: Monitoring, Research, and Training*). Moreover, in recent years, the attention and resources for sexual and reproductive health and rights have weakened, largely due to political forces that influence the allocation of aid (Glasier et al., 2006). Both within and outside the health sector, gender inequity means reduced voice, decision-making power, authority, and recognition for women relative to men. Fig. 13.2 shows that the proportion of women who have a final say in decision-making on their own health care varies strongly across low- and middle-income countries, from below 20% in Burkina Faso to around 88% in Jordan.

Even in places where gender inequities are less obvious, women usually still have less access to political power and lower participation in political institutions, from the local municipal council or village to the national parliament and the international arena (UN, 2006b; WGEKN, 2007).

Gender inequities can be reduced. In fact, the position of women has changed dramatically over the last century in many countries, although progress has been uneven. Legislation, technology, and structural changes have contributed to the empowerment of women in many countries. Use of modern contraceptives has given women, in many cases, more control over their bodies and reproductive lives, and declining fertility rates have substantially reduced the time women spend on bearing and raising children. Literacy and educational attainment among girls and women have risen, and there has been a steady increase in the proportion of women in the labour force (UNICEF, 2006b). However, much remains to be done.

Education, training, and skills development are important for the empowerment of women. In addition, gender inequities in the labour market, including the pay gap, must be addressed. Furthermore, it is important that the political and financial commitment to reproductive and sexual health and rights are strengthened. The intergenerational effects of gender inequity make the imperative to act even stronger. Acting now, to improve gender equity and empower women is critical for reducing the health gap in a generation.

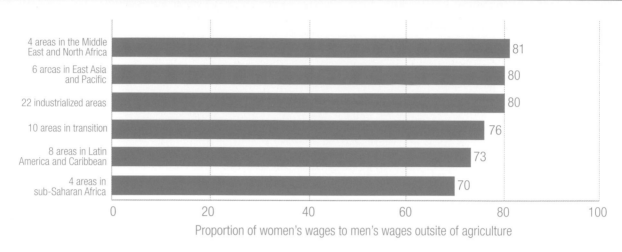

Figure 13.1: Level of wages for women compared with men in selected areas.

Reprinted, with permission of the author, from UNICEF (2006).
Middle East and North Africa: Bahrain, Egypt, Jordan, West Bank and Gaza Strip. East Asia and Pacific: Malaysia, Myanmar, Philippines, Republic of Korea, Singapore, Thailand. Industrialized countries: Australia, Austria, Belgium, Cyprus, Denmark, Finland, France, Germany, Greece, Hungary, Iceland, Ireland, Japan, Luxembourg, Malta, Netherlands, New Zealand, Norway, Portugal, Sweden, Switzerland, the United Kingdom.Countries in transition: Bulgaria, Croatia, Czech Republic, Georgia, Kazakhstan, Latvia, Lithuania, Romania, Turkey, Ukraine. Latin America and Caribbean: Brazil, Colombia, Costa Rica, El Salvador, Mexico, Panama, Paraguay, Peru. Sub-Saharan Africa: Botswana, Eritrea, Kenya, Swaziland.

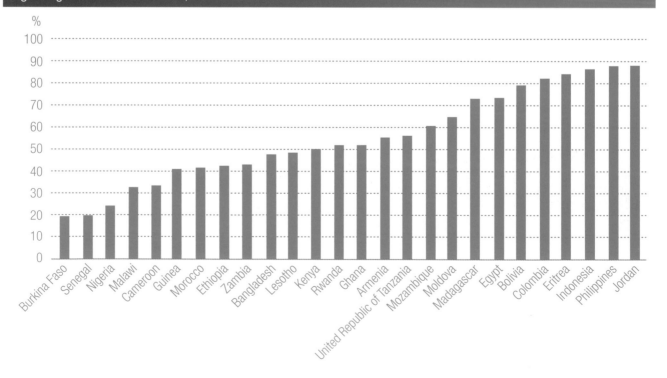

Figure 13.2: Percentage of women who have a final say in decision-making regarding their own health care, 2001–2005.

ACTION TOWARDS IMPROVING GENDER EQUITY FOR HEALTH

Legislation

The Commission recommends that:

13.1 Governments create and enforce legislation that promotes gender equity and makes discrimination on the basis of sex illegal (see Rec 14.1).

The success of interventions to improve gender equity – whether to increase access to education, to reduce all types of violence against women, or to protect women and girls from discrimination and exploitation in labour markets – is dependent on a legislative environment that protects and promotes gender equity. This may require legislative reform: repealing discriminatory laws, developing and implementing laws and regulations that protect and promote gender equity, and harmonizing legislation with human rights treaties (WHO, 2005a) (Box 13.1). Among other things, governments must guarantee women and girls equal property and inheritance rights (Grown, Gupta & Pande, 2005). In sub-Saharan Africa, for instance, these rights are important in enabling girls and women to manage the strains of being heads of households and primary caregivers for those living with HIV/AIDS (WGEKN, 2007).

Effective implementation requires addressing the judicial capacity to interpret and use such laws and sensitizing legal and justice systems (including police forces, investigators, lawyers, judges), community leaders, and health-care workers to the particular needs of women (WHO, 2005a; WHO, 2007b). It includes, for example in the case of violence, ensuring that women who bring complaints of violence are treated professionally and respectfully, protecting their safety as witnesses and taking measures to deter further violence (WHO, 2005a).

Effective enforcement and implementation of laws that support gender equity requires appropriate budgeting. Budgeting must be sufficient to reach the entire target population and address the magnitude of the problem (Box 13.2). Resource allocation that is mainstreamed into government budget line items, rather than depending on discretionary funds, is essential to successful implementation.

Effective implementation of laws that promote gender equity also requires that women know of and are empowered to claim their rights and challenge gender inequity – by means of expanding their capabilities, particularly through education and paid employment (WGEKN, 2007). Civil society organizations and national governments can play an important role in raising awareness among women about their legal rights (WGEKN, 2007) (Box 13.3).

BOX13.1: CORRECTING GENDER BIAS IN FAMILY LAW IN KENYA

In Kenya, the International Commission of Jurists, on the basis of an investigation revealing the extent of bias against women in family law, successfully lobbied for and established a Family Division within the High Court of Kenya to focus on arbitration of divorce, maintenance, and family property, and to undertake training to correct gender bias within the judicial system. Subsequent efforts have focused on using the Convention on the Elimination of All forms of Discrimination Against Women as a guiding instrument in judicial practice, to align national policy with international human rights standards.

Source: WGEKN, 2007

BOX13.2: BUDGETING FOR IMPLEMENTATION OF LAWS ON DOMESTIC VIOLENCE IN LATIN AMERICA

A study by the International Center for Research on Women in 2002 compared budgetary allocations and spending to implement laws on domestic violence in a sample of Latin American and Caribbean countries. It showed that funding for domestic violence programmes is typically insufficient to reach the entire target population and address the magnitude of the problem. Moreover, much of the funding was discretionary, from ministries' budgets and international donors (Luciano et al., 2005).

Source: WGEKN, 2007

GENDER EQUITY : ACTION AREA 13.1

Address gender biases in the structures of society – in laws and their enforcement, in the way organizations are run and interventions designed, and the way in which a country's economic performance is measured.

There can be powerful organized opposition to changes that seek to promote gender equity. Usually, reform will take a long period of preparation, especially if there is an organized opposition that can use the threat of change as a way to mobilize fears on cultural or religious grounds. Local groups of advocates, especially women's organizations or human rights groups, can play a strong role in this struggle. In Pakistan, for example, civil society organizations have played an important role in legislative changes that make it easier for women to prove a rape allegation (Box 13.4). Therefore, support should be provided to local women's organizations for the long term (WGEKN, 2007).

Some practices, like female genital mutilation, may change more readily as a result of community-level interventions than through legislation and policing (Box 13.5). Legislation against female genital mutilation alone is insufficient. Indeed, if not well designed and implemented in consultation with community leaders and civil society organizations, legislation and sanctions can have negative consequences, such as driving the practice underground (WHO, 2008b).

Changing societal norms regarding gender inequity and practices that harm girls and women requires working with boys and men, as the example on female genital mutilation illustrates. Lessons from programmes that seek to challenge gender stereotypes and inequitable normative systems include: offering young men opportunities to interact with gender-equitable role models in their own community setting and promoting more gender-equitable attitudes in small group settings and in the wider community (Box 13.6) (see Chapter 5: *Equity from the Start*).

Gender mainstreaming

The Commission recommends that:

13.2   Governments and international institutions set up within the central administration and provide adequate and long-term funding for a gender equity unit that is mandated to analyse and to act on the gender equity implications of policies, programmes, and institutional arrangements (see Rec 10.2; 15.2).

Not only bias in the design and implementation of legal systems needs to be addressed. Gender discrimination and bias in the way organizational structures of governments and institutions and the mechanisms through which strategies and policies are designed and implemented need attention too (Ravindran & Kelkar-Khambete, 2007). This requires a systematic integration of a gender perspective at all levels – as opposed to an add-on activity – in the way organizations are structured and function and in the way policies, programmes, and services are designed and implemented, that is, gender mainstreaming (Ravindran & Kelkar-Khambete, 2007). This is the process of assessing the implications for women and men of any planned action so that women and men benefit equitably (ECOSOC, 1997; Ravindran & Kelkar-Khambete, 2007).

Whereas gender mainstreaming is increasingly recognized as important, implementation requires substantial strengthening. Gender mainstreaming must be understood properly, owned institutionally, funded adequately, and implemented effectively, and needs to be supported by a catalytic gender unit with strong institutional positioning, authority, and budget (WGEKN, 2007). The Commission recommends that national governments and international institutions, with

---

BOX13.3: CIVIL SOCIETY RAISING AWARENESS ABOUT PROPERTY RIGHTS IN THE UNITED REPUBLIC OF TANZANIA

The Women's Legal Aid Centre in United Republic of Tanzania raises awareness among women about how to acquire, dispose of, and mortgage land, to have title deeds of land owned, and to participate in land-related decision-making, while providing legal aid

services. In addition, the Centre provides training to police, magistrates, and judges about women's rights to property.

Source: WGEKN, 2007

BOX 13.4: CHANGING JURISDICTION OVER RAPE CASES IN PAKISTAN

According to the Human Rights Commission of Pakistan, there is a rape every 2 hours and a gang rape every 8 hours in the country. The small but articulate women's movement together with the human rights movement in Pakistan has been struggling for change in a political situation made increasingly complicated by the wars in Afghanistan and Iraq. Their efforts have recently borne fruit with the passing by the National Assembly and Upper House of the 2006 Protection of Women Bill, which

transfers the jurisdiction over rape cases from sharia to civil courts. It also makes it easier for a woman to prove a rape allegation without being charged for adultery. Although consideration of the Bill had to be postponed earlier because of Islamist opposition, it has been signed into law. Yet, more will be needed for it to be fully implemented and endorsed.

Source: WGEKN, 2007

assistance from, among others, WHO, set up a gender unit that supports the consideration of gender equity implications of policies, programmes, and institutional arrangements across the organization. In Sweden, for example, the Division of Gender Equality within the central administration is responsible for the coordination of gender mainstreaming activities (Box 13.7).

There are a variety of other strategies for mainstreaming gender within organizations, policy-making processes, and design of programmes and interventions (Ravindran & Kelkar-Khambete, 2007) (Box 13.8). Effective organizational mainstreaming is facilitated by placing responsibility for mainstreaming gender with senior management, and by

allocating adequate financial and human resources for a central unit with gender expertise.

When planning for gender mainstreaming, it is useful to examine whether enabling conditions are present. If not, preparatory work will be required to create these conditions, even while work is being initiated for mainstreaming gender (Ravindran & Kelkar-Khambete, 2007). Enabling conditions include the presence of political will, the establishment of legal and constitutional frameworks that support gender equity, and the presence of a strong women's movement (Ravindran & Kelkar-Khambete, 2007) (Box 13.9).

BOX 13.5: CHANGING NORMS REGARDING FEMALE GENITAL MUTILATION

Multi-pronged education approaches have succeeded in changing attitudes and norms regarding female genital mutilation in some cases. Examples of success include the Senegal project that is now a regional model endorsed by UNICEF. Its success involves public declaration of intent to abandon the practice, and a slow but steady human rights education programme that encourages villagers to make up their own minds about the practice. More generally, effective programmes typically have the following features: (i) inclusion of men in interventions that attempt to change attitudes; (ii) careful selection of

the right group leaders/facilitators for projects, and agreement on criteria for selection of participants; (iii) reproductive health and rights education classes that lift the taboo on talking about health problems associated with female genital mutilation; (iv) collaboration with the community to design an alternative rite of passage; and (v) education with a focus that is much wider than female genital mutilation to include rights, health, and development.

Source: WGEKN, 2007

BOX 13.6: 'STEPPING STONES', SOUTH AFRICA

Stepping Stones is a behavioural intervention programme that seeks to reduce HIV transmission through building stronger, more gender-equitable relationships. Using both men's and women's groups, the programme applies principles of participatory learning and skill building, including critical reflection and drama. Rigorous evaluations of the programme

in South Africa have shown a reduction in STIs in women, changes in men's sexual risk-taking behaviour, and a reduction in their use of violence against women.

Source: WGEKN, 2007

BOX13.7: MAINSTREAMING – SWEDEN'S GENDER EQUALITY STRATEGY

The main goal of gender mainstreaming in Sweden is to tackle the structural roots of gender inequity in society at large. Having such a goal is far from being the norm even within the EU. In Sweden, it involves taking gender relations into account in all activities by public, private, and voluntary organizations through systematic gender analysis in the design and delivery of all policies and services. This has been made possible by the key role played by technical experts in defining objectives and methods. This has, however, been stronger at the central government

level than at the municipal level. A second important success factor in Sweden is effective coordination across sectors and different bodies. Coordination is provided by the Division of Gender Equality within the central administration. Yet most important has been the forging of a broad social consensus across the political spectrum that insulates gender mainstreaming to some extent from the vagaries of democratic politics.

Source: WGEKN, 2007

Including women's economic contribution in national accounts

The Commission recommends that:

13.3 Governments include the economic contribution of household work, care work, and voluntary work in national accounts and strengthen the inclusion of informal work (see Rec 8.3).

National accounts provide data on economic activities within a country and measure a nation's production, income, and wealth. The UN System of National Accounts (UNSNA), set up as guide for countries to develop their national accounting systems and to facilitate cross-country comparisons, defines economies in terms of market transactions (Waring, 2003).

Unpaid work, mostly done by women – in the home and as caregivers – remains excluded from national accounts, thus making these activities invisible in national statistics. Unpaid work in Canada has an estimated value of 33% of GDP, with nearly two thirds of this unpaid work being done by women (data for 1998) (Hamdad, 2003). "Lack of visibility of women's economic contribution to the economy results in policies which perpetuate economic, social and political inequities between women and men. If you are invisible as a producer in a nation's economy, you are invisible in the distribution of benefits", such as credit facilities or training (Waring, 2003). It is critical that women and girls who function as 'shock absorbers' for families, economies, and societies through their responsibilities in caring for people are supported through resources, infrastructure, and effective policies and programmes (WGEKN, 2007). Making them visible in national accounts is an important first step (Waring, 1988; Waring, 1999).

Women's contributions to the global, national, and local economy need to be recognized and made visible through new accounting systems (Waring, 2003). While in 1993 the UNSNA rules were revised, they still did not account for activities both produced and consumed within the same household (Waring, 2003). Several techniques of measuring and valuing unpaid work have been proposed, and some countries, such as Canada (Box 13.10), are using these techniques to estimate the value of unpaid work. The various methods available have their advantages and disadvantages, and further work on the development and use of techniques is necessary.

Apart from household work, care work, and voluntary work, many women have paid informal work. The inclusion of paid informal work in national accounts needs to be strengthened as it remains inadequately covered. There are methodologies to include such work within the existing accounting systems (Delhi Group on Informal Sector Statistics, nd).

BOX 13.8: GENDER MAINSTREAMING IN THE CHILEAN GOVERNMENT – MANAGEMENT IMPROVEMENT PROGRAMME

The Management Improvement Programme in Chile works as a group incentive linked to institutional performance: all staff in a public institution receive a bonus of up to 4% of their salaries if the institution attains programme management targets that have been approved by the Ministry of Economics. The Management Improvement Programme of each institution is prepared considering a group of common areas for all institutions in the public sector. One of these areas is gender planning. The proposal is presented yearly, together with the proposed budget, to the Ministry of Economics. The incorporation of a gender planning component implies the introduction of the gender approach in the budgetary cycle. This makes it possible to integrate gender considerations in the routine and habitual procedures of public administration, permanently introducing modifications into the daily dynamics of the institutions and their standardized procedures. Thus, public institutions need to incorporate this dimension into all their strategic products, making it possible to allocate the public budget in a way that responds better to men's and women's needs and contributes to the reduction of gender inequities. The implementation of this incentive mechanism constitutes an important innovation: for the first time a concept of gender equity is integrally associated with budgetary management in Chile.

Source: WGEKN, 2007

BOX13.9: ADVOCACY FOR GENDER EQUITY

Organized efforts by feminist movements across the globe in the 1970s demanded changes in legislation, policies, programmes, and services affecting women's health. Women's health centres were established in many countries of the North and also in some countries of the South. Grassroots activism to promote women's control over their fertility and sexuality, to demystify medical knowledge, and to advocate women-centred policies and programmes was widespread in many developing countries. All these contributed to the emergence of an International Women's Health Movement in the early 1980s, providing further impetus to women's health advocacy. One outcome of advocacy was the development of women's health policies in some countries.

Source: Ravindran & Kelkar-Khambete, 2007

Education and training

The Commission recommends that:

13.4 Governments and donors invest in expanding girls' and women's capabilities through investment in formal and vocational education and training (see Rec 5.4).

Promoting gender equity and empowering women is a key development strategy and is embedded within the framework of the MDGs (MDG 3). Expanding girls' and women's capabilities through education underpins the empowerment of women. A number of initiatives improve girls' enrolment and retention rates in schools and address the barriers to education for girls, as discussed in Chapter 5 (*Equity from the Start*). At the same time there is a pressing need to expand formal and vocational educational opportunities to the millions of adult women who have received little or inadequate education.

Existing initiatives were considered insufficient to achieve the Education for All goal of halving adult illiteracy rates by 2015 (UNESCO, 2007b). In response UNESCO has launched the Literacy Initiative for Empowerment, a framework for literacy development that will be implemented in 35 countries with literacy rates lower than 50% or with more than 10 million illiterate people (UNESCO, 2007b). The initiative stresses respect for learners and their needs and the importance of engaging learners as partners in learning. It is a partnership between governments, civil society, development agencies, international organizations, the private sector, universities, the media, and learners themselves.

Engaging people in assessing their own needs is integral to the social determinants of health approach. An innovative model that takes a literacy-based approach to alleviating poverty in Bangladesh, particularly among rural women, is outlined in Box 13.11.

BOX 13.10: MEASURING THE CONTRIBUTION OF UNPAID WORK – STATISTICS CANADA

Statistics Canada is one of the leading country agencies in development and use of techniques to measure and value unpaid work. Canada's General Social Survey includes time-use surveys every six years. It collects information on the time spent on households' unpaid work. This time-use information is combined with imputed hourly cost to estimate the value of unpaid work. There are different methods to impute the hourly cost of unpaid work, including the opportunity cost method (i.e. forgone employment income) and the market replacement method (i.e. costs if replacement labour had to be bought on the open market). The estimated value of unpaid labour can vary widely according to the method used. In Canada, it varied from 33% to 52% of GDP (in 1998) depending on the method used.

Source: Hamdad, 2003

GENDER EQUITY : ACTION AREA 13.2

Develop and finance policies and programmes that close gaps in education and skills, and that support female economic participation.

BOX 13.11: GANOKENDRAS – PEOPLE'S LEARNING CENTRES IN BANGLADESH

Despite improvements in recent years following a range of initiatives to expand education in Bangladesh, women's literacy rate overall is low (UNESCO, 2007a). The Ganokendra-based programme was set up in 1992 by the Dhaka Ahsania Mission, a Bangladesh NGO, and now operates in over 800 communities, benefiting more than 400 000 people. Ganokendras take a literacy-based approach to alleviating poverty and empowering women. Ganokendras are organized and run by the local community, with strong participation by women, and develop their range of activities in response to locally identified needs. Men, women, and children participate in Ganokendra activities, but the majority of members are women. In addition to developing women's literacy skills and providing basic education for illiterates, the Ganokendras act as community centres for training and for discussing important issues. They develop activities linked with social and environmental programmes, and many provide micro-credit services. In addition, Ganokendras act to bring people in the community together, providing opportunities to network with each other and with NGOs and government agencies, enabling improved access to available services.

Source: Alam, 2006; UNESCO, 2001

Initiatives to make vocational training available to women can provide them with skills to enhance their income-generating ability. A number of such initiatives have been set up across the world. In the United Kingdom, for example, an education programme has been set up in recent years in response to the report of the Women and Work Commission (2006) (Box 13.12).

Economic participation

The Commission recommends that:

13.5 Governments and employers support women in their economic roles by guaranteeing pay-equity by law, ensuring equal opportunity for employment at all levels, and by setting up family-friendly policies that ensure that women and men can take on care responsibilities in an equal manner (see Rec 7.2).

Improving girls' enrolment and retention rates at all levels of education is often insufficient to address the next level of constraints, that is, economic participation. Where strong gendered norms persist, even those girls who do attend school may eventually take up gender-stereotyped roles (WGEKN, 2007). Breaking these barriers requires action to remove labour market biases and barriers (WGEKN, 2007).

Guaranteeing pay-equity by law

Across the world, women earn between 30% and 60% less then men, due to a combination of so-called women's jobs, wage differentials, and differences in participation in the labour force (UNICEF, 2006). Even for equivalent work, women generally

earn less then men (Cohen, 2007; Hartmann, Allen & Owens, 1999). This has important consequences for poverty levels, for example among children of single mothers (Hartmann et al., 1999). Differences in accumulated earnings can also result in large gender gaps in pension benefits (Cohen, 2007; US Social Security Administration, 2004). Poverty and low pension benefits are associated with worse health outcomes (see Chapter 8: *Social Protection across the Lifecourse*), while income in the hands of women can be particularly beneficial for the health of their children (UNICEF, 2006).

Action at all levels is required to tackle this unjust situation. Laws that oblige employers to achieve and maintain pay equity can be powerful instruments to help eliminate the pay gap. The ILO adopted the "Resolution concerning the promotion of gender equality, pay equity and maternity protection", which calls on all governments and social partners (trade unions and the employers or their representative organizations) to take specific actions to address the gender wage gap (ILO, 2004a). More specifically, the resolution proposes that social partners negotiate the introduction of gender neutral job evaluation schemes, statistical indicators, and gender and race reviews at the workplace (Box 13.13).

Unions are powerful vehicles in pressing for 'equal pay for work of equal value' laws. They can gather information to gauge the extent of the problem using, for example, the Code of Practice on the Implementation of Equal Pay for Work of Equal Value issued by the European Commission (European Commission, 1996; Gender Promotion Programme ILO, 2001).

BOX 13.12: SUPPORTING WOMEN IN DEVELOPING SKILLS AND CAREERS – UNITED KINGDOM

As part of an action plan in response to the Women and Work Commission's report, the United Kingdom government has piloted skills coaching schemes aimed at helping low-skilled women return to work. In addition, they have developed a programme to broker links between employers and training providers. A Women's Enterprise Task Force has been set up to

work with Regional Development Agencies to pilot various approaches to supporting women in setting up businesses.

Source: Department for Communities and Local Government, 2006

BOX 13.13: THE RIGHT TO EQUAL PAY IN QUEBEC, CANADA

In Quebec, as in the rest of Canada, women earn about 70% of men's pay for equivalent work. Trade unions in Quebec have committed themselves to the 'equal pay for work of equal value' struggle and were involved in a long lobbying effort that led to the adoption of a law on pay equity. After women mobilized and the unions lobbied, the Quebec Government brought in a law that obliges employers to achieve and maintain pay equity within their enterprises. Under the law, all enterprises with 50 or more employees must draw up a pay equity

programme. It includes four stages: (1) identifying the predominantly female and predominantly male job categories within the enterprise; (2) describing the method and tools for assessment (of the job categories); (3) assessing the job categories, comparing them, estimating the wage gaps, and calculating the necessary pay adjustments; and (4) determining how the wage adjustments are to be paid.

Adapted, with permission of the publisher, from Côté (2002/3).

Ensuring equal opportunity for employment at all levels

In addition, measures are needed to support women to equally progress in work, to be on a par with men. Governments and employers need to use a multi-pronged approach, including enforcement of anti-discrimination legislation at the workplace and ensuring that women are not penalized financially for motherhood (ILO, 2004b). It will also include providing management training, mentors, and role models at the highest levels, and admittance to formal and informal networks and channels of communication at work (ILO, 2004b). Some countries use quotas as an instrument to help women break through the glass ceiling. In Norway, for example, at least 40% of board members in state-owned enterprises must be women. Equal employment opportunity policies – including recruitment, job assignment, career planning, grading, wages, transfer, and promotion – should be closely monitored. The procedures should be transparent, objective, and fair (ILO, 2004b).

The quality and conditions of work matter as much as gender inequities in work opportunities. One key element of improving the quality of work is the implementation of sexual harassment policies and provision of education about sexual harassment to create a climate of respect in the workplace (ILO, 2004b).

Family-friendly policies

Family-friendly policies are important to ensure equal opportunities for employment for women and men (see Chapter 7: *Fair Employment and Decent Work*). Governments and employers should take measures that allow women and men to take on work and care responsibilities in an equal manner. These include the provision of quality childcare facilities, policies on flexible working hours and parental leave for men

and women, and programmes to transform male and female attitudes to caring work so that men begin to take an equal responsibility in such work (WGEKN, 2007; ILO, 2004b). Quality childcare, irrespective of ability to pay, not only allows women to enter the labour market, it also prevents young children being left home alone or in the care of older siblings – which can have serious health consequences (Heymann, 2006) – and allows girls to go to school instead of looking after younger siblings (UNICEF, 2006). Even in poor countries, childcare facilities are feasible, as illustrated in Box 13.14.

Sexual and reproductive health and rights

The Commission recommends that:

13.6 Governments, donors, international organizations, and civil society increase their political commitment to and investment in sexual and reproductive health services and programmes, building to universal coverage (see Rec 9.1; 11.3).

Gender inequities have a strong bearing on the reproductive and sexual health and rights of women. Critical problems related to gender inequity, such as intimate partner violence, can remain invisible in the process of service delivery for reproductive health. For example, intimate partner violence during pregnancy, which is more common than hypertension or pre-eclampsia – for which pregnant women are routinely assessed during antenatal visits – is rarely addressed by reproductive health services (Glasier et al., 2006). Reproductive and sexual health programmes and services can and should be structured such that they empower women to make informed sexual and reproductive choices across the lifecourse, giving them autonomy over their reproductive lives. Strengthening

BOX 13.14: PROVIDING CHILDCARE SERVICES IN INDIA

SEWA is a trade union of poor, self-employed women. Its members expressed the need for childcare, which would allow them to work without jeopardizing their children's safety and development. Working closely with the government, SEWA's 100 childcare centres are managed by cooperatives of childcare providers, which have been formed with SEWA's support. Each serves 35 children, ranging from birth to 6 years of age. They focus on the overall development of the children, including their physical and intellectual growth. The teachers hold regular meetings with the mothers, where they discuss and give suggestions for the child's development. Children are regularly weighed and records of their growth are properly maintained. The childcare centres double as centres for childhood immunization and antenatal and postnatal care. SEWA's studies show important

impacts of childcare provision: mothers reported income increases of over 50%, with spin-offs to, among others, child nutrition. They said that for the first time they could bring vegetables and lentils to feed their children. They also reported 'peace of mind', knowing that their children were well looked after while they were at work. Furthermore, older siblings, especially girls, entered school for the first time as they were released from childcare responsibilities. Also, the physical growth of young children improved significantly with the nutrition at the centres, as did their cognitive skills. All children started primary school at the age of 6 years and the majority continued until high school.

Adapted, with permission of the author, from SEWA Social Security (nd).

GENDER EQUITY : ACTION AREA 13.3

Reaffirm commitment to addressing sexual and reproductive health and rights universally.

political and financial commitment to the goal of universal sexual and reproductive health is critical, including funding of relevant research.

The first decades of the second half of the 20th century saw a strong focus on population control. Family planning programmes were set up and carried out with more concern for targets and macroeconomic outcomes than for the welfare and rights of individual women. The UN Conference on Population and Development in 1994 in Cairo marked a paradigm shift, from population control to reproductive health and rights. Central to the concept of reproductive health and rights is the, "recognition that advancement of gender equality and equity and the empowerment of women, the elimination of all kinds of violence against women, and ensuring women's ability to control their own fertility, are cornerstones of population and development-related programmes" (Glasier et al., 2006). As such, reproductive health is an empowering concept, emphasizing sexual and reproductive rights and seeking to enable women to achieve autonomy over their reproductive lives. The reproductive health paradigm emphasizes the importance of seeking to understand women's individual experiences and constraints and the social factors that influence sexual and reproductive health across the lifecourse (Langer, 2006). It is an integral part of the social determinants of health agenda.

In 1994, delegates from 179 countries and 1200 NGOs agreed to provide universal access to reproductive health by 2015 (Glasier et al., 2006) and, more recently, this was agreed as a target for the MDGs. Progress towards the goal of universal access to reproductive health has, however, been uneven. While the lifetime risk of maternal death in Ireland is only 1 in 47 600, it is 1 in 8 in Afghanistan (UNICEF, 2007c). Also within countries, inequities are huge. In Indonesia, for example, maternal mortality is three to four times higher among the poor compared to the rich (Graham et al., 2004). In low- and middle-income countries, 65% of the births without a skilled birth attendant occur among the rural poor (Houweling et al., 2007). Providing access to reproductive health services to internally displaced women and, more generally, women in countries of conflict and other crises also remains a critical challenge (Hargreaves, 2000; Petchesky et al., 2007).

In the 21st century, attention has been distracted by new global priorities (Fathalla, 2006). Delinked from HIV/AIDS, sexual and reproductive health has failed to attract the financial resources that were expected from the donor community, especially in fields of family planning, unsafe abortion, and STIs (Langer, 2006). The success of family planning programmes in reducing fertility rates led to reduced investment in family planning services, "with disastrous consequences in countries with still low contraceptive rates" (Glasier et al., 2006). In addition, there have been attempts to roll back agreements made in Cairo (Fathalla, 2006). Ideological resistance to the sexual and reproductive health and rights paradigm, in particular to issues related to sexuality, abortion, and services to adolescents, has had detrimental impacts on access to services that particularly benefit women (Langer, 2006; Fathalla, 2006).

It is crucial that governments and donors reaffirm their commitment to reproductive health and rights and re-establish sexual and reproductive health as a key health and development priority (Glasier et al., 2006; Fathalla, 2006). There are movements in a positive direction. In 2004, all WHO Member States (only the United States disassociated itself from the strategy) endorsed the WHO global reproductive health

strategy to accelerate progress towards international goals and targets relating to reproductive health (Glasier et al., 2006). In 2007, at the World Summit review of the MDGs at the UN, world leaders reaffirmed commitment to, "achieving universal access to reproductive health by 2015", as set out in the Cairo conference (Fathalla, 2006). While initially omitted from the MDG framework, a specific target on reproductive health ("achieve, by 2015, universal access to reproductive health") was included in the 2007 revision. Strengthened political and financial commitment is needed to implement the sexual and reproductive health target under the MDGs. This includes financing civil society organizations that are committed to taking forward reproductive health and rights.

The knowledge and technologies for achieving the target of sexual and reproductive health for all are available (Glasier et al., 2006). "Five core components of sexual and reproductive health care are improvement of antenatal, peri-natal, postpartum and newborn care, provision of high-quality services for family planning, including infertility services, elimination of unsafe abortions, prevention and treatment of sexually transmitted infections, including HIV, reproductive tract infections, cervical cancer and other gynaecological morbidities, and promotion of healthy sexuality" (Glasier et al., 2006). The reduction of sexual and intimate partner violence is also a critical area for intervention. While the availability of high-quality sexual and reproductive health services is obviously crucial (Glasier et al., 2006) (see Chapter 9: *Universal Health Care*), they should be embedded in an approach that also tackles the underlying societal and cultural roots of gender inequity.

Gender inequities are socially governed and can be changed to improve the health of millions of girls and women worldwide. Action includes ensuring that laws protect and promote gender equity and addressing gender biases in organizational structures and policies. In some regions, education and training of women is a priority; in other regions, alleviating the constraints on their economic, social, and political participation at all levels has become a higher priority. Finally, it is crucial that governments and donors reaffirm their commitment to addressing sexual and reproductive health and rights, as this commitment is weakening.

CHAPTER 14
Political empowerment – inclusion and voice

"People all over the world resent loss of control over their lives, over their environment, over their jobs, and, ultimately, over the fate of the Earth. Thus, following an old law of social evolution, resistance confronts domination, empowerment reacts against powerlessness, and alternative projects challenge the logic embedded in the new global order, increasingly sensed as disorder by people around the planet"

Castells 1997:69 (Oldfield & Stokke, 2004)

THE RELATIONSHIP BETWEEN POWER AND HEALTH INEQUITIES

Being included in the society in which one lives is vital to the material, psychosocial, and political aspects of empowerment that underpin social well-being and equitable health. In this chapter we consider the role of power as a major structural driver of health inequities. Any serious effort to reduce health inequities will involve political empowerment – changing the distribution of power within society and global regions, especially in favour of disenfranchised groups and nations.

The manifestation of power imbalance

The right to the conditions necessary to achieve the highest attainable standard of health is universal (UN, 1948). However, the risk of having one's rights violated is not universal and this inequity in risk of violation results from entrenched

structural inequities (Farmer, 1999). Manifesting across a range of intersecting social categories – class, education, gender, age, ethnicity, disability, and geography – social inequity reflects deep and entrenched inequities in the wealth, power, and prestige of different people and communities. People who are already disenfranchised are further disadvantaged with respect to their health.

Health equity depends vitally on the empowerment of individuals and groups to represent their needs and interests strongly and effectively and, in so doing, to challenge and change the unfair and steeply graded distribution of social resources (the conditions for health) to which all men and women, as citizens, have equal claims and rights (CS, 2007). Underlying the structural drivers of inequity in daily living conditions addressed throughout this report is the unequal distribution of power. Inequity in power interacts across four main dimensions – political, economic, social, and cultural – together constituting a continuum along which groups are, to varying degrees, excluded or included. The *political dimension* comprises both formal rights embedded in legislation, constitutions, policies, and practices and the conditions in which rights are exercised including access to safe water, sanitation, shelter, transport, energy, and services such as health care, education, and social protection. The *economic dimension* is constituted by access to and distribution of material resources necessary to sustain life (e.g. income, employment, housing, land, working conditions, livelihoods). The *social dimension*

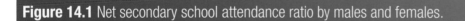

Figure 14.1 Net secondary school attendance ratio by males and females.

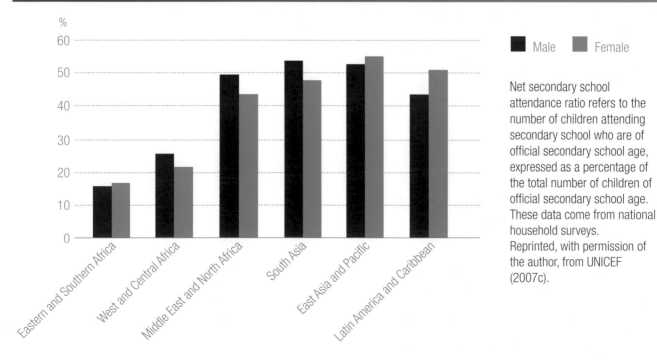

Net secondary school attendance ratio refers to the number of children attending secondary school who are of official secondary school age, expressed as a percentage of the total number of children of official secondary school age. These data come from national household surveys.
Reprinted, with permission of the author, from UNICEF (2007c).

Figure 14.2 Age-adjusted mortality among men and women of
the Republic of Korea by educational attainment, 1993–1997.

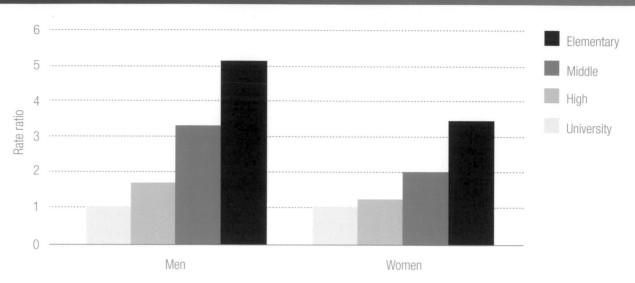

Source: Son et al., 2002

Figure 14.3 Full immunization rates among the poorest and richest population quintiles (regional averages).

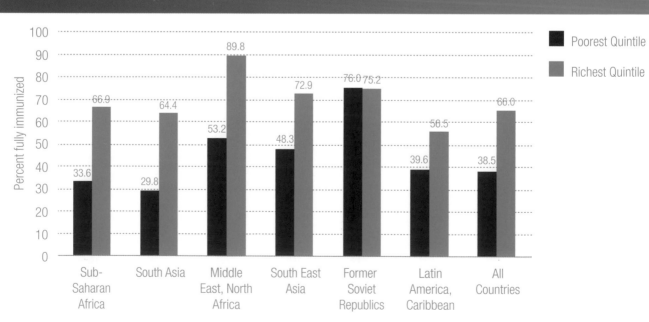

Reprinted, with permission of the publisher, from Gwatkin & Deveshwar-Bahl (2001).

is constituted by proximal relationships of support and solidarity (e.g. friendship, kinship, family, clan, neighbourhood, community, social movements) and the *cultural dimension* relates to the extent to which a diversity of values, norms, and ways of living contribute to the health of all and are accepted and respected (SEKN, 2007).

Having the freedom to participate in economic, social, political, and cultural relationships has intrinsic value (Sen, 1999). Inclusion, agency, and control are each important for social development and health (Marmot, 2004). Restricted participation also results in deprivation of fundamental human capabilities, setting the context for differentials in, for example, employment, education, and health care. For instance, differential access to education (Fig. 14.1) leads to inequity in all-cause mortality (Fig. 14.2).

Underdevelopment of potential leads to other inequities. Lack of access to quality education can lead to exclusion from the labour market or inclusion on appallingly poor terms, leading to relatively low income and poor household conditions (such as living space, nutrition, and other contributors to ill health). The global growth in precarious employment and child and bonded labour both reflects and reinforces a disempowerment of workers and their industrial and political representatives. The political, economic, financial, and trade decisions of a handful of institutions and corporations are having a profound effect on the daily lives of millions of people (EMCONET, 2007) whose own voice and aspirations are not listened to or are dismissed by more powerful interests.

There are major social inequities, too, in the enjoyment of technical and biomedical advances. Analysis of the DHS for 42 countries (Gwatkin & Deveshwar-Bahl, 2001) illustrates the marked socioeconomic inequalities in full immunization, with higher rates among the rich compared to the poor virtually everywhere (Fig. 14.3).

Identity and agency

The differential status some groups enjoy and the differential opportunities for participation by specific populations is clearly manifested in the treatment of indigenous cultures – their world views, values, and aspirations – on the part of governments and those who deliver direct services (Indigenous Health Group, 2007). The persistent inequity in the health conditions of Indigenous populations goes to the heart of the relationship between health and power, social participation, and empowerment (Indigenous Health Group, 2007). Regaining personal and cultural continuity has massive implications for the health and well-being of these communities, as shown in youth suicide rates among First Nations youth in Canada (Fig. 14.4).

Unfair denial of participation and disempowerment can also lead to conflict. In conflict settings, people suffer a range of physical and social deprivations including lack of security, displacement and loss of social networks and family structure, loss of livelihood, and food insecurity and poor physical and social environments (Watts et al., 2007). The disempowerment of individuals, communities, and even countries that is associated with conflict brings a multitude of health concerns. As with other dimensions of inequity, the needs of people in conflict must be represented in the construction and strengthening of economic and social policy and systems.

Issues of power imbalance relate not only to individuals and communities. Some countries remain profoundly disempowered through lack of resources relative to others. National poverty combines with and exacerbates unequal capacity in multilateral negotiating environments, leading to treaties and agreements that do not consistently represent their best interests (see Chapter 15: *Good Global Governance*). This has major implications for how nations can create conditions that support health and health equity.

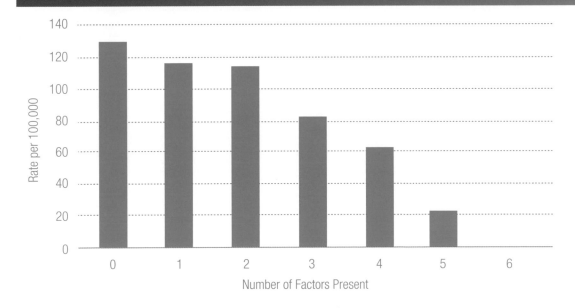

Figure 14.4 First Nations youth suicide rates, by cultural continuity factors.

Proxy measure of cultural continuity factors: land claims, self-government, education services, police and fire services, health services, and cultural facilities.
Reprinted, with permission of the publisher, from Chandler & Lalonde (1998).

ACTION TOWARDS FAIRNESS IN VOICE AND INCLUSION

Political empowerment for health and health equity requires strengthening the fairness by which all groups in a society are included or represented in decision-making about how society operates, particularly in relation to its effect on health and health equity. Such fairness in voice and inclusion depends on social structures, supported by the government, that mandate and ensure the rights of groups to be heard and to represent themselves – through, for example, legislation and institutional capacity – and on specific programmes supported by those structures, through which active participation can be realized. Beyond these, fairness depends on the growth of civil society organizations, networks, and movements and their progressive ability to challenge inequity and push for the installation of equity – in general and in relation to health – in the centre of all existing and emerging political debates.

Legislation for political empowerment – rights and agency

The right to the conditions necessary to achieve the highest attainable standard of health – Article 12 of the International Covenant on Economic, Social and Cultural Rights – is principally concerned with disadvantaged groups, participation, and accountability and lies at the heart of the health and human rights movement (Hunt, 2007). General Comment 14 (2000) is a substantive instrument which confirms that the right to the conditions for health not only encompasses access to health care, but also includes the underlying determinants of health, such as safe water, adequate sanitation, a healthy environment, health-related information, and freedom from discrimination (UN, 2000a). Fundamental to the progressive realization of this right is the ratification, operationalization, and monitoring of General Comment 14 and associated actions. WHO, in collaboration with other international agencies and the UN Special Rapporteur on the Right to the Highest Attainable Standard of Health (see Chapter 15: *Good Global Governance*), supports states in the adoption and implementation of General Comment 14.

Central to fair participation is the right to a legal civic identity. People cannot claim their rights – access to education and social assistance, health care, or civic participation and human security – without a legalized identity (Box 14.1) (Acosta, 2006). It is important therefore that countries, supported by international agencies and donors, strengthen the legal and institutional framework to ensure the right to a legal civic identity (see Chapter 16: *Social Determinants of Health: Monitoring, Research, and Training*).

Underpinning the realization of rights, fair participation, and inclusion in decision-making and action that affects health and health equity are transparent, accountable, and participative

---

POLITICAL EMPOWERMENT : ACTION AREA 14.1

Empower all groups in society through fair representation in decision-making about how society operates, particularly in relation to its effect on health equity, and create and maintain a socially inclusive framework for policy-making.

political and legal systems that build on and reinforce authentic participation.

The Commission recommends that:

14.1 National government strengthens the political and legal systems to ensure they promote the equal inclusion of all (see Rec 13.1; 16.1).

Gender

One of the most equitable and inclusive political reforms is that which addresses the marked global gender inequities. This requires the participation of women in policy and decision-making processes and will increase the probability of gender-sensitive planning and delivery. For example, national-level legislative reform in India that ensured a minimum number of women in village council seats proved critical to the political empowerment of women and, subsequently, to action at the local level that was responsive to local needs (Box 14.2).

Autonomy

Indigenous Peoples' lives continue to be governed by specific and particular laws, regulations, and conditions that apply to no other members of civil states. Indigenous People continue to live on bounded or segregated lands and are often at the heart of jurisdictional divides between levels of governments, particularly in areas concerning access to financial allocations, programmes, and services. As such, Indigenous Peoples have distinct status and specific needs relative to others.

The Commission recommends that:

14.2 National government acknowledges, legitimizes, and supports marginalized groups, in particular Indigenous Peoples, in policy, legislation, and programmes that empower people to represent their needs, claims, and rights

As noted by the UN, Indigenous People have the right to, "special measures for immediate and continuing improvement of their economic and social conditions, including in the areas of employment, vocational training and retraining, housing, sanitation, health and social security". In addition, the Declaration of Indigenous Peoples, which was recently passed by the UN Human Rights Council, states that, "Indigenous People have the right to determine and develop all health, housing and other economic and social programs affecting them and, as far as possible, to administer such programs through their own institutions". These realities imply Indigenous Peoples' rights to autonomy and self-determination. It is important that the UN finalizes the Declaration on the Rights of Indigenous Peoples and obtains ratification from and encourages implementation by all Member States.

How the Declaration on the Rights of Indigenous Peoples is operationalized for health and health equity within different sociopolitical contexts will require careful consideration, led by Indigenous Peoples. The example of the British Columbia Tripartite Health Plan – including elements of legislation, participatory governance, and responsive health services – offers

---

BOX 14.1: IDENTITY AND RIGHTS IN BOLIVIA

Of Bolivia's population, 55% is of Quechua or Aymara origin. It is estimated that nearly 9 out of 10 people in Bolivia's rural and indigenous communities do not possess identity cards, while more than half do not have the birth certificates needed to acquire one. Without a birth certificate, children cannot go to school – closing off a potential escape route from poverty. Without an identity card, people cannot vote, have limited legal rights, and are effectively excluded from accessing social and health services. These services include Bolivia's national health insurance for mothers and pregnant women, which was introduced

to combat the country's high maternal and child mortality rates and yet is closed to women who cannot produce their identity cards.

Through the Right to Identity project, the United Kingdom DFID is working with Bolivia's National Electoral Court, nongovernmental organizations, and communities to make it easier for people to register and receive their identity cards and to raise awareness of their rights as citizens.

Source: DFID, 2008

BOX 14.2: INDIAN LEGISLATIVE SUPPORT FOR WOMEN

Through the Indian national parliament, the 73rd Amendment to the Indian Constitution, enacted in 1993, legislated that one third of village council seats be for women. This is considered one of the strongest reform measures to change the pre-existing norm whereby women had very little representation in political bodies. Women's organizations have been

active in training elected women. There are over 1 million elected women representatives on village councils, exercising authority over budgets and setting local policy priorities.

Source: Indian Government, 1992

one participative framework for moving forward (Box 14.3). The apology issued by the new Australian Labour Government in February 2008 to Indigenous Peoples who were stolen from their families as children and forced to live with foster parents or in group homes was an example of a government recognizing the unique history of colonization on Indigenous Peoples and the need for special measures (The Age, 2008). The apology was accompanied by a pledge to reduce the gap in LEB between indigenous and other Australians in a generation (25 years).

Fair participation in policy-making

Good governance is the foundation for successful action and requires attention to trust, reciprocity, and social accountability mechanisms (KNUS, 2007). For this to happen, fair participation in governance is essential. Indeed, an integral feature of the right to health is the active and informed participation of individuals and communities in health decision-making that affects them.

> *"The difference between tokenism and meaningful participation is some kind of follow up and being included from beginning to end." (Landon Pearson Resource Centre for the Study of Childhood and Children's Rights, 2007)*

The Commission recommends that:

14.3 National- and local-level government ensure the fair representation of all groups and communities in decision-making that affects health, and in subsequent programme and service delivery and evaluation (see Rec 6.1; 7.1; 9.1; 11.6).

All members of society – including the most disadvantaged and marginalized – are entitled to participate in the identification of priorities and targets that guide the technical deliberations underlying policy formulation. Moreover, participation should not be limited to the design of programme delivery, but rather be seen as the contextual process itself, through which policy is made, converted into programmes and services, delivered, experienced, and evaluated.

The recommendations for ISA in Chapter 10 (*Health Equity in All Policies, Systems, and Programmes*) offer processes and mechanisms through which different social groups and communities can participate in policy development, implementation, and evaluation. Much can be learned from existing practices. The establishment of a governance support network, perhaps through the Economic and Social Council, operating at the global, regional, and national levels would facilitate the identification and sharing of successful practices (e.g. Alliance for Healthy Cities, European Network of Healthy Cities, Municipalities Network, and the Pan-American Health Organization [PAHO]).

The mandatory representation of civil society within a whole-of-government mechanism, as in Uganda for example, is an important element of coherent and needs-driven policy for health and health equity (Box 14.4).

The Social Inclusion Initiative from South Australia (Box 14.5) illustrates the value of political recognition and strong commitment to inclusion and health equity. It demonstrates the merit of having an independent unit that facilitates, rather

---

BOX 14.3: CANADA: THE BRITISH COLUMBIA TRIPARTITE HEALTH PLAN – FIRST NATIONS

The British Columbia Tripartite Health Plan is an unprecedented agreement signed on 11 June 2007 by the Government of Canada, the Province of British Columbia, and the First Nations Leadership Council of British Columbia. The Plan commits the parties to collaborate in developing practical and innovative solutions that will support fundamental improvements in the health of First Nations in British Columbia. It reflects a shared vision of partnership to develop, test, and implement new ways of planning and delivering

health programmes and services. Central to the Plan is a commitment to create a new governance structure that will enhance First Nations' control of health services and promote better integration and coordination of services to ensure improved access to quality health care by all First Nations living in British Columbia.

Source: Government of Canada, 2007

BOX 14.4: UGANDAN CONSTITUTION AND CITIZEN'S PARTICIPATION

Uganda now actively encourages participation in health decision-making. The Constitution underlines the importance of, "active participation of all citizens at all levels" and civil society organizations have been involved in the preparation of Uganda's Poverty Eradication Action Plan.

Uganda has a new policy of decentralization in the health sector. Within district health systems, there

are four levels of organization and administration, the lowest being Village Health Teams, also known as Village Health Committees. From the right-to-health perspective, these Village Health Teams play a pivotal role in providing grassroots community participation in the health sector.

Source: Hunt, 2006

than manages, the processes of engagement required for social inclusion, and of having a strategic plan and setting targets for change.

Societal fairness is rooted not just in an equity focus in central national policy-making. That focus is stimulated by, and feeds into, local conditions of inclusion and fair representation. One way to support this is to make building a healthy and equitable community a local statutory requirement. This can be done through the development of a democratically sanctioned, statutory, strategic local development plan that is regularly monitored and reviewed (Box 14.6). The provision of statutory funding to support community engagement and participation in the process is critical. Annual monitoring and reporting will help measure progress against a set of specific targets including health equity impact (LHC, 2000).

BOX 14.5: SOUTH AUSTRALIA'S SOCIAL INCLUSION INITIATIVE

The Social Inclusion Initiative is the Government of South Australia's response to addressing social exclusion through: facilitating joined-up implementation of programmes across government departments, sectors, and communities; sponsoring/employing innovative approaches; developing partnerships and relationships with stakeholders; and focusing on outcomes.

The Social Inclusion Initiative works across government and nongovernment sectors using a model that reflects the Government of South Australia's and the public's concern for a particular issue, or for a particular group whose circumstances currently or potentially exclude them from living healthy and fulfilled lives.

The Social Inclusion Board consists of the Chair and 9-10 Board members who are generally well-known community members or high-level experts in their field. The Chair and Social Inclusion Board are independent of government but strongly embedded in a process that is supported by, and closely linked to, government. There is a close working relationship between the Chair of the Social Inclusion Board and the Premier (head of state), and also between the Chair and the Executive Director of the Social Inclusion Unit (SIU). The Social Inclusion Board has stated terms of reference and is responsible for:

providing leadership to the work of the SIU to ensure that government receives expert policy advice on identified social policy issues and a coordinated and integrated approach to developing, implementing, and reviewing the directions of government to reduce social exclusion;

providing recommendations, information, and advice to the Premier and Cabinet, including advice on potential priorities for government funding consideration;

providing guidance, support, and advice to the SIU in addressing issues identified by the Premier and Cabinet;

developing strategies to deal with the causes of social exclusion and to provide leadership to influence and shape national social justice policy;

assisting the SIU to develop and maintain appropriate engagement mechanisms across government, the community, and stakeholders;

providing advice and information to the SIU to assist in research activities;

reporting on a quarterly basis to the Premier.

Source: Newman et al., 2007

BOX 14.6: STATUTORY PARTICIPATORY PLANNING IN THE UNITED KINGDOM

In London, the Greater London Authority Act 1999 instituted the Greater London Authority (GLA). This Act confers the responsibility for developing and delivering an overarching spatial development plan (the London Plan), plus associated strategies for air quality, biodiversity, ambient noise, municipal waste, culture, transport, and economic development. The Act also includes a statutory responsibility for the Mayor and the GLA to promote health, address equity, and ensure sustainable development.

The GLA provides a good platform for partnership working at a city level as it brings together the

Mayor, a separately elected Assembly, the London Development Agency, the London Fire and Emergency Planning Authority, the Metropolitan Police, and Transport for London. London also has a specific partnership body to improve health and reduce inequities in the form of the London Health Commission, which brings together all the statutory, public, private, academic, and voluntary agencies that can influence the social determinants of health.

Source: LHC, 2000

Financial support for fair participation

An essential element of a supportive and inclusive governance structure for health equity is financial support for communities and local governments to partner in building healthier and more equitable societies. The example from Porto Alegre in Brazil illustrates the significant effect on population health of a participatory budgeting programme, instituted by the municipal government in an attempt to utilize citizens' unique knowledge and perspective in solving the many problems facing the city (Box 14.7).

Similarly, the example from Venezuela (Box 14.8) illustrates a model of participatory governance underpinned by principles of participatory budgeting and legislative support for community participation.

Bottom-up approaches to health equity

While the empowerment of social groups through their representation in policy-related agenda-setting and decision-making is critical, so too is empowerment for action through bottom-up, grassroots approaches (Sibal, 2006). The struggles against the injustices encountered by the most disadvantaged in society, and the process of organizing these people, builds local people's leadership. It is empowering. It gives people a greater sense of control over their lives and future. This empowerment permeates all aspects of their lives. If they have a sick child, for example, they seek care rather than leaving it to 'fate'. Better still, they take early action such as immunizing the child, so that sickness is prevented in the first place.

Evidence from interventions for youth empowerment, HIV/AIDS prevention, and women's empowerment suggest that, "the most effective empowerment strategies are those that build on and reinforce authentic participation ensuring autonomy in decision-making, sense of community and local bonding, and psychological empowerment of the community members themselves" (WGEKN, 2007).

The Commission recommends that:

14.4. Empowerment for action on health equity through bottom-up, grassroots approaches requires support for civil society to develop, strengthen, and implement health equity-oriented initiatives.

The enactment of legal changes to recognize and support community empowerment initiatives will ensure the comprehensive inclusion of disadvantaged groups in action at global, national, and local levels concerned with improving health and health equity. The support of women's efforts to coordinate through resourcing – by donors and governments – of women's organizations is also important for gender equity (Box 14.9).

As the SEWA example illustrates, building their own organizations has been one of the ways that women have chosen to promote solidarity, offer support, and collectively work for change. These organizations are of various sizes, from small village-based or neighbourhood groups to large movements. It is imperative to support and encourage such

---

BOX 14.7: PARTICIPATORY BUDGETING IN PORTO ALEGRE, BRAZIL

Porto Alegre instituted participatory budgeting and allowed all citizens to vote on the municipal budget. The city provided training sessions so that community members could understand and engage in budgetary discussions. This training was invaluable for members of society who directly represented larger communities in the Regional Plenary Assemblies. Government officials and community representatives jointly ran these assemblies, which met twice annually. Cooperation between officials and civilians led to a proposed budget, which would then be put to a vote in the communities at large. While city officials provided guidance and helped settle difficult budgetary issues, the proposed and finalized budgets were created by the citizens of Porto Alegre.

The participatory budgeting programme spurred greater civil society activity, community input, and tangible improvements in city life. Of the city's total population, 8% (100 000 people) directly participated in budgeting; 57.2% of citizens assert that the population always or almost always "really decides" upon public works. The new budget allowed the housing department to offer assistance to 28 862 families, against 1714 for the comparable period of 1986-1988. The rubbish collection system reaches virtually all households and has included a separate collection of recyclables since 1990. Virtually all the people of Porto Alegre have water piped to their homes and most have good-quality sanitation and drainage. Participatory budgeting devolved power from the city council and provided citizens with tools for change. Porto Alegre now has the highest standard of living and the highest LEB of any Brazilian metropolitan centre.

Source: KNUS, 2007

POLITICAL EMPOWERMENT : ACTION AREA 14.2

Enable civil society to organize and act in a manner that promotes and realizes the political and social rights affecting health equity

organizations and movements in a way that preserves and protects their autonomy and promotes their long-term sustainability, including self-reliance. This could be done in a number of ways:

- providing resources as seed money, revolving funds, and matching funds to women's organizations; combinations of these could be used;

- providing platforms for exposure and networking;

- providing capacity-building support through training courses, funds for leadership, and management development.

An example from Japan shows how a partnership of people organizing themselves to solve their own public health issues and other concerns with government and nongovernmental organizations can work well, providing the community leads the agenda and is adequately resourced (Box 14.10). This

BOX 14.8: BARRIO ADENTRO – THE RIGHT TO HEALTH AND SOCIAL INCLUSION IN BOLIVARIAN REPUBLIC OF VENEZUELA

The Venezuelan Constitution firmly establishes the right to health and the citizen's duty to take an active part in the management of health. The draft bill of the new General Health Law declares that participation and social control in health is a constitutional right of all citizens and that they have the right to make decisions, intervene, and exercise direct control, with autonomy and independence, in all matters related to the formulation, planning, and regulation of health-sector policies, plans, and projects, as well as the evaluation, control, and monitoring of health-sector management and financing.

Mission Barrio Adentro is a key element in the proposal for social inclusion embodied in the 1999 Constitution of the Bolivarian Republic of Venezuela. The Mission, established in 2003, has become a national public health programme committed to wiping out the national health-care deficit. Mission Barrio Adentro promotes specific actions for the intervention and participation of community leaders in the design and control of health management. Since January 2004, the main purpose of Mission Barrio Adentro has been to provide the population with complete primary health-care coverage.

In the administrative structure of Mission Barrio Adentro, individuals are responsible for coordinating brigades of physicians by parishes, municipalities, and regions in collaboration with neighbourhood health committees, which participate integrally in the drafting of health policies, plans, projects, and programmes, as well as execution and evaluation of the Mission's management. In 2006, there were 150 registered committees associated with Barrio Adentro and the other Social Missions. The mandate of the health committees is to identify the priority health problems in the community, prioritize these, and decide on the main actions that the community should take to address them. Operation of the health committees is regulated by the Community Councils Law of 6 April 2006, which mandates that the health committees work in concert with other community organizations affiliated with the community council. Among other responsibilities, the community councils administer the budgets allocated to each community, including the budgets of the health committees.

Source: PAHO, 2006

BOX 14.9: LEGAL SUPPORT FOR COMMUNITY EMPOWERMENT – SEWA, INDIA

Like other poor self-employed women, the vegetable sellers of Ahmedabad, India, live in poor conditions. SEWA, a union of almost 1 million workers, is an example of collective action by these women to challenge and change these conditions.

Frequently harassed by local authorities, the vegetable sellers campaigned with SEWA to strengthen their status through formal recognition in the form of licences and identity cards and representation on the urban boards that govern market activities and urban development. That campaign, started within Gujarat, subsequently went all the way to the Supreme Court of India.

To strengthen control over their livelihoods, all SEWA members linked together to set up their own wholesale

vegetable shop, cutting out exploitative middlemen. SEWA also organizes childcare, running centres for infants and young children, and campaigns at the state and national level for childcare as an entitlement for all women workers. Further, SEWA members are improving their living conditions through slum upgrading programmes to provide basic infrastructure. This happens in partnerships with government, civil society organizations, and the corporate sector. In order to solve the problem of access to credit, the SEWA Bank provides small loans and banking facilities to poor self-employed women. The bank is owned by its members, and its policies are formulated by an elected board of women workers.

Source: SEWA Bank, nd

requires the development of mechanisms to bring together public, private, and civil society sectors, and the definition of roles and mechanisms for international and national actors to support popular action.

While it is critical that community members share control over processes that affect their lives, without political commitment and leadership and allocation of resources such initiatives can be short lived, as the Bangladesh example illustrates (Box 14.11).

There are notable examples where an explicit rights agenda has been successfully applied to global governance. In the case of TRIPS and AIDS medicines, civil society-driven action from South Africa, with worldwide take-up, created a 'norm cascade' leading to immediate and structural changes not only in the market accessibility of life-saving drugs, but in the global understanding of questions of intellectual property and the application of appropriate norms for global health equity (Box 14.12).

BOX 14.10: JAPAN – THE POWER OF THE COMMUNITY

The population of the Kamagasaki district is estimated at 30 000 people, of which approximately 20 000 people are day labourers and the rest are general households or self-employed workers. The most significant problem for the workers is that they are not assured prerequisites of health such as food, housing, employment, and social inclusion.

A movement of regeneration began in 1999, with nongovernmental organization support groups appearing alongside longstanding church initiatives and increased activity by labour unions. At the same time, the Kamagasaki Community Regeneration Forum – the first grassroots group for community development in the area – was established. This group began to create and build community bonds and encourage new businesses. The Forum has been working to rebuild the Kamagasaki district, which was once seen as a socially excluded community, through, "rediscovering local assets and (human) resources, empowering the assets and resources by networking them, and developing the capability of living".

The Forum has achieved a number of milestones. Since it held the first political debate and voter drive in Kamagasaki in 2003, the district registered the only increase in electoral participation in Nishinari Ward and Osaka as a whole in the general election of that year. Politicians have begun to canvass for support in the district. The increased registration was partly the result of private initiatives to increase provision of permanent accommodation for workers in former lodges. In 2000, the Forum created the opportunity for labourers/homeless people to obtain public livelihood assistance after some owners of cheap lodging hotels converted their hotels into 'Supportive Houses' – small-room apartments adjusted to people in special need and providing support services to help residents maintain their self-reliance. This arrangement made it possible for day labourers and homeless people to apply for public assistance. The 10-year national homeless law, which clarifies the responsibility of city and state authorities for the problem, should also prove a positive development.

Source: KNUS, 2007

BOX 14.11: COMMUNITY PARTICIPATION IN BANGLADESH

Government initiatives have sought to promote community participation in the delivery of essential services. For example, the government's 5-year (1998-2003) Health and Population Sector Programme included a component to motivate service users to monitor the performance of public providers at the local level. Selected nongovernmental organizations formed local stakeholder committees and provided training/capacity building in participation and deliberation for service users. Women and men, elite and landless people were transparently recruited to participate in committees. There was strong and varied participation and diverse membership; awareness about public health facilities was raised; community demand for public health was increased and doctors were pressured to be present during working hours and not to levy illegal fees. However, more negatively, community awareness about the committees and the opportunities they offered to

provide feedback to the health-care system was low. The committees lacked the authority and political capability to enact decisions and, with the implementation of the new health-sector programme in 2003, which did not continue these stakeholder committees, most have disbanded. The 5-year plan for 1998-2003 also experimented with community ownership of health facilities. The community was expected to donate the land, and construction costs were shared between the local community and central government. However, membership of the community groups was biased towards the local elite and relatives of the chairperson. Leadership was poor and, in the absence of defined structures, unequal relationships between rich and poor and men and women were reproduced, and little value was attached to the voices of those with low status.

Source: SEKN, 2007

Social movements

For changes in power, there also needs to be space for challenge and contest by social movements. Although social movements and community organizations tend to mobilize around concrete issues in local everyday life, their actions are clearly rooted in and address structures and processes that extend far beyond this local realm. These movements tend to take one of three forms: political societies (e.g. political parties, pressure groups, lobbying groups), which seek influence within the political arena; civil societies such as trade unions, peasant organizations, and religious movements; and civil-political societies that combine or link the activities of political and civil societies (e.g. labour movements, women's movement, anti-apartheid movement).

The People's Health Movement (**http://phmovement. org/**) is a large global civil society network of health activists supportive of the WHO policy of Health for All and organized to combat the economic and political causes of deepening inequities in health worldwide and to call for the return to the principles of Alma Ata. Support for People's Health Movement and other similar civil society organizations such as the global antipoverty movement and labour movement will help to ensure that action on the social determinants of health is developed, implemented, and evaluated.

A society concerned with better and more equitably distributed health is one that challenges unequal power relations through participation, ensuring all voices are heard and respected in decision-making that affects health equity. Being more inclusive requires social policies, laws, institutions, and programmes to protect human rights. It requires inclusion of individuals and groups to represent strongly and effectively their needs and interests in the development of policy. And it requires active civil society and social movements. It is clear that community or civil society action on health inequities cannot be separated from the responsibility of the state to guarantee a comprehensive set of rights and ensure the fair distribution of essential material and social goods among population groups (Solar & Irwin, 2007). Top-down and bottom-up approaches are equally vital.

BOX 14.12: TAKING ACTION ON RIGHTS AND TRADE: THE CASE OF AIDS MEDICINES

"The human right to health requires the provision of essential medicines as a core duty that cannot be traded for private property interests or domestic economic growth. This right may provide a means of achieving a more public health-oriented formulation, implementation and interpretation of trade rules by domestic courts, governments and the WTO alike. The growing power of this right is similarly reflected in an emerging jurisprudence where medicines have been successfully claimed under human rights protections".

A decade ago, the high cost of AIDS medicines led WHO and UNAIDS to advise that treatment was not a wise use of resources in poorer countries. Prevention of HIV/AIDS was preferred over treatment. There was no international funding for developing countries to purchase drugs and companies gave extremely limited price concessions. A dramatic battle for AIDS medicines ensued that peaked in 2001 in the Pharmaceutical Manufacturer's Association case in South Africa. Between 1997 and 2001, the United States and 40 pharmaceutical companies used trade pressures and litigation to prevent the South African government from passing legislation to access affordable medicines. Industry claimed that the legislation (and the parallel importing it authorized) breached TRIPS and South Africa's Constitution and threatened industry's incentive to innovate new medicines. The pharmaceutical companies went to

court in South Africa. An extraordinary level of public action accompanied the case, attracting global censure against the corporations. In April 2001, the pharmaceutical companies withdrew their case.

A norm cascade followed, with a sharp upsurge at the UN in international statements on treatment as a human right and articulations of state obligations on antiretroviral therapy. The same year saw the WTO issue its Declaration on TRIPS and Public Health. These rhetorical commitments were matched by considerable policy and price shifts. Antiretroviral therapy prices in many low-income countries dropped from US$ 15 000 to US$ 148-549 per annum. New global funding mechanisms were created, such as the Global Fund to Fight HIV/AIDS, Tuberculosis and Malaria, the United States PEPFAR and the World Bank Multi-Country HIV/AIDS Program for Africa. In 2002, WHO adopted the activist goal of placing 3 million people on antiretroviral therapy and, in late 2005, shifted upwards to the goal of achieving universal access to treatment by 2010, a goal similarly adopted by the UN General Assembly and by the G8. In 5 years, access to antiretroviral therapy in sub-Saharan Africa has increased from under 1% to current levels of 28%.

Source: Forman, 2007

CHAPTER 15
Good global governance

"We are indeed witnessing, and living in, a new and very important stage in global history."

Kemal Dervis (2005)

GOOD GLOBAL GOVERNANCE AND HEALTH EQUITY

Dramatic differences today in the health and life chances of peoples around the world reflect a deep, longstanding, and growing imbalance in the power and prosperity of nations. In 2000, the average member of the world's top wealth decile owned nearly 3000 times the mean wealth of the bottom decile (Davies et al., 2006). From the poorest to the richest nations, the difference in LEB is over 40 years - four decades of life denied. The costs of information and communication technologies – vital aspects of globalization's growth – are 170 times higher in some low-income countries than in high-income ones. While the risks associated with globalization – related to health, trade and finance, or human security – are increasingly transnational and disproportionately experienced in low- and middle-income countries, the benefits remain profoundly unequally distributed in favour of high-income regions. It is imperative that the international community recommits to a multilateral system in which all countries, rich and poor, engage with an equitable voice. It is only through such a system of global governance, placing fairness in health at the heart of the development agenda and genuine equity of influence in the centre of its decision-making, that coherent attention to global health equity, realizing the rights of all people to the conditions that create health, is possible.

Opportunities and threats

Globalization has brought new opportunities for equitable health. But it has also brought threats and risks. "Global markets have grown rapidly without the parallel development of economic and social institutions necessary for their smooth equitable functioning. At the same time, there is concern about the unfairness of key global rules ... and their asymmetric effects on rich and poor countries" (World Commission on the Social Dimension of Globalization, 2004). The current picture of globalization includes 'winners' and 'losers' among the world's countries. In order to address the risks of inequity in globalization, and to manage the potential of globalization for better and fairer health, there is the need now for new forms of global governance. Globalization offers unprecedented opportunities for the realization of health equity through effective governance. But what it offers as opportunity, improperly managed it equally offers as threat (Box 15.1).

Aspects of globalization, such as trade liberalization and market integration between countries, have brought major shifts in countries' national productive and distributive policies. 'Structural adjustment' – a core global programmatic and policy influence from the 1970s onwards – framed the emergence of a dominant (sometimes referred to as 'neoliberal') orthodoxy in global institutions. Designed to reduce inflation in indebted developing countries, decrease public spending, and promote growth – all strongly oriented towards supporting debt repayment – adjustment policies promoted trade liberalization, privatization, and a reduced role for the public sector. This had a severe adverse impact on key social determinants of

---

BOX 15.1: GLOBALIZATION – POLICY INFLUENCES THAT CAN ENDANGER HEALTH EQUITY

The policy influences that can endanger health equity include:

technological advances, leading to rapidly decreasing costs for transportation, communication, and information processing that, alongside institutional changes such as trade liberalization, facilitate the global reorganization of productive activity in ways that can enhance inequity;

an increase in the value of foreign direct investment relative to trade, reflecting the growing interchangeability of direct investment and trade in the production and provision of goods and services;

an increase in the importance of 'off-shored' or 'out-sourced' production, often undertaken by independent

contractors rather than subsidiaries or affiliates of a parent firm, frequently giving rise to poorer working conditions;

a drastic increase in flows of hypermobile portfolio investment ('hot money'), increasing the risk of currency crises;

increased competition for investment and a consequent shift of power from local and national authorities to decision-makers in international financial markets, creating policy influence that may harm health equity.

Source: GKN, 2007

health – including health care and education – across most participating countries. Many countries, without doubt, stood to benefit from reducing runaway inflation and improving fiscal management. But it is not clear that the harsh degree and policy straitjacket that structural adjustment imposed produced the anticipated benefits, much less whether the health and social costs were warranted (Jolly, 1991).

Persisting poverty

While debate may continue about the relationship between trade liberalization and growth, it is clear that increasing trade on improved terms is desirable – assuming it is within the ecological imperatives of sustainable resource use. However, the relationships among globalization, growth, and poverty reduction are deeply problematic. Overall, the number of people living at or under US$ 1/day dropped by 414 million between 1981 and 2003. However, much of this was caused by sharp reductions in poverty in China (Chen & Ravallion, 2004). Globalization's rising tide has not lifted all boats, or lifted them very far – nor has it kept pace with population growth. In sub-Saharan Africa during this period, the number of people living on US$ 1/day or less doubled, and the number living on US$ 2/day or less almost doubled.

Global health inequity

Growth in global wealth and knowledge has not translated, either, into increased global health equity. Rather than convergence, with poorer countries catching up to the OECD, there has instead been a dispersion of life expectancies across countries and regions, with some improving, others stagnating, and others getting worse (Fig. 15.1).

While LEB continues to converge and plateau across high-income countries, and is rapidly converging towards high-income country levels in middle-income countries, in many countries of sub-Saharan Africa and in the transition

economies, LEB in 2006 was lower than in 1990. Much of this is due to dramatic reversals in the transition economies of the former Soviet Republics and the HIV/AIDS pandemic (although very recently, since 2005, estimated mortality due to HIV/AIDS has been declining in sub-Saharan Africa). However, regression analysis undertaken by the GKN suggests that other factors, such as those driven by dominant market-oriented economic policies, have contributed to the dispersion of regional performances in LEB. While OECD countries saw a net increase of around 3 years in LEB, sub-Saharan Africa saw a loss of around 6 years.

As well as increasing inequity in health between countries, the recent phase of globalization has exacerbated health inequity within them, too. Trade liberalization and market integration, contributing to the emergence of a global labour market, have increased the requirement for labour flexibility, resulting in increasing job insecurity (see Chapter 7: *Fair Employment and Decent Work*). Increasing demand for labour, while providing new opportunities for women's participation in the labour force, has also maintained inequitable gender differentials in conditions of employment, contributing at the same time to a double burden of labour for women who remain responsible for the family and household (see Chapter 13: *Gender Equity*). Gains in income through expanded markets and increased productivity have not flowed equally through societies. The World Bank concedes that, "labour market changes will lead to increased economic inequality in countries accounting for 86% of the developing world's population over the period until 2030, with the 'unskilled poor' being left further behind" (World Bank, 2007).

The effects of globalization on health inequity within countries can also be detected in trade agreements that restrict the use of tariffs, reducing income to the public purse in poor countries with weak direct tax capacities, thus reducing public sector spending in key social determinants such as health and

Figure 15.1 Life expectancy at birth (in years) by region, 1950–2005.

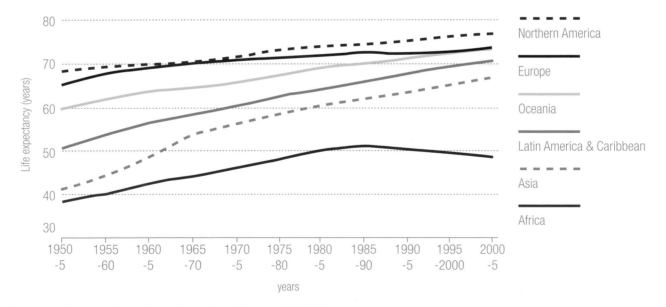

Reprinted, with permission of the publisher, from Dorling et al. (2006).

Globalization points to the interdependence of nation-states and peoples, and the proportional benefit, not to say necessity, of cooperation in areas of common interest. A concept of global public goods has emerged – the shared management of conditions and resources vital to all people, and which lie outside the capacity of individual countries to control. So far it has encompassed issues such as climate change and environmental controls, peace and security, disease control, and knowledge. Beyond these – and arguably underpinning them all – is the concept of social justice, of equity and hence of health equity, not simply within countries, but between them too.

ACTIONS FOR GOOD GLOBAL GOVERNANCE

The Commission recommends that:

15.1 By 2010, the Economic and Social Council, supported by WHO, should prepare for consideration by the UN the adoption of health equity as a core global development goal, with appropriate indicators to monitor progress both within and between countries (see Rec 10.1; 10.3; 16.3).

Health equity – a global goal

Reducing health inequities between and within countries requires policy coherence at the global level, just as it does at the national level (see Chapter 10: *Health in All Policies, Systems, and Programmes*). By adopting health equity between, as well as within, countries as a core measure of development, the Economic and Social Council can use its coordinating function to improve coherence of actions on the social determinants of health across UN agencies (Box 15.7).

Multilateral coherence

The 61st session of the UN General Assembly, "Strengthening the Economic and Social Council" (14 November 2006), presented an opportunity for the Economic and Social Council to lead on globally coherent action for development and health equity. First, the Council can direct its standing Commission for Social Development to adopt health equity as a theme for the 2009-2010 biennial review, focusing on the development of a multilateral framework for action on the social determinants of health. Second, it can ensure a standard report-back on progress in health equity to the Annual Ministerial Review process. Third, although it appears primarily focused on

---

BOX 15.6: TIME TO RETHINK GLOBAL ECONOMIC INFLUENCE

Representation in decision-making on the Executive Boards of the IMF and the World Bank is based on the economic contribution (and thus, to a large extent, the wealth) of Member States. Developed countries, accounting for 20% of IMF members and 15% of the world's population, have a substantial majority of votes in both institutions. Developing countries, by contrast, are seriously underrepresented. The weighted voting system gives the United States alone, and any four other G7 members acting together without the United States, the ability to block policy decisions in the 18 areas requiring a qualified majority of 85% of the votes. The Chief Executive Officers of the World Bank and the IMF are effectively appointed by the United States and the EU, respectively, and Executive Board discussions and decision-making remain secretive. Despite efforts to engage with a broader range of stakeholders, improve public information systems, and provide fuller reporting of activities, the transparency of key decision-making processes remains inadequate.

Source: GKN, 2007

GOOD GLOBAL GOVERNANCE : ACTION AREA 15.1

Make health equity a global development goal, and adopt a social determinants of health framework to strengthen multilateral action on development.

BOX 15.7: THE ECONOMIC AND SOCIAL COUNCIL

The Economic and Social Council is the principal organ to coordinate the economic, social, and related work of the 14 UN specialized agencies, functional commissions, and five regional commissions. It also receives reports from 11 UN funds and programmes. The Council serves as the central forum for discussing international economic and social issues, and for formulating policy recommendations addressed to Member States and the UN system. It is responsible for: promoting higher standards of living, full employment, and economic and social progress; identifying solutions to international economic, social, and health problems; facilitating international cultural and educational cooperation; and encouraging universal respect for human rights and fundamental freedoms.

Source: ECOSOC, nd

improving multilateral response to humanitarian crises, the Development Cooperation Forum, established to meet every other year from 2008, can usefully serve to raise key emerging areas of global health concern, including issues around equity.

The Millennium Development Goals

The MDGs are a profound statement of the concerted will of the global community to act decisively. They offer a strong platform on which the Commission sees its agenda building. The MDGs reflect a growing consensus on the need for global actors to work together for coherent social and economic development. Unfortunately, the MDGs also reflect an inattention to health equity within countries. There is a clear opportunity here, both for leadership from WHO and coherent collaboration for equity across the multilateral system, to look again at the MDGs and advance equity as a core marker of achievement (Box 15.8).

Multilateral agencies are already playing vital roles in the development of global standards for policy and action across a range of social determinants of health, through global, international, and regional agreements and governance mechanisms, including ILO's Global Campaign on Social Security and Coverage for All and the Decent Work agenda, the UNDP Poverty Reduction Programmes, the Economic Commission of Latin America and the Caribbean Social Cohesion Contract, the PAHO Health Exclusion Initiative, the UN Commission on Human Rights Special Rapporteur

on the Right to Health, and the EU Annual Joint Reports on Social Protection and Social Inclusion (SEKN, 2007). But there are greater opportunities still to be gained from closer policy and programme planning between relevant multilateral agencies, strengthening their own collective governance.

The Commission urges the relevant global agencies to take a further step. Improving global governance for health equity depends on multilateral agencies working more coherently to a common set of overarching objectives, underpinned by a common vision of issues to be addressed and shared indicators by which to measure the impact of their actions. For this, the agencies would benefit from a more systematic, shared set of data (combining the data sets they already use, but adding measures of health equity) (see Chapter 16: *Social Determinants of Health: Monitoring, Research, and Training*).

The Commission proposes that the multilateral community revise existing global development frameworks to incorporate health equity and social determinants of health indicators more coherently. Such a revised framework would require global credibility and buy-in from Member States, much in the way the Human Development Index and the Common Country Assessment have achieved, or are achieving, common recognition and use. The Commission's proposed framework would incorporate indicators of progress on the social determinants of health and on health equity. Jointly developed and rigorously tested, this framework of social development

BOX 15.8: HEALTH EQUITY AT THE HEART OF GLOBAL HEALTH GOVERNANCE – THE MILLENNIUM DEVELOPMENT GOALS

The MDGs are a set of eight poverty alleviation goals set out by the UN at the Millennium Summit in 2000. All the MDGs relate to action on social determinants of health. The global consensus represented by the MDGs is a new point of departure for the development community. The UN Millennium Project and scores of other decision-makers, activists, bilateral aid organizations, and communities are already deeply immersed in efforts to achieve the MDGs. Yet this

global effort could still benefit from explicit and systematic commitment to equity at the country level. Well-defined, equity-sensitive targets – linked to relevant data sources – are necessary to ensure that poor, marginalized, and vulnerable groups are given opportunities for improved health and access to health services.

Source: Wirth et al., 2006

BOX 15.9: SOCIAL EXCLUSION – THE EUROPEAN UNION 'OPEN METHOD OF COORDINATION'

At the 2000 Lisbon European Council, heads of state formulated a strategy to combat social exclusion in the EU and have an impact on the eradication of poverty by 2010. The strategy underlined the need to improve the understanding of social exclusion and to organize policy cooperation across member states based on an 'Open Method of Coordination'. All member states were to adopt common objectives in the fight against poverty and social exclusion and produce biannual National Action Plans on Social Inclusion,

providing data on poverty and social exclusion in their countries. Common social inclusion indicators – the Laeken Indicators – would be used. New member states agreed to produce mandatory Joint Inclusion Memoranda outlining their country situation and political priorities on poverty and social exclusion prior to full membership.

Source: SEKN, 2007

and health equity could be supported by the planned global health observatory (WHO) and would constitute the basis for regular, periodic global report-back to the Economic and Social Council. This is covered in more detail in Chapter 16 (*Social Determinants of Health: Monitoring, Research, and Training*). A similar adaptable framework could also be used by participating countries to formulate their own national social determinants of health plans, indicators, and reporting, strengthening health and health equity objectives – and thus coherence of aid allocations – within the wider Poverty Reduction Strategy Process (see Chapter 11: *Fair Financing*).

This will be a progressive process. By agreeing fundamental goals – including health equity as central among these – global agencies can build towards shared indicators. The regional example of social exclusion indicators agreed progressively, under opt-in mechanisms, among EU Member States provides a possible model of how a cross-agency focus on health equity as a core developmental objective and shared marker of progress might be built (Box 15.9).

The Commission recommends that:

15.2 By 2010, the Economic and Social Council, supported by WHO, prepare for consideration by the UN the establishment of thematic social determinants of health working groups – initially on early child development, gender equity, employment and working conditions, health-care systems, and participatory governance – including all relevant multilateral agencies and civil society stakeholders, reporting back regularly (see Rec 5.1; 6.2; 9.1; 13.2).

By adopting social determinants of health as targets for collaborative action, relevant multilateral agencies could form working groups, reporting regularly on progress in their determinant field, under an umbrella framework of social determinants of health and health equity indicators (as above). There are examples of this kind of cross-agency working group – such as the UN system Standing Committee on Nutrition (see Chapters 5, 6, and 7: *Equity from the Start; Healthy Places*

BOX 15.10: THE WORLD HEALTH ORGANIZATION AND UN-HABITAT

UN-HABITAT and WHO have identified three relevant interventions to jumpstart a response from the health sector for healthy urbanization: an urban health equity assessment and response tool (Urban HEART) that enables ministries of health to track areas of rapid urbanization and monitor health inequity; a global report on urban health; and a joint UN-HABITAT/WHO global meeting on healthy urbanization to coincide

with the biannual World Urban Forum of UN-HABITAT, possibly in 2010. There are also tools for reducing health inequity in urban settings, that is, a 'social technology grid' and a training module (the Healthy Urbanization Learning Circle) to link public health and community efforts at the municipal level.

KNUS, 2007

BOX 15.11: THE PAN-AMERICAN HEALTH ORGANIZATION AND INTERNATIONAL LABOUR ORGANIZATION

ILO and PAHO are jointly developing a strategy for the, "extension of social protection in health". The strategy to extend social protection to heath is defined by PAHO and ILO as, "public interventions oriented to guarantee all citizens access to effective health care and to reduce the negative impact, both economic and social, of (i) adverse personal circumstances (including for example, disease and unemployment) (ii) collective risks such as natural disasters and over population and/or (iii) the specific risks experienced by vulnerable social groups." Unlike policies directed at

the social management of risk, PAHO conceptualizes social protection in health as a human right not only an economic risk. As proposed by PAHO, the right to social protection in health has three components: (i) guaranteed access to health services with the elimination of economic, social, geographic, and cultural barriers; (ii) guaranteed financial security of households; and (iii) guaranteed quality of health care that is respectful of human dignity.

Source: SEKN, 2007

Healthy People; Fair Employment and Decent Work). The working groups could also build on existing interagency collaborations. WHO, for example, works with a range of major UN agencies (such as UNICEF, UN-HABITAT, ILO, and the World Bank) (Boxes 15.10 and 15.11).

Such working groups could further strengthen the coherence of programmes and delivery at country level by complementing in-country frameworks for unified action (Box 15.12).

Champions for global health governance

If social, economic, and political justice are central concerns of the growing apparatus of global governance, health equity must be a core marker of the success of such governance. Installing health equity as a shared concern and a key indicator of action across the community of multilateral actors requires global leadership – champions to maintain global focus on progress towards health equity.

A Special Envoy for Global Health Equity

The appointment of Special Envoys can be interpreted as the tipping point at which an issue becomes fully acknowledged as global, urgent, and possible to address. A central objective in the appointment of a Special Envoy is to drive all relevant actors towards more concerted multilateral action (Box 15.13).

A Permanent Special Rapporteur on the Right to Health

There are clear links between a 'rights' approach to health and the social determinants of health approach to health equity. The Universal Declaration of Human Rights points to the interdependence of civil, cultural, economic, political, and social rights – dimensions of social exclusion highlighted in the social determinants of health framework. The right to health, as set out by the existing Special Rapporteur, Professor Paul Hunt, presents a compelling case for action on the social determinants of health (Box 15.14).

BOX 15.12: THE FRAMEWORK OF UNIFIED UN ACTION

From the global to the national level, the Framework of Unified UN Action seeks to bring together the work of disparate UN agencies at country level to reduce duplication and increase the synergies across agencies and donors. Pilot work in eight countries is currently testing a model in which

UN agencies operate through a single 'resident coordinator' providing support for the development and implementation of comprehensive National Development Plans aimed at achieving the MDGs.

Source: SEKN, 2007

BOX 15.13: THE SPECIAL ENVOY ON HIV/AIDS IN AFRICA

Canada's former ambassador to the UN, Stephen Lewis, was named Secretary-General Kofi Annan's Special Envoy for HIV/AIDS in Africa in 2001. In this role, Lewis was described as, "one of our most powerful weapons in the war against the epidemic". The Special Envoy's role has been one of advocacy, raising issues of attention to gender as a key driver in the pandemic, the condition of orphans, access to treatment, and the quantity of aid being directed towards action on HIV/AIDS.

"The world has been terribly delinquent," in responding to the AIDS crisis in Africa, he said, as were some African leaders. Even in the late 1990s, "a lot of them simply weren't engaged ... and their countries were clearly in terrible trouble. To be fair to

them, the world wasn't engaged either.... Everybody was ... frozen in time, while all around us this pandemic was wreaking havoc."

Underlying it all, Mr. Lewis asserted, has been an exponential increase in understanding of the scope and nature of the AIDS crisis in Africa – most critically its links to gender oppression. "Finally the world seems to understand that [in Africa] this is a gender-based pandemic. Unless there is recognition that women are most vulnerable ... and you do something about social and cultural equality for women, you're never going to defeat this pandemic."

Reproduced, with permission of the publisher, from UN (2001).

The Commission recommends that:

15.3 WHO institutionalizes a social determinants of health approach across all working sectors, from headquarters to country level (see Rec 10.5; 16.8).

There is evidence of fragmentation and competition among major global actors with significant roles in the social determinants of health (from the World Bank, WTO, and major UN agencies, through G8, to other groupings of countries) and national social development initiatives (Deacon et al., 2003). International funding for global health has also diversified in recent decades, with corresponding changes in processes and structures of accountability. The budget of the Gates Foundation, for example, has at times exceeded WHO's core budget (Kickbusch & Payne, 2004). The Commission strongly supports WHO in renewing its leadership in global health and its stewardship role across the multilateral system. Central to this renewed leadership, however, is the need for WHO itself to achieve institutional renewal through installing a social determinants of health approach across its programmes and departments.

This work is already under way. One of the Commission's Knowledge Networks, working on priority public health conditions (PPHCKN), was convened from within WHO itself, reaching across all major offices and health condition programmes as well as involving academia and field researchers, projects, and nongovernmental organizations working in countries. The PPHCKN collaboration has adopted and utilized an analytical framework, applying it to many of the main public health conditions that the WHO works on starting at the conventional level of health outcomes, but working upstream to analyse deeper, more structural causal factors and

thus identifying a wider field of entry points at each of the five levels of the framework (Fig. 15.2). WHO has also appointed regional focal points for action on the social determinants of health, to work closely with Member States, supporting the Commission's country work stream and stimulating policy and action for health equity.

Condition-specific programmes have significant appeal and thus the ability to raise funding. About two thirds of WHO's budget is devoted to these programmes; on a global scale, programmes focusing on a single or a very limited number of diseases are flourishing. The PPHCKN is developing action points for programmes to elaborate a social determinants of health approach. The work started by the PPHCKN has already shown potential to engender support for change across WHO (Box 15.15).

Institutionalization of social determinants of health action across WHO will require significant investments in organizational capacity building (see Chapter 16: *Social Determinants of Health: Monitoring, Research, and Training*).

Globalization is a fact. It has the potential to generate considerable benefits, including great advances in global health. As things stand, however, that benefit is not in evidence. Instead, what we see is growing inequity both across and within regions and countries. Increased integration between peoples in the economic domain has not been balanced by commensurate attention to the wider imperatives of fair social development. For this to happen, the architecture of global governance needs to be reformed and extended – opening its forums of policy-making more equitably to all, and setting at the heart of its concerns the equitable health and well-being of all.

BOX 15.14: THE RIGHT TO HEALTH – THE RIGHT TO THE CONDITIONS FOR HEALTH

"The right to health includes the right to health care – but it goes beyond health care to encompass adequate sanitation, healthy conditions at work, and access to health-related information, including on sexual and reproductive health. It includes freedoms, such as the right to be free from forced sterilization and discrimination, as well as entitlements, such as the right to a system of health protection. The right to health has numerous elements, sort of sub-rights, including maternal, child and reproductive health. Like other human rights, the right to health has a particular preoccupation with the disadvantaged, vulnerable, and those living in poverty. Although subject to progressive realization, the right imposes some obligations of immediate effect, such as the obligations of equal treatment and non-discrimination. It demands indicators and benchmarks to monitor the progressive realization of the right."

Reprinted, with permission of the author, from Hunt (2003).

GOOD GLOBAL GOVERNANCE : ACTION AREA 15.2

Strengthen WHO leadership in global action on the social determinants of health, institutionalizing social determinants of health as a guiding principle across WHO departments and country programmes.

Figure 15.2 Priority public health conditions – causal pathways for health action.

Flow of Analysis

We are attempting to establish the causal pathways that lead to observed differential health outcomes, i.e. to explain – therefore the analysis would naturally start with the outcome [1]. As the consequences could feed back to both social position and vulnerability, it is natural to analyse consequences next [2]. There after conduct an explanatory inquiry 'up-the-stream'. i..e. [3, 4, 5]

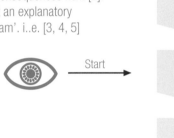

Start

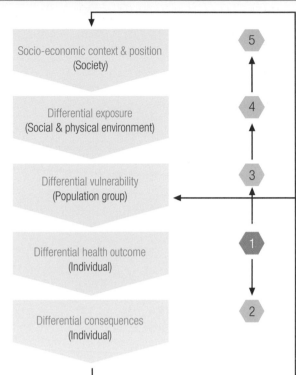

BOX 15.15: INSTITUTIONAL CHANGES IN SOCIAL DETERMINANTS ACROSS THE WORLD HEALTH ORGANIZATION

Progress on social determinants of health action, embodied in the PPHCKN, is already under way in WHO, including:

leading a conceptual shift in WHO, through review of technical guidelines on diseases and determinants, and reviewing other aspects of priority national programmes showing how health promotion and prevention activities, coupled with disease-specific programmes, have successfully addressed social determinants of health and health equity;

influencing condition-specific programmes to better do what they are currently doing (prevent, detect, treat, cure), but also to advocate social change as a means for sustainable improvement of population health to figure more prominently across WHO;

encouraging WHO to take an even stronger political leadership role to position health and health equity as intrinsic global values and not merely a means to economic growth;

measuring sustainability and institutional commitment to the social determinants of health collaboration across WHO and within programmes by resource allocation and staff profiles – commitment to social determinants action, to more programmatic work linked to social patterns of disease, and to change at country-level working, including the adoption of a social determinants of health action framework by countries.

Source: PPHCKN, 2007c

KNOWLEDGE, MONITORING, AND SKILLS: THE BACKBONE OF ACTION

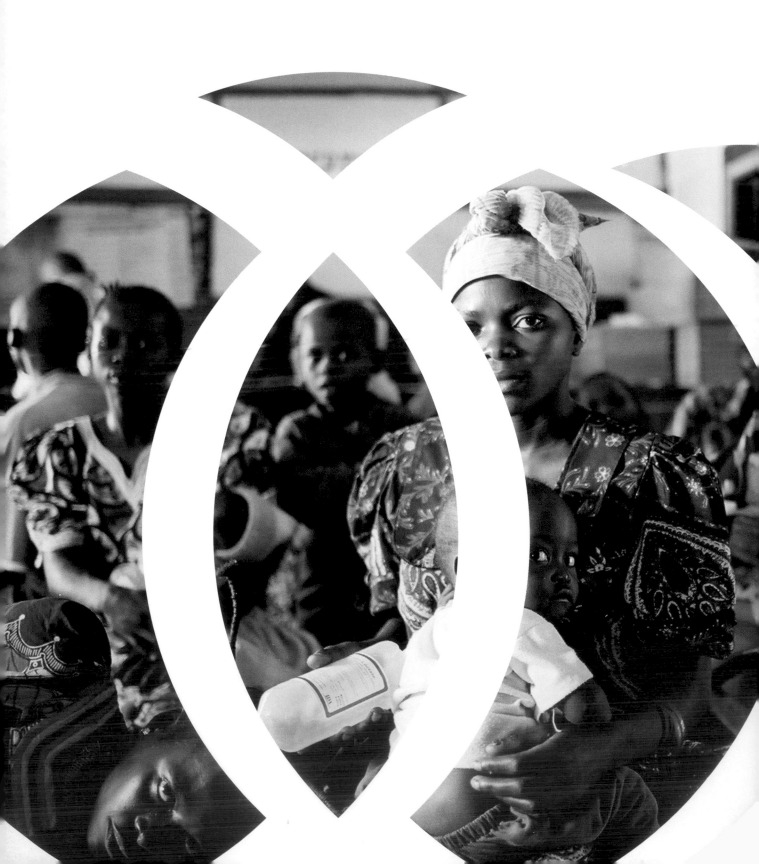

The third of the Commission's three principles of action is:

Measure the problem, evaluate action, expand the knowledge base, develop a workforce that is trained in the social determinants of health, and raise public awareness about the social determinants of health.

A society that is concerned with health and health equity acknowledges the existence of all its citizens and the importance of their well-being. It measures the extent of health problems and health inequity, and their determinants, and uses evidence to design and adjust policies and programmes to maximize health benefit for all.

The world is changing fast and often it is unclear the impact that social, economic, and political change will have on health in general and on health inequities within countries and across the globe in particular. Action on the social determinants of health will be more effective if basic data systems, including vital registration and routine monitoring of health inequity and the social determinants of health, are in place and there are mechanisms to ensure that the data are understood and applied to develop more effective interventions.

Creating the organizational space, mandate, and capacity to act effectively on health inequity depends on a better understanding – among political actors, practitioners, and the general public – of how population health is affected by social determinants. WHO needs to help build capacity at the international, national, and local level and assert its leadership role by increasing its capacity to advise on policies for health equity and provide technical support on the social determinants of health. There is definitely enough evidence to act now. Dedicated efforts to strengthen, and share, the global evidence base on health equity and the social determinants of health are needed to improve our capacity to act.

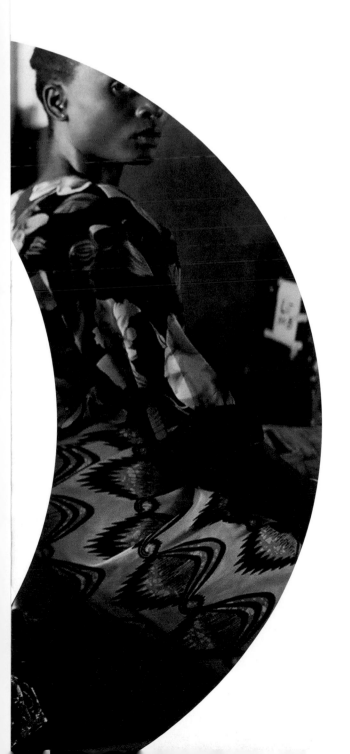

needed to improve the quality and comparability of vital statistics, such as through the Health Metrics Network (Setel et al., 2007; Mahapatra et al., 2007; Health Metrics Network, nd). Support for civil registration also needs to be built into projects funded by international agencies (Mahapatra et al., 2007). The World Bank, for example, can build this into its financing of health systems development and reform, while UNICEF could more actively promote death registration in addition to its efforts to improve birth registration (Mahapatra et al., 2007).

National health equity surveillance systems

The Commission recommends that:

16.2 National governments establish a national health equity surveillance system, with routine collection of data on social determinants of health and health inequity (see Rec 10.3).

A health equity surveillance system routinely collects, collates, and disseminates information on health, health inequities, and health determinants in a coherent fashion. Many countries and international organizations already collect data on the social determinants of health in one form or another. National and global health equity surveillance systems can build on these existing efforts, and would add two important things. First, while most existing data systems only present country averages, a health equity surveillance system would present data stratified by social groups within countries, and would include measures of inequity in health and determinants between these groups. Second, while data on different social determinants of health are currently dispersed across a multitude of information systems, a health equity surveillance system would bring together in one place data on a broad range of social determinants of health.

Building a minimum health equity surveillance system

It is recommended that all national governments build towards a comprehensive health equity surveillance system (see Box 16.3), where necessary with technical assistance from WHO. Such a surveillance system can be built progressively, depending on a country's stage of development and existing health information system. The first requirement is that governments ensure the availability of basic mortality and morbidity data, stratified by socioeconomic group and by regions within countries. Experience from work for the EU shows consistently that countries without basic data on mortality and morbidity by socioeconomic indicators are incapable of moving forward on the health equity agenda (Mackenbach &

Bakker, 2003); the same is arguably true for countries outside the EU. A framework for a minimum health equity surveillance system is presented in Box 16.2.

In order to build a minimum health equity surveillance system, all countries need to:

- immediately build routine health statistics where they do not exist; even in areas of conflict/emergency, cluster sample health and living conditions surveys can be feasible (Burnham, 2006; UNDP & Ministry of Planning and Development Corporation, 2005), albeit difficult;

- improve routine health statistics in such a way that it will be possible to follow health and mortality trends separately for men and women and for different social strata, using nationally representative data;

- where reliant on surveys, improve:

  - representativeness – nationally representative while also addressing the problem of missing data for vulnerable groups such as the homeless, mobile groups, Indigenous Peoples;

  - statistical power – sufficient to disaggregate the majority of health outcomes and determinants for relevant social strata, and to monitor time-trends in health inequity;

  - data quality and methods – reliability, validity, sample and estimation methods, statistical techniques;

  - consistency/comparability of data collection – to allow for comparisons over time and across countries;

  - geo-referencing – to facilitate data linking;

  - frequency with which surveys are conducted –ideally at least every five years;

- improve knowledge about health and mortality across all ages and social strata in poor countries. Survey data, in particular the DHS, have been invaluable for the description of inequities in childhood mortality and its determinants in low- and middle-income countries. Their widespread use shows that such surveys are feasible in these countries. It is important to set up systems that will provide information on adult health as well, for example by extended DHS.

The health equity surveillance system should be coordinated nationally so that it can be useful for national and local health policy-makers. Governments, where necessary with help from donors, should provide sufficient long-term core funding to a central agency that coordinates national health equity

---

BOX 16.1: VITAL STATISTICS – CRUCIAL FOR POLICY-MAKING

"In Africa, South Africa is one of the best-documented cases in which the absence of good data for cause of death allowed-for a time-poor national policies to continue, and the improved use of existing data for vital events has led to changes in policy and programme priorities. ...In the early 2000s, this country's available data for vital events pointed unambiguously at a huge increase in adult deaths. Absent information about the causes of those deaths, however, provided an opportunity for a government

that was officially sceptical of AIDS to persist in casting doubt on the true effects of the epidemic in their country. Authorities in Cape Town participated in analysis of existing information about cause of death, particularly about AIDS and homicide, and gained an appreciation of the value of locally generated data for local decision making."

Reproduced, with permission of the publisher, from Setel et al. (2007).

surveillance. WHO should play a crucial role in supporting health equity surveillance systems at the Member State level. This should include providing technical support for systems improvement; improving quality and comparability of data (across countries and over time); and building capacity at the country level to use the data for policy-making, public health programme development, and analysis. Initiatives such as the Health Metrics Network could also support building technical capacity for health equity surveillance (Health Metrics Network, nd). In addition, experience could be drawn from existing initiatives to monitor health equity, such as the EU Health Monitoring Programme (EU, 1997).

Towards a comprehensive health equity surveillance system

Data on the most important social determinants of health should be collected and analysed together with health data. The surveillance system should provide data on a range of social determinants of health along the causal pathway, ranging from daily living conditions to more structural drivers of health inequities (Solar & Irwin, 2007). The system should be structured so that it is possible to follow time-trends on social determinants of health separately for men and women and for different social strata.

Box 16.3 provides an example of what a framework for health equity surveillance could look like. It should include information on health inequities and determinants and the consequences of ill-health. Health information should be presented in a stratified manner, using both social and regional stratifiers. While health information for specified social groups should be included, the absolute level of health of disadvantaged groups in particular is an important indicator for policy-makers. In addition, measures that summarize the magnitude of health inequity between population groups should be included. It is advisable to include both a measure of

relative and a measure of absolute health inequity, as these types of measure are complementary and findings can depend on which type is used. When interpreting inequality patterns and trends, policy-makers, planners, and researchers should be clear about which type of summary measure they are using. Simple measures of health inequity – such as the rate ratio and rate difference – can, for research purposes, be complemented with more complex measures of health inequity (such as the relative index of inequality) (Kunst & Mackenbach, 1994; Mackenbach et al., 1997; MEKN, 2007b; Vågerö, 1995). Information on the distribution of the population across social and regional groups needs to be included in the surveillance system as the size of the groups will determine the population impact of the health inequities.

The framework in Box 16.3 shows broad categories of health outcomes and determinants for which indicators will need to be developed using a participatory process at the international and national level. The broad categories are derived from the work of the Commission, as laid out in this report. The framework clearly describes the importance of monitoring beyond the health-care sector (CW, 2007). Ideally, a core set of indicators that are comparable across countries should be developed, under the stewardship of WHO and in consultation with stakeholders at the country and international level (see Chapter 15: *Good Global Governance*, recommendation 15.1). These should include human rights-based health indicators to enable monitoring and evaluation of progressive realization of the right to the conditions for health (UN, 2000a). At the country level, modules and specific indicators for national- and local-level adaptation could be developed within this coherent framework.

BOX 16.2: A MINIMUM HEALTH EQUITY SURVEILLANCE SYSTEM

A minimum health equity surveillance system provides basic data on mortality and morbidity by socioeconomic and regional groups within countries. All countries should, as a minimum, have basic health equity data available that are nationally representative and comparable over time. Ideally, mortality is estimated on the basis of complete, good-quality registries of vital events, while morbidity data could be collected using health interview surveys (Kunst & Mackenbach, 1994). In many low- and middle-income countries, health surveys will remain an important source of information on mortality in the near future.

Health outcomes:

mortality: infant mortality and/or under-5 mortality, maternal mortality, adult mortality, and LEB;

morbidity: at least three nationally relevant morbidity indicators, which will vary between country contexts and might include prevalence of obesity, diabetes, undernutrition, and HIV;

self-rated mental and physical health.

Measures of inequity:

In addition to population averages, data on health outcomes should be provided in a stratified manner including stratification by:

sex;

at least two social markers (e.g. education, income/ wealth, occupational class, ethnicity/race);

at least one regional marker (e.g. rural/urban, province);

Include at least one summary measure of absolute health inequities between social groups, and one summary measure of relative health inequities between social groups (see Box 16.3).

Good-quality data on the health of Indigenous Peoples should be available, where applicable.

BOX 16.3: TOWARDS A COMPREHENSIVE NATIONAL HEALTH EQUITY SURVEILLANCE FRAMEWORK

HEALTH INEQUITIES

Include information on:

health outcomes stratified by:

- sex
- at least two socioeconomic stratifiers (education, income/wealth, occupational class);
- ethnic group/race/indigeneity;
- other contextually relevant social stratifiers;
- place of residence (rural/urban and province or other relevant geographical unit);

the distribution of the population across the sub-groups;

a summary measure of relative health inequity: measures include the rate ratio, the relative index of inequality, the relative version of the population attributable risk, and the concentration index;

a summary measure of absolute health inequity: measures include the rate difference, the slope index of inequality, and the population attributable risk.

HEALTH OUTCOMES

mortality (all cause, cause specific, age specific);

ECD;

mental health;

morbidity and disability;

self-assessed physical and mental health;

cause-specific outcomes.

DETERMINANTS, WHERE APPLICABLE INCLUDING STRATIFIED DATA

Daily living conditions

health behaviours:

- smoking;
- alcohol;
- physical activity;
- diet and nutrition;

physical and social environment:

- water and sanitation;
- housing conditions;
- infrastructure, transport, and urban design;
- air quality;
- social capital;

working conditions:

- material working hazards;
- stress;

health care:

- coverage;
- health-care system infrastructure;

social protection:

- coverage;
- generosity.

Structural drivers of health inequity:

gender:

- norms and values;
- economic participation;
- sexual and reproductive health;

social inequities:

- social exclusion;
- income and wealth distribution;
- education;

sociopolitical context:

- civil rights;
- employment conditions;
- governance and public spending priorities;
- macroeconomic conditions.

CONSEQUENCES OF ILL-HEALTH

economic consequences;

social consequences.

In some countries, there are already initiatives to monitor health inequities and the social determinants of health in a comprehensive way (CW, 2007) (Box 16.4).

The role of communities in health equity surveillance

Involving local communities is an integral part of the overall health equity surveillance process. This is especially important because, if the ground realities with regard to equity are to be assessed accurately, then it is those who are excluded who can provide evidence of changes, if any. Community-based monitoring can, for example, expose various conditions at the grassroots level, such as lack of services and resources for HIV-related treatment (Box 16.5). Another example is the issue of sex determination tests and declining female sex ratio in India. It was community health and women's groups who exposed the

practice of sex determination followed by abortion, as they had been monitoring changes in births by gender at the local level.

Not only can community monitoring provide authentic and reliable data, it can also be empowering for local people (Boxes 16.5 and 16.6). Building capacity to collect and analyse data is often a precursor to community action on the social determinants of health and can enable communities to make choices and decisions on issues affecting their lives. Giving communities access to or even control over their own data and monitoring can facilitate action on the social determinants of health. Typically, data are collected locally but go up to administrators and policy-makers and are rarely given back to local people. They do not see changes, if any, nor how their community fares compared to others. This need not be the case (Box 16.6).

BOX 16.4: MONITORING THE SOCIAL DETERMINANTS OF HEALTH IN ENGLAND

As part of monitoring progress since the Acheson inquiry in 1997, the Department of Health is reviewing trends in health inequity and the social determinants of health. The review includes a number of health outcomes by social class, together with data on a broad range of social determinants ranging from health behaviours, through health systems and

health-care use, to material conditions, employment arrangements, and social and economic policies, following broadly the framework laid out in Box 16.3.

Source: Health Inequalities Unit, 2008; Department of Health, 2005

BOX 16.5: AN EQUITY GAUGE APPROACH TO MONITORING

GEGA seeks to reduce health inequities through an equity gauge approach that includes assessment and monitoring, advocacy, and community empowerment. In at least 10 countries, an equity gauge is active. A diverse set of societal actors can be involved in an equity gauge, including communities, civil society organizations, researchers, policy-makers, the media, health workers, and local government. Monitoring of health inequities is linked to social and political

mobilization. The HIV Gauge in South Africa, for example, uses community monitoring and evaluation to assess whether or not key services and resources for HIV-related treatment are present. The findings of this monitoring activity are used in community advocacy and to develop local solutions to factors impeding the take-up of HIV-related services.

Sources: GEGA, nd; Health Systems Trust, nd

BOX 16.6: ENGAGING COMMUNITIES IN THE IMPLEMENTATION, INTERPRETATION, AND FOLLOW-UP OF HOUSEHOLD SURVEYS

Nongovernmental organizations can play an important role in community monitoring. For example, the Dutch nongovernmental organization Connect International funds and facilitates local partner organizations to carry out community development programmes in several African countries. The partners conduct household surveys on health and the social determinants of health in the communities in Mozambique, United Republic of Tanzania, and Zambia in which they work. The surveys serve to evaluate the community development programmes

and provide insight into the strengths and weaknesses of health and social determinants in each involved village. Local health workers in the villages and staff of the local partner organizations are trained to conduct the surveys. The results of the surveys are presented back to and discussed with the communities, which are actively involved in discussing progress made and setting priorities for further improvement based on the outcome of the surveys.

Source: Connect International, nd

A global health equity surveillance system

The Commission recommends that:

16.3 WHO stewards the creation of a global health equity surveillance system as part of a wider global governance structure (see Rec 15.1).

A global health equity surveillance system would systematically collate and make publicly accessible, for all countries globally, data on health inequities and determinants. Such a surveillance system is an important element of good global governance (see Chapter 15: *Good Global Governance*). A global health equity surveillance system would build on, and add to, national health equity surveillance systems. It could be based on a similar framework to that laid out in Box 16.3 for national surveillance systems. In addition to within-country inequities, the global surveillance system should monitor inequities in health outcomes between countries (Box 16.7), and the determinants of these inequities. These determinants can, among others, be found at the level of the global environment, such as between-country wealth differences, the amount of global funds spent on social determinants of health work (compared with disease-specific funds), WHO allocation to health equity and social determinants of health work, the extent to which overseas aid spending commitments are met, and the scale of debt relief. These are illustrations of determinants of between-country health inequities. A coherent framework with core indicators for global health equity surveillance needs to be developed, under the stewardship of WHO and involving stakeholders at the country level as well as from international organizations and research institutes (see Chapter 15: *Good Global Governance*).

BOX 16.7: MEASURES OF GLOBAL HEALTH INEQUITY

Several methods for measuring global health inequity have recently been developed. These include the dispersion measure of mortality (Moser, Shkolnikov & Leon, 2005), cluster analysis (Ruger & Kiml, 2006), and application of the slope index of inequality – generally used for measuring within-country health inequities – to measure inequities between countries (Dorling, Shaw & Davey Smith, 2006). Using the dispersion measure of mortality, for example, it has been shown that global mortality convergence (from 1950-55 to 1985-90) has been replaced by divergence since the mid-1980s (Moser, Shkolnikov & Leon, 2005) (Fig. 16.1). Further research into ways to measure global health inequity and its determinants is needed. It is important to develop targets globally for reduction of health inequities between and within countries, with regular monitoring of progress.

Figure 16.1 Trend in the dispersion measure of mortality for life expectancy at birth, 1950–2000.

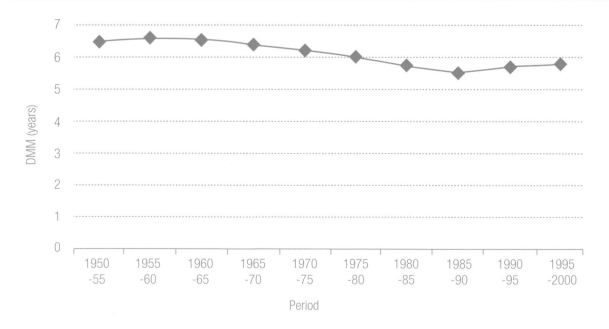

DMM = dispersion measure of mortality.
Reprinted, with permission of the publisher, from Moser, Shkolnikov & Leon (2005).

The role of WHO and the UN system

Monitoring and surveillance of population health worldwide is one of the core functions of WHO. The Commission endorses the establishment of a global health observatory that would, "collect, collate and disseminate data on priority health problems" (WHO, 2008a). It is critical that global health equity surveillance is a key component of such an observatory. While involving stakeholders from Member States, international organizations, and research institutes, the specific global health equity component of a global health observatory could perform several key activities: development of a coherent monitoring framework with core indicators that are comparable across countries; provision of standards and guidelines for health equity surveillance; development of interactive and rapidly updated national, regional, and global profiles on inequities in health and the social determinants of health tailored to different target audiences; and provision of a transparent data and evidence platform that can be used and improved by all stakeholders as inputs for policies, programmes, or advocacy.

As part of a wider UN process for more coherent planning (see Chapter 15: *Good Global Governance*), WHO can steward improvements in coordination and cooperation between countries and international agencies to reduce fragmentation and duplication of requests to countries in data collection and reporting (UNICEF, 2007c). This includes facilitating interagency discussions on technical and methodological issues, such as the standardization of indicators; identifying key gaps in data availability; and developing strategies to overcome these. Such a role requires that WHO builds internal capacity to monitor health equity and the social determinants of health.

A global health equity surveillance system, to be most effective, will need to be UN-system wide and invite partners in civil society, the private sector, and all levels of government (see Chapter 15: *Good Global Governance*). Championing the collection and monitoring of stratified data on health outcomes and the social determinants of health across the UN system is an important role of WHO. Importantly, within the UN system, the General Assembly and national PRSPs could focus

on health equity, and the MDGs could include a health equity component. The Common Country Assessment, which is a common instrument across the UN system to monitor and analyse countries' development, could become an important monitoring device by inclusion of indicators on health equity and the social determinants of health. The UN Country Teams, made up of specialized organizations including WHO, could provide a mechanism to implement this. As part of the global health equity surveillance system, it is recommended that the UN system creates a process towards a comprehensive set of globally agreed long-term health equity targets with interim benchmarks (see Chapter 17: *Sustaining Action Beyond the Commission on Social Determinants of Health*).

Using surveillance data for policy-making

As part of global and national surveillance systems, data on health inequities and determinants should be made publicly available and accessible and disseminated widely for advocacy purposes and to support coherent policy-making. This requires that results are made accessible for a non-technical audience on a routine basis. Raw data need to be made publicly accessible for research purposes. National health equity surveillance data need to be reported to, among others, national policy-makers and WHO. Global health equity surveillance data need to be reported to the Economic and Social Council, other international bodies, and back to national governments (see Chapter 15: *Good Global Governance*).

There should be a clear process, with a feedback loop, from data on health inequities to policy-making, such that data are drawn upon in the development of national and sub-national policies and in the design of public health programmes (Box 16.8). The policy implications of observed health patterns and trends (Braveman, 1998) for all sectors, not just the health-care sector, should be assessed on an ongoing basis. Key constituencies should be involved in this process, including policy-makers, practitioners from different sectors, researchers from a variety of disciplines, civil society, and community organizations. Their knowledge and experience can aid the interpretation of the data, and their involvement is key for mobilization to implement policy and create and sustain political will (Braveman, 1998).

BOX 16.8: MEXICO – USING EVIDENCE TO REFORM THE NATIONAL HEALTH SYSTEM

At the time of the health system reform in Mexico in 2000, half of Mexican families, most of them poor, had no protection against the financial consequences of ill-health. The reform of the Mexican health system invested heavily in the generation and application of knowledge. National health accounts showed that more than half of all health expenditure in Mexico was out-of-pocket. As a consequence, many households were driven below the poverty line or forced deeper into poverty. This evidence created public awareness of a reality that had hitherto been outside the policy debate – namely, that health care itself could become a direct cause of impoverishment. Major legislative reform was undertaken to establish a system of

protection in health and was approved by all political parties in the Mexican Congress. The new public voluntary scheme, called Seguro Popular, came into effect on 1 January 2004. It will expand until universal coverage is achieved in 2010.

Periodic national income and expenditure survey analyses show a reduction in the number of households affected by catastrophic health-care payments and a major increase in the use of early detection services for several non-communicable diseases.

Source: MEKN, 2007a

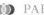
Expanding the knowledge base

The Commission recommends that:

16.4. Research funding bodies create a dedicated budget for generation and global sharing of evidence on social determinants of health and health equity, including health equity intervention research.

The scope of public health research

The work of the Commission clearly shows the importance of broadening the scope of public health research to include a stronger emphasis on the social determinants of health. It requires that funding bodies, including national health, medical, and social research councils, invest more in research on the social determinants of health and in the multi- and interdisciplinary research that this entails, rather than the disease-specific biomedical focus of research funding that currently prevails (Global Forum for Health Research, 2006; Sanders et al., 2004; McCoy et al., 2004).

The themes of all the chapters in this report require more research on what works to reduce health inequities (see Chapter 17: *Sustaining Action Beyond the Commission on Social Determinants of Health*). Three broad areas need particular investment. First, research on determinants of health inequities, rather than determinants of average population health, need further study. Second, more research is needed on what works to reduce health inequities in what circumstances, and how best to implement interventions such that they contribute to a reduction of these inequities (Box 16.9). This research should take into account the complexity of these interventions. There is some experience with the evaluation of complex interventions (such as Head Start and Moving to Opportunity in the United States and Health Action Zones in the United Kingdom). But compared to biomedical science, funding in the development of appropriate methods

for these types of evaluation has been negligible. The global Healthy Cities movement has been most important for a broad approach to improving health, but there has been little systematic evaluation. The third area for investment is the development of methods for measuring and monitoring health inequities and for evaluating the impact of population-level interventions (MEKN, 2007b). WHO could lead a process to bring together, from a range of disciplinary backgrounds, researchers experienced in using methods to evaluate complex interventions. WHO could also lead investment by national governments in multinational intervention studies that use context-appropriate methods but that can be compared across national borders.

Broadening the definition of evidence

Action on the social determinants of health is best served through developing a rich and diverse evidence base. This should include evidence from multiple disciplines and methodological traditions (Box 16.10), as well as systematic collection of knowledge and experience from key stakeholders involved, especially from practitioners and the planned beneficiaries of the interventions. This is particularly important as evidence on the social determinants of health is often context dependent. Evaluations of social determinants of health interventions require rich qualitative data in order to understand the ways in which context affects the intervention and the reasons for its success or failure. What counts as legitimate evidence should be determined on the basis of 'fitness for purpose' rather than on a single hierarchy of evidence (which traditionally puts randomized controlled trials and laboratory experiments at the top) (MEKN, 2007a). Whereas no single approach to the generation of evidence or data should be privileged over others, all types of evidence can be assessed using the following criteria: making explicit the specific research questions the evidence seeks to answer within the broader field of social determinants of health research;

BOX 16.9: MEXICO – EVALUATING POPULAR HEALTH INSURANCE (SEGURO POPULAR)

The reform of the Mexican health system invested heavily in the generation and application of knowledge. The impact assessment and evaluation experience established under Mexico's conditional cash transfer programme Oportunidades is being applied to the health system reform, which saw the introduction of a popular health insurance, Seguro Popular. In addition to its technical aspects, rigorous evaluation has political value to assure the continuity of innovations through changes in administration. In the case of Oportunidades, scientific evidence persuaded the government not only to continue with the programme, but also to expand it. The encouraging results shown by the continuing assessment of Seguro Popular may serve once again to maintain the reform through future changes of government.

Source: MEKN, 2007a

MONITORING, RESEARCH, AND INTERVENTION   ACTION AREA 16.2

Invest in generating and sharing new evidence on the ways in which social determinants influence population health and health equity and on the effectiveness of measures to reduce health inequities through action on social determinants.

transparency (especially making all forms of potential bias explicit); and relevance for different population groups and contexts (MEKN, 2007a).

Addressing gender biases in research

Medical research may not always deal objectively with gender issues (Begin, 1998). Much research is gender biased – both in terms of what is studied, as well as in terms of how the research is done (Williams & Borins, 1993; Eichler, Reisman & Borins, 1992). Health problems that particularly affect women, for example, tend to be more slowly recognized. Some of women's health complaints are brushed away as psychological, without including them as objects of research (Begin, 1998). Interaction between gender and other social factors is often not recognized and sex-disaggregated data are often not collected (Iyer, Sen & Östlin, 2007). Methods used in medical research and clinical trials for new drugs can lack a gender perspective and exclude women from study populations. Biases also include a gender imbalance in ethical committees and research-funding and advisory bodies, and differential treatment of women scientists (WGEKN, 2007).

Mechanisms and policies need to be developed to ensure that gender biases in both the content and processes of health research are avoided and corrected (WGEKN, 2007). These mechanisms and policies include:

- ensuring collection of data disaggregated by sex and other stratifiers in individual research projects as well as through larger data systems;

- including women in clinical trials and other health studies in appropriate numbers;

- analysing data generated from clinical trials and other health studies using gender-sensitive tools and methods;

- strengthening women's role in health research, among others by redressing the gender imbalances in research committees and funding, publication, and advisory bodies.

Strengthening global generation, sharing, and accumulation of evidence

The production and synthesis of evidence and the production of evidence-based guidance on the social determinants of health is resource intensive. There is a need for international collaboration to ensure knowledge accumulation and to prevent unnecessary duplication of effort. Mechanisms for global knowledge sharing and accumulation need to be improved, for example, by creating a 'clearing house' for evidence on interventions on the social determinants of health. Creating such a clearing house could, for example, be a function of the global health observatory. Building on the experience of the Commission, this should include not just technical information, but also learning from practice, policy-makers, and civil society. A clearing house could also help translate findings on the effectiveness of interventions from one setting to another. For this to happen, dialogue and exchange of experience between governments, donors, development partners, and civil society should be facilitated. The importance for all countries of knowledge accumulation and exchange on health equity justifies international investment (EUROTHINE, 2007).

BOX 16.10: THE POWER OF QUALITATIVE DATA IN UNDERSTANDING THE SOCIAL DETERMINANTS OF HEALTH

Statistical data are essential to describe the extent of a public health problem but do little to explain the experience of that problem or its impact on people's lives. Yet providing a sense of the lived experience is important for explanatory purposes, as well as for advocacy and giving politicians and others the rich story that can turn hearts and minds (Baum, 1995). For example, policy-makers are often at a loss to explain why people smoke despite the evidence of its negative impact on health. Graham (1987) used qualitative research to show that for poor women smoking can be a coping mechanism in response to the demands of living in poverty and being a mother. Qualitative evidence can also help explain counterintuitive findings from statistical analyses. Some research on social capital and health, for example, found that participation in community life can be a predictor of poorer health status. The statistical analysis that reveals this pattern says nothing of the reasons for it. The complementary qualitative data provided accounts of participation and suggested that a likely factor was the conflict that not infrequently occurs when people are involved in community groups (Ziersch & Baum, 2004).

Training and education on the social determinants of health

Training of medical and health professionals

The Commission recommends that:

16.5 Educational institutions and relevant ministries make the social determinants of health a standard and compulsory part of training of medical and health professionals (see Rec 9.3).

Medical and health professionals, including physicians, nurses, auxiliary personnel, and community workers, need to be aware of health inequities as an important public health problem. They also need to understand the importance of social factors in influencing the level and distribution of population health. Unfortunately, in most medical and health curricula, there is too little place for training on the social determinants of health.

Ministries of health and education, in collaboration with medical, nursing, public health, and health management schools, need to make the social determinants of health a standard and compulsory part of the curriculum of medical and health practitioners. All health professionals need to receive such training at a basic level as a minimum. In addition, dedicated groups of people can be trained at a more specialist level such that they, as members of the public health community, can take the issue forward.

The health-care sector has an important stewardship role in ISA for health equity (see Chapter 10: *Health Equity in all Policies, Systems, and Programmes*). This requires an understanding among policy-makers and professionals in the health-care sector of how social determinants influence health. Health professionals also need to understand how the health-care

sector – depending on its structure, operations, and financing – can exacerbate or ameliorate health inequities. They need to understand their role in the equitable provision of quality care. Health workers and other professionals, for example, need to be trained in good communication and listening skills and in how to tailor their communication to meet their patients' needs (Kickbusch, Wait & Maag, 2006). They also need to be aware of how gender influences health outcomes and health-seeking behaviour. This requires the integration of gender into the curriculum of health personnel as part of training on the social determinants of health (Box 16.11).

The recommended reorientation of the health-care sector towards a greater importance of prevention and health promotion (see Chapters 9 and 10: *Universal Health Care; Health Equity in All Policies, Systems, and Programmes*) requires a reorientation in the skills, knowledge, and experience of the health personnel involved and an enhancement of the professional status and importance of these areas. Prevention and health promotion should certainly be given a more prominent place in the medical curriculum.

Making the social determinants of health a standard and compulsory part of medical training and training of other health professionals requires that textbooks and teaching materials are developed for this purpose. There is an urgent need to develop, among other things, a virtual repository of teaching and training materials on a broad range of social determinants of health that can be downloaded without cost. Furthermore, opportunities for interdisciplinary professional training and research on social determinants of health are needed. In low-income countries this can be done, for example, through regional centres of excellence and/or distance education models (Box 16.12).

MONITORING, RESEARCH, AND INTERVENTION   **ACTION AREA 16.3**

Provide training on the social determinants of health to policy actors, stakeholders, and practitioners and invest in raising public awareness.

BOX 16.11: INTEGRATING GENDER INTO THE MEDICAL CURRICULUM

Over the past decade there have been efforts to integrate gender into the medical curriculum in training institutions in a range of developed and developing countries including the Netherlands, Sweden, Australia, Canada, the United States, the Philippines, and India.

In the Netherlands, for example, a countrywide initiative to integrate gender into the medical curriculum of the eight medical schools was undertaken in 2002. A review of the initiative found that the integration was largely successful. Key obstacles included the continued low priority accorded to gender within the medical curriculum and lower levels of support for the initiative among male medical educators.

In India, the Gender Mainstreaming in Medical Education project is an important initiative that not only focuses on medical schools, but also takes a broader view of gender mainstreaming through collaboration with health professionals and nongovernmental organizations. The project is intended to gender-sensitize medical students by incorporating the gender perspective into textbooks as well as by training a core group of medical educators in gender issues.

Source: Govender & Penn-Kekana, 2007

The Commission recommends that:

16.6 Educational institutions and relevant ministries act to increase understanding of the social determinants of health among non-medical professionals and the general public (see Rec 10.2).

Training of other practitioners and policy actors

Training and education on the social determinants of health needs to be extended to other practitioners, policy actors, and stakeholders. Professionals, such as urban planners, transport planners, teachers, and architects, are in a privileged position to act on the social determinants of health. Improving the understanding of what affects population health and the social gradient in health prepares the ground so that the evidence can be understood and acted on, providing a basis for ISA. Training of non-medical practitioners requires that schools of social work and faculties of education collaborate in making training on the social determinants of health a standard part of the curriculum. There is an urgent need to develop training and learning resources that demonstrate the central messages about how population health is improved not through action on high-risk individuals but mainly through action that addresses the characteristics of entire societies (Rose, 1985) and about the implication of the health gradient for improving population health (Graham & Kelly, 2004).

Raising awareness about the social determinants of health

The understanding of the social determinants of health among the general public needs to be improved as a new part of health literacy. Health literacy is the, "ability to access, understand, evaluate and communicate information as a way to promote, maintain and improve health in a variety of settings across the life-course" (Rootman & Gordon-El-Bihbety, 2008). "It is

a critical empowerment strategy to increase people's control over their health, their ability to seek out information and their ability to take responsibility" (Kickbusch, Wait & Maag, 2006). Poor health literacy is prevalent, even in high-income countries, and is likely to contribute to health inequities between social groups (Kickbusch, Wait & Maag, 2006) (Box 16.3).

The scope of health literacy should be expanded to include the ability to access, understand, evaluate, and communicate information on the social determinants of health. Improving health literacy is an important element of strategies to reduce health inequity. This requires good, reliable, accessible information tailored to the needs and circumstances of different social groups (Kickbusch, Wait & Maag, 2006).

Health literacy is not just about the individual's ability to read, understand, and act on health information, but also the ability of public and private sector actors to communicate health-related information in relevant and easy-to-understand ways. This requires improving awareness and knowledge of health literacy among health professionals. Also, policies need to be developed on the use of clear language and visual symbols in health communications (Rootman & Gordon-El-Bihbety, 2008).

Health literacy initiatives are ideally developed, funded, and implemented through coordinated countrywide strategies (Rootman & Gordon-El-Bihbety, 2008). This requires long-term investment (Kickbusch, Wait & Maag, 2006). Countries can create a multi-stakeholder 'Council on Health Literacy', at arm's length from government, to monitor and assess progress, facilitate partnerships between organizations, and provide strategic direction for health literacy (Rootman & Gordon-El-Bihbety, 2008).

BOX 16.12: CAPACITY BUILDING ON EARLY CHILD DEVELOPMENT – THE EARLY CHILDHOOD DEVELOPMENT VIRTUAL UNIVERSITY (ECDVU)

The ECDVU is an innovative approach to building leadership and capacity on ECD. It is a North-South institution currently working closely with academic institutions in Ghana, Malawi, and United Republic of Tanzania and with academic, governmental, and nongovernmental groups in other parts of sub-Saharan Africa and the Middle East and North Africa. International and local partner funds have allowed the

delivery of a combination of web-based and face-to-face leadership courses designed to advance country-identified, intersectoral ECD initiatives. An external evaluation at the conclusion of a pilot delivery noted that the ECDVU has been, "singularly successful in meeting and exceeding all of its objectives".

Source: ECDKN 2007b

BOX 16.13: POOR HEALTH LITERACY – ALSO A PROBLEM IN RICH COUNTRIES

One in five adults in the United Kingdom has problems with the basic skills needed to understand simple information that could lead to better health. Poorer groups are less likely to seek information or help for health problems.

Amended, with permission of the publisher, from Kickbusch, Wait & Maag (2006).

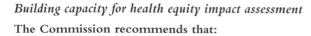
Building capacity for health equity impact assessment

The Commission recommends that:

16.7. Governments build capacity for health equity impact assessment among policy-makers and planners across government departments (see Rec 10.3; 12.1)

Raising awareness of the importance of social determinants of health and health equity among policy actors is important but, in itself, not enough. Implications for health and health equity need to be routinely considered in policy-making and practice. Health equity impact assessment is one of the tools recommended by the Commission (see Chapters 10 and 12: *Health Equity in All Policies, Systems, and Programmes; Market Responsibility*). It is a tool to help decision-makers to systematically assess the potential impact of policies, programmes, projects, or proposals on health equity in a given population with the aim of maximizing the positive health equity benefits and minimizing the potential adverse effects on health equity (MEKN, 2007b).

Health equity impact assessment is important for several reasons. First, the extent to which the health sector achieves its objectives is strongly influenced by other sectors. It is therefore crucial that the health and health equity impact of policies and programmes in all sectors, not just the health sector, are assessed. Second, with the best intentions, policies and programmes can have unintended effects that may be prevented following systematic health equity impact assessment. And finally, solutions to improve health and reduce health inequities cannot be universally applied to all contexts. Proposed policies and programmes must therefore be reviewed in context (MEKN, 2007a).

Health equity impact assessment of policies and programmes must happen as a matter of course – that is, it should be a routine procedure in policy development. Considerable

learning from the environmental sector and review of environmental policies provides a sound basis that health equity impact assessment can provide a concrete tool to enable all actors to work together to develop more equitable policies and programmes.

There are three important elements of strengthening capacity for health equity impact assessment.

- *Investment in training, tools, and resources.* Routine consideration of health and health equity impacts in policy development requires capacity building among policy-makers and planners across all sectors, not just the health sector, locally, nationally, and internationally. Currently, there are too few people able to assess health equity impact to allow for such routine consideration. Training of health equity impact assessment practitioners is therefore a matter of urgency (Wismar et al., 2007). Training opportunities need to be expanded and tools and resources need to be developed (Harris, 2007) (see Box 16.15). Equity considerations need to be systematically included in training on health impact assessment. Health equity impact assessment could also be included in public health courses (Wismar et al., 2007).

- *Creation of national and regional support centres.* National or regional centres can be created or strengthened to support health equity impact assessment with technical leadership, advice, and guidance (Wismar et al., 2007). In addition, organizational commitment to health impact assessment can be promoted through general education and communication strategies that raise awareness of the scope and purpose of such assessment among users and key stakeholders (Wismar et al., 2007). WHO can be instrumental in creating or strengthening these support centres.

- *Ensuring budgeting for health equity impact assessment across departments.* Routine consideration of health equity impacts requires that such assessment is adequately resourced through

BOX 16.14 HEALTH EQUITY IMPACT ASSESSMENT

The Australian Better Health Initiative is part of a Council of Australian Governments Reform Package, which aims to improve health for all Australians. As part of the development of the Implementation Plan for New South Wales, a Rapid Equity Focussed Impact Assessment was conducted. Eight initiatives were assessed on their potential equity impacts, looking

at inequities by age, gender, place of residence, ethnicity, and socioeconomic status. Concrete recommendations were formulated on how to improve the equity focus and potential positive impacts on health equity of the Initiative.

Source: Harris, Harris & Kemp, 2006

BOX 16.15 EXPANDING CAPACITY FOR HEALTH EQUITY IMPACT ASSESSMENT

An example of capacity building for health impact assessment is the 'Learning by Doing' approach that was part of the New South Wales Health Impact Assessment Project. Learning by Doing includes formal training, access to resources and technical support, and continued building of consensus on the

scope of health impact assessment. An equity focus needs to be incorporated into all training on health impact assessment.

Source: Harris, 2007

factoring it into every department's work plans (Wismar et al., 2007), with separate funding for health equity impact assessment support centres. There are indications that the benefits of health equity impact assessment far exceed the costs (Wismar et al., 2007).

Strengthening capacity at WHO

The Commission recommends that:

16.8. WHO strengthens its capacity to provide technical support for action on the social determinants of health globally, nationally, and locally (see Rec 5.1; 9.1; 10.5; 15.3).

WHO plays a key stewardship role in action on the social determinants of health and health equity. In order to fulfil this role effectively, WHO needs to strengthen its institutional capacity – at global, regional, and country levels – relating to the social determinants of health. Member States can strengthen WHO and other UN agencies with mandates related to the social determinants of health through core (regular budget) funding. Within WHO, it is important that this priority is reflected by allocating substantial and commensurate core funding support. This commitment should extend to an increase in the proportion of staff with social science and other disciplinary backgrounds (PHM, Medact & GEGA, 2005). WHO's stewardship role with regard to action on the social determinants of health implies specific action affecting WHO's core functions:

- Provide leadership to Member States and global and local actors on actions to promote effective public policies that will address the social determinants of health.

- Articulate evidence-based initiatives to mainstream the social determinants of health approach across governments and within WHO's programmes.

- Stimulate the development, synthesis, dissemination, and translation of new knowledge to support cross-sectoral implementation of actions on the social determinants of health at country level.

- Develop standards and guidelines for policy implementation of the social determinants of health approach for achieving health equity.

- Provide technical support and build sustainable institutional capacity of governmental and nongovernmental institutions to implement a social determinants of health agenda (see Chapter 10: *Health Equity in all Policies, Systems, and Programmes*).

- Monitor health inequities at global, regional, and country levels and assess their trends as related to the social determinants of health (see also recommendation 16.3).

Some mechanisms that may facilitate the achievement of strengthened WHO capacity include the establishment of:

- groups consisting of WHO Member States to guide policy coherence in WHO on the social determinants of health closely linked with broader strategies such as PHC, human rights, MDGs, and health and poverty reduction;

- external expert groups to advise WHO on evidence-based policies;

- cross-sectional internal technical groups to steer effective institutional mainstreaming of social determinants of health, such as the PPHCKN (see Chapter 15: *Good Global Governance*) (PPHCKN, 2007c).

Promotion of development through a social determinants of health approach that particularly addresses health equity implies specific action concordant with WHO's agenda. WHO should:

- work with Member States to strengthen health systems such that they provide equitable and accessible primary and tertiary health care across communities and support people and organizations to act on the conditions that affect health;

- harness research, information, and evidence on the social determinants of health in order to guide policy and programmatic decisions at national and local levels;

- enhance partnerships between UN agencies and other international organizations, donors, civil society, the private sector, and community members to take evidence-based action to address the social determinants of health needs articulated by countries and communities;

- improve performance of its own work in promoting the social determinants of health approach and its technical work with countries through comprehensive programme monitoring and performance measures.

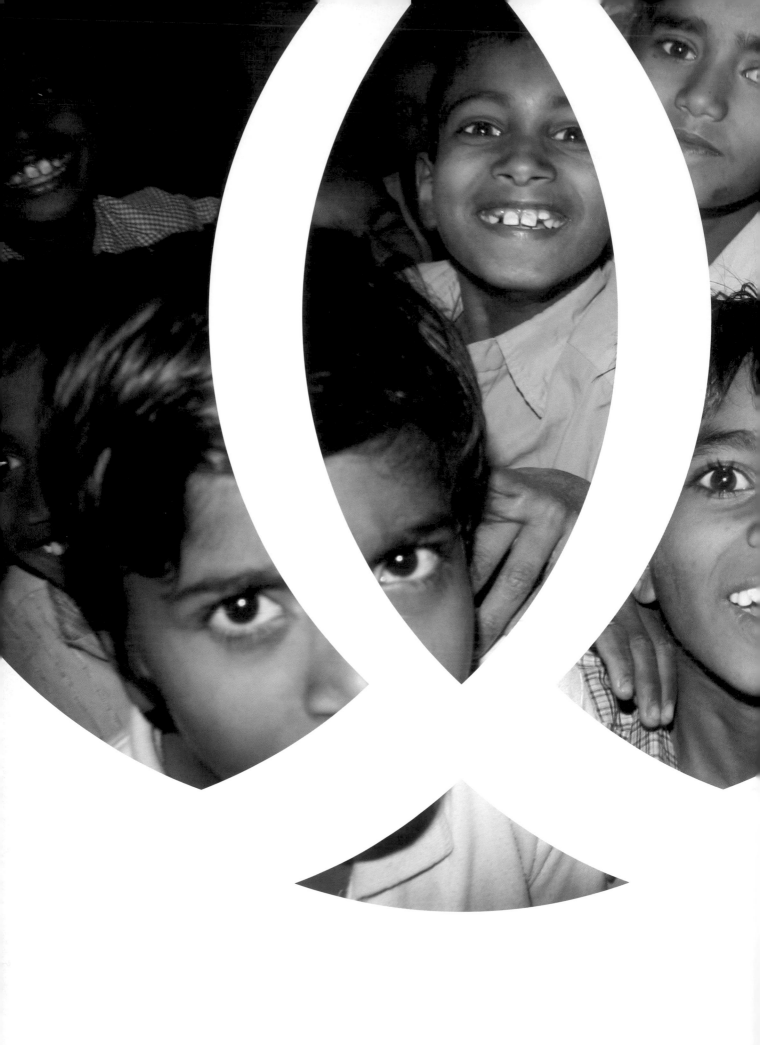

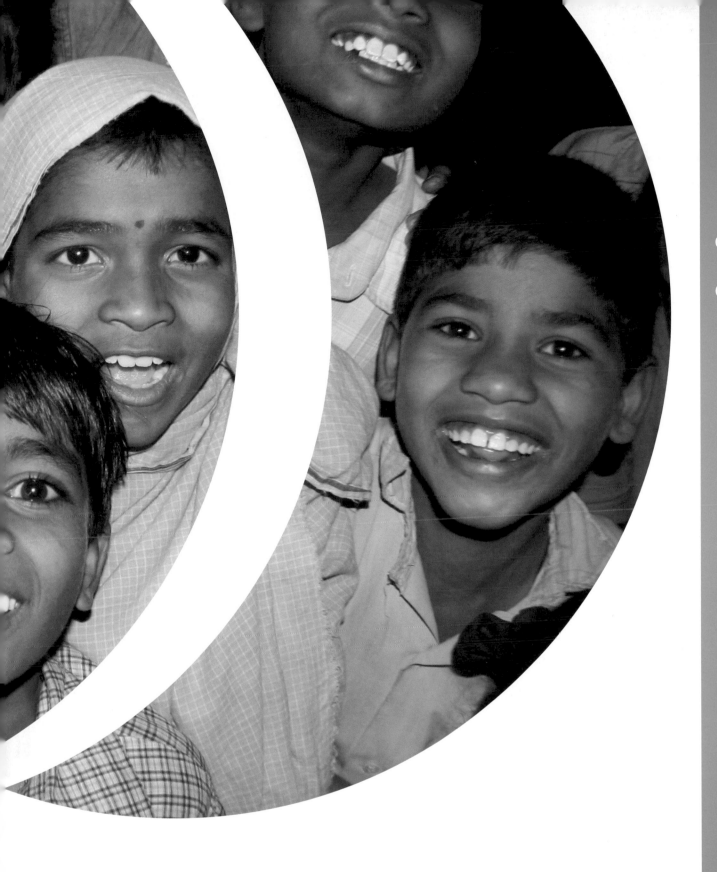

CHAPTER 17

Sustaining action beyond the Commission on Social Determinants of Health

Taking action on the social determinants of health and health equity is an ambitious agenda that needs global champions, committed leadership, and bold action at all levels. The foundations have been laid. The Commission was designed with the intention that it would be a broad partnership of those who do research, those who devise policy, those who implement policy, and those who advocate and act. The effect of top-down political commitment and policy action combined with bottom-up action from communities and civil society groups has been called 'the nutcracker effect' (Fig. 17.1) (Baum, 2007).

Foundations for sustained action

Global leaders

It is vital that the international and global policy environment supports action on the social determinants of health and health equity. To this end, the Commissioners – including former heads of government, government ministers, national policy-makers, and international advisors; leaders in international organizations; leading academics; and representatives of civil society – are a vital resource. Together they constitute a small but powerful caucus of global champions, advocating the adoption of a social determinants approach to health and health equity. Building leadership within the UN system – in global governance, policy-making, and development financing – and through global social movements will help to establish health equity as a priority on the global agenda for the 21st century.

WHO

The Commission worked closely with WHO at country, regional, and global levels. Although the judgements reached by the Commission are independent of WHO's decision-making process and governing bodies, it is of course critical that WHO, the UN body mandated to provide leadership in global health, takes the recommendations forward.

And there are positive signs. Already WHO is taking steps to institutionalize the social determinants of health approach across all its working sectors. This is laid out in WHO's Medium Term Strategic Plan for 2008-2013 (MTSP) (WHO, 2007a) – which includes the strategic objective, "to address the underlying social and economic determinants of health through policies and programmes that enhance health equity and integrate pro-poor, gender-responsive, and human rights-based approaches" – and the organization-wide expected results that are being used to measure accomplishment of the objective (Box 17.1). According to the MTSP, the objective is underpinned by an approved budget of almost US$ 66 million for the 2008-2009 biennium.

Figure 17.1 Cracking the nut of health equity.

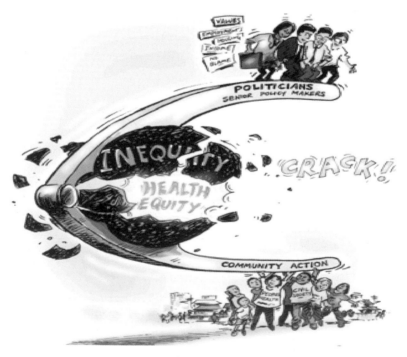

Cartoon by Simon Kneebone. Reprinted, with permission of the publisher, from Baum (2007).

To implement these expected results at a technical level, WHO has followed three strategies: mainstreaming health equity across programmes, strengthening cross-cutting functions related to health equity, and enhancing its existing monitoring capacities. As part of mainstreaming, WHO began a review of the potential for programmes to improve efficiency and equity in 2006 under a cross-programmatic network, the PPHCKN, which is looking at ways to incorporate social determinants of health approaches and address equity more directly through global and national health programmes. WHO has appointed regional focal points to coordinate action on the social determinants of health and supported analysis and dissemination of existing data at the national and regional level from an equity perspective.

The Commission supports the aims of these various processes and calls on all countries to initiate the development of action plans on social determinants of health to improve health equity.

Country partners

Action at country level is one of the primary vehicles for using the Commission's global evidence base, implementing the recommendations of the Commission, and sustaining awareness and understanding of social determinants of health among political leaders, ministers of health, and other major stakeholders.

The Commission collaborated with a number of partner countries, supporting the development of national policies aimed at reducing health inequities through a variety of mechanisms. Brazil, Canada, Chile, Islamic Republic of Iran, Kenya, Mozambique, Sri Lanka, Sweden, and the United Kingdom each became a Commission 'country partner', through a formal process of a written letter of commitment to making progress on the social determinants of health to improve health equity. As the work of the Commission gained momentum, other supportive countries added both to the accumulation of technical work on tackling social determinants for health equity (e.g. Norway provided case studies on ISA) and to sharing experiences and advice on improving policy coherence in this field (e.g. Thailand).

The Commission's formal country partners continue to create momentum for change in different ways, which has been documented (for more on the Country work stream, see CW, 2007). Some countries focused on generating political interest in social determinants of health. Others, such as Brazil, Canada, and Chile, established new mechanisms and institutional structures to promote intersectoral policy development. Brazil, for instance, launched a National Commission on Social Determinants of Health in March 2006. The Public Health Agency of Canada set up the Canadian Reference Group, an influential advisory group making real political progress in advancing the social determinants of health agenda in Canada and internationally. In England, the Scientific Reference Group advises on policy and has developed indicators to measure health inequities.

Another approach countries used was to explore processes for inter-country sharing of lessons and joint research initiatives (e.g. Canada, Chile, Sweden; in the United Kingdom: England and Scotland). A Nordic reference group, set up with representatives from five countries, fed the Commission evidence on national policies from that region. A similar group was established in East Asia. These models of collaboration between countries of similar sociopolitical context could be utilized elsewhere.

Joint efforts by all the various Commission country partners have amplified the call to tackle the social determinants of health inequities in different regional and global public health and human development fora. More countries will follow – Argentina, Mexico, New Zealand, Poland, and Thailand have all expressed enthusiasm. In Australia, a social determinants of health approach has been established as a central element in the government's plan, announced in 2007, to close the LEB gap between Indigenous Peoples and the overall population within a generation (COAG, 2007). The aim for the future is that more countries will engage politically with the approach set out in this report and that this political process will translate into policies and programmes that measurably improve population health and reduce health inequities.

BOX 17.1: WORLD HEALTH ORGANIZATION STRATEGIC OBJECTIVE (SO) NUMBER 7 AND RELATED ORGANIZATION-WIDE EXPECTED RESULTS

SO7: "To address the underlying social and economic determinants of health through policies and programmes that enhance health equity and integrate pro-poor, gender-responsive, and human rights-based approaches."

Expected Result 7.1: Significance of social and economic determinants of health recognized throughout the organization and incorporated into normative work and technical collaboration with Member States and other partners.

Expected Result 7.2: Initiative taken by WHO in providing opportunities and means for intersectoral collaboration at national and international levels in order to address social and economic determinants of health and to encourage poverty reduction and sustainable development.

Expected Result 7.3: Social and economic data relevant to health collected, collated, and analysed on a disaggregated basis (by sex, age, ethnicity, income, and health conditions such as disease or disability).

Expected Result 7.4: Ethics- and rights-based approaches to health promoted within WHO and at national and global levels.

Expected Result 7.5: Gender analysis and responsive actions incorporated into WHO's normative work and support provided to Member States for formulation of gender-sensitive policies and programmes.

Cities

In addition to the cities represented in the KNUS, the cities of New York, Glasgow, London, and New Orleans have all made links with the Commission and are working to take the agenda forward through a sharing of practice-based evidence. The Healthy Cities movement (coordinated by the WHO Regional Office for Europe) and the WHO Kobe Centre's healthy urbanization programme are both strong allies.

Civil society

Civil society groups are powerful protagonists in the global health equity agenda. From the beginning, the Commission actively sought the involvement of representatives of civil society groups in Africa, Asia, the Americas, and Europe. Members of civil society groups were engaged in the Commission's knowledge-gathering processes. They helped to shape the Commission's thinking and will be active partners for change in the future (for more on the Civil Society work stream, see CS, 2007).

Building and sharing knowledge

The Commission has built a global evidence base for understanding the social determinants of health and establishing effective action to promote health equity. To support that process, the Commission created nine Knowledge Networks – including academics and practitioners from universities and research institutions, government ministries, and international and civil society organizations around the world. These networks, in a variety of forms, will continue to generate global knowledge for action. The Commission built further evidence-gathering partnerships through two continuing regional networks (the Nordic and Asian networks) and with researchers in additional key thematic areas, such as ageing, Indigenous Peoples, food and nutrition, violence and conflict, and the environment. The reports produced by the Knowledge Networks and all other background papers and reports, including reports from the Country and Civil Society work streams, are available on the Commission's website: **www. who.int/social_determinants/en**.

An unfinished agenda

The list of determinants of health inequities explored by the Commission was not exhaustive. Other areas of vital global importance, such as climate change, were not addressed in detail. The Commission recognizes this critical agenda, and the amount of work already ongoing to address it, and aligns itself with the goals of equitable and sustainable development.

Climate change

Climate change stands out as a priority area for attention in relation to health inequities. Climate change, urbanization, rural development, agriculture, and food security are intertwined determinants of population health and health equity. It is critical to ensure that economic and social policy responses to climate change and other environmental degradation take into account health equity. But much more analysis of the relationship between social determinants, environmental change, and health inequities is needed to inform the necessary development of policy and practice. The Stern report demonstrated compellingly that if action is not taken, the overall costs of climate change will be equivalent to losing at least 5% of global GDP each year (Stern, 2006). Therefore, the investment that takes place in the next 10-20 years will have a profound and long-lasting effect not only on the climate but on the health of our children and our children's children. It is likely that effects will be stronger among those at socioeconomic disadvantage.

Research agenda

The Commission has brought together an unprecedented global evidence base on social determinants of health and action for health equity. There is a need, though, to expand the scope of evidence across thematic areas and across country contexts. In addition, the social and economic drivers of health inequities are dynamic, changing over time. A regular review of key research gaps can help to identify the most pressing research needs. Some of the overarching research needs that have emerged from the work of the Commission are:

1. The determinants of health inequities in addition to the determinants of average population health:

   - understanding reasons for the relationship between social stratification and health outcomes;

   - understanding the interaction between aspects of stratification (for example, gender, ethnicity, and income) and health inequities;

   - quantifying the impact of supra-national political, economic, and social systems on health and health inequities within and between countries.

2. Interventions, global to local, to address the social determinants of health and health equity:

   - evaluating the impact of societal-level action (policies and programmes) on health inequities;

   - research on the social, economic, and health costs and benefits of reducing health inequities.

3. Policy analysis:

   - analysing policy processes towards health equity-related interventions;

   - understanding contextual barriers and enablers to ISA and coherence in national and local governance and policy-making;

   - identifying current good practice and developing tools for ISA.

4. Monitoring and measurement:

   - developing new methodologies for measuring and monitoring health inequities, and for assessing the impact of population-level interventions.

Goals and targets for health equity

The Commission has made its recommendations and has set global challenges. Progress towards health equity requires goals and measurable objectives along the way. Goals and targets can redirect policy, improve resource allocation, and improve development outcomes. Regular public reporting, and the development of data systems, globally and nationally, ensure that the world can see which targets are being met and where further efforts are needed.

This has been seen with the MDGs. The MDGs have also brought into focus the importance of good statistics in setting and monitoring major targets in development policy. Achieving the health-related MDGs and targets at the country level implies a reduction of absolute between–country health inequities. Currently, these goals do not embody a perspective of health equity within countries. Indeed, the MDGs for health outcomes are formulated in terms of population averages, rather than including the distribution of health outcomes within and between countries.

Extending beyond the current focus of the MDGs and their timeline of 2015, the Commission concerns itself certainly with the health inequity between countries, but also with the social gradient in health within high-, middle-, and low-income countries, and with the impact on adult mortality due to communicable and non-communicable diseases and violence/injury.

The goal that the Commission would like to see the world – its leaders, international organizations, national governments, and civil society groups – aspire to is:

Close the health gap in a generation

Progress towards this aspirational goal requires a narrowing of the gap between the worst off and the best off over time. It also involves a progressive flattening of the health gradient by improving the health of all social groups to a level closer to that of the most advantaged.

It is for international agencies and national governments to develop detailed goals and targets for health equity and the social determinants of health through consultative processes and to institute action plans that demonstrate clearly how the targets are to be achieved and what resources will be required. As a starting point, the Commission proposes three targets (below). They are challenging and illustrate the scale of the problem. However, if pursued through action as recommended by the Commission, much will be done towards closing the health gap in a generation. The Commission urges WHO to develop these health equity targets in consultation and to take the lead in achieving them.

Target 1: *Reduce by 10 years, between 2000 and 2040, the LEB gap between the one third of countries with the highest and the one third of countries with the lowest LEB levels, by levelling up countries with lower LEB.*

Halve, between 2000 and 2040, the LEB gap between social groups within countries, by levelling up the LEB of lower socioeconomic groups.

Target 2: *Halve, between 2000 and 2040, adult mortality rates in all countries and in all social groups within countries.*

In effect, achieving this target means reducing the gap in adult mortality between and within countries by half.

Target 3: *Reduce by 90%, between 2000 and 2040, the under-5 mortality rate in all countries and all social groups within countries, and reduce by 95%, between 2000 and 2040, the maternal mortality rate in all countries and all social groups within countries.*

In effect, achieving this target means reducing the gap in under-5 mortality between and within countries by 90%, and reducing the gap in maternal mortality between and within countries by 95%.

As stated in Chapter 1, while we do not anticipate the absolute abolition of health differences in a generation, we do see the potential to reduce – dramatically – inequity within and between countries. In order to define the targets set out here, past trends of well-performing groups of countries were projected forward. In the case of Target 1 (LEB), the trend between 1950 and 1980 was considered – a period when there was a reduction in the global LEB gap. In some cases, in particular in the case of within-country inequities in LEB, few data were available to use as a basis to define the target. Target 3 roughly projects MDGs 4A and 5A[11] to 2040. Targets 2 and 3 are based on the principle that decreases in mortality should be at least proportional across countries and across social groups within countries. More specifically, countries and social groups with the highest mortality levels should achieve at least the same proportional mortality decline as countries and social groups with lower mortality levels. Achieving these targets, with the above principle, will assure that absolute mortality inequities between countries and between social groups within countries will decline. Relative inequities will either stay the same or, if a more than proportional mortality increase is achieved, will decline. More ambitiously, the Commission would like to see accelerated improvement within social groups and countries with worse health outcomes.

Achieving the targets will be challenging. First, it is well known that the world is having serious difficulty with achieving MDGs 4 and 5, in particular in sub-Saharan Africa but also in countries in other regions. India, for example, is not on track to meet MDG 4 (Countdown Group, 2008). Similarly, these countries and regions will face great challenges achieving the magnitude of mortality reductions laid out above. It is, however, a global responsibility to achieve these goals, not least because of the global-level determinants of health inequities between and within countries. The strong declines in childhood mortality between 1950 and 1980 suggest that it should be feasible to achieve MDG 4 and Target 3 for under-5 mortality. Indeed, there are countries that are performing well on MDGs 4 and 5. Indonesia and Peru, with their 6.2% and 7.1% average annual reduction in under-5 mortality, for example, are on track to reach MDG 4 (Countdown Group, 2008) as well as Target 3 for under-5 mortality. Reduction in under-5 mortality in India (less then 3% per year) is, however, insufficient to meet MDG 4 (Countdown Group, 2008).

Achieving these Targets will require commitment to sustained investment in the social determinants of health, and will only be realistic if very strong and focused efforts are made – with particular attention to those countries and regions that are currently not expected to meet the MDGs. Yet while highly ambitious, achieving the Targets is possible with sufficiently proactive measures. In India maternal mortality in 2005 was 450 per 100 000 live births; in China the rate is one tenth that in India, namely 45 per 100 000 live births (Countdown Group, 2008). Target 3 means that maternal mortality in India in 2040 – more than three decades from now – should be 22.5 per 100 000 live births, in absolute terms not much less than China's maternal mortality rate today.

These Targets are proposed for consultation and further development. The process of setting targets, if carried out in a consultative fashion, can itself build collaborative partnerships

---

11 MDG 4A: Reduce by two thirds, between 1990 and 2015, the under-5 mortality rate. MDG 5A: Reduce by three quarters, between 1990 and 2015, the maternal mortality ratio.

that support achievement of the intended outcomes (Kickbusch, 2003). Steps towards achieving and, importantly, monitoring the targets can be taken now, as outlined in the recommendations throughout this report. Countries and international organizations are invited to reassess existing targets and incorporate an equity component within them. The general principle of at least proportional mortality decline across countries and social groups may be applied across a number of existing targets.

It is critical that international organizations and countries integrate measures of health equity and the social determinants of health in their existing monitoring systems. Targets for the social determinants of health and health equity will need to be defined on the basis of the framework laid out in Chapter 16 (*The Social Determinants of Health: Monitoring, Research, and Training*).

Milestones towards health equity – short- to medium-term deliverables

Having proposed recommendations for action and suggested targets, it is also important that milestones be set. Using these, it will be possible to monitor the progress of action on the social determinants of health and health equity within the global and national arenas and also help to ensure international institutions, national governments, civil society, and the private sector are held to account. To initiate such a process, the Commission outlines below a timeline of key but partial deliverables.

Table 17.1: Milestones towards health equity

Date	Milestone
November 2008	Global conference: "Closing the Gap in a Generation: Health Equity through Action on the Social Determinants of Health".
2008–09	Creation of post-Commission global alliance to take forward the social determinants of health agenda in partnership with WHO.
2008–09	Economic and social costing of Commission recommendations and costs of not taking action.
2009	Meetings of Commissioners and social determinants of health champions to advance global plan for dissemination and implementation of Commission recommendations.
2009	World Health Assembly resolution on social determinants of health and health equity.
2008–13	Research funders progressively dedicate more resources to research on social determinants of health, especially in areas highlighted by the Commission.
2008–13	Increasing numbers of countries adopt a social determinants of health approach to health equity and develop and implement social determinants of health policies, so that by 2013 at least 50% of all low-, middle-, and high-income countries have a committed plan for action to reduce health inequity through action on the social determinants of health, with evidence that they are implementing the plan.
2009–10	The Economic and Social Council, supported by WHO, set up a UN interagency mechanism for social determinants of health with working groups dedicated to specific thematic areas, initially on ECD, gender equity, employment and working conditions, health-care systems, and participatory governance, including all relevant multilateral agencies and civil society stakeholders.
2010	The Economic and Social Council, supported by WHO, prepare for consideration by the UN the adoption of health equity as a core global development goal, with appropriate indicators to monitor progress both within and between countries.
2010	1st Report on Health Equity (report on global and national health equity surveillance framework indicators and targets) to 1st Global Forum of UN Member States on social determinants of health and health equity.
2013	Review of progress on WHO social determinants of health targets.
2015	MDG target date; review of progress from health equity perspective: second 5-yearly global health equity report and Global Forum.
2020–2040	5-yearly reviews of progress on reducing health inequities within and between countries.

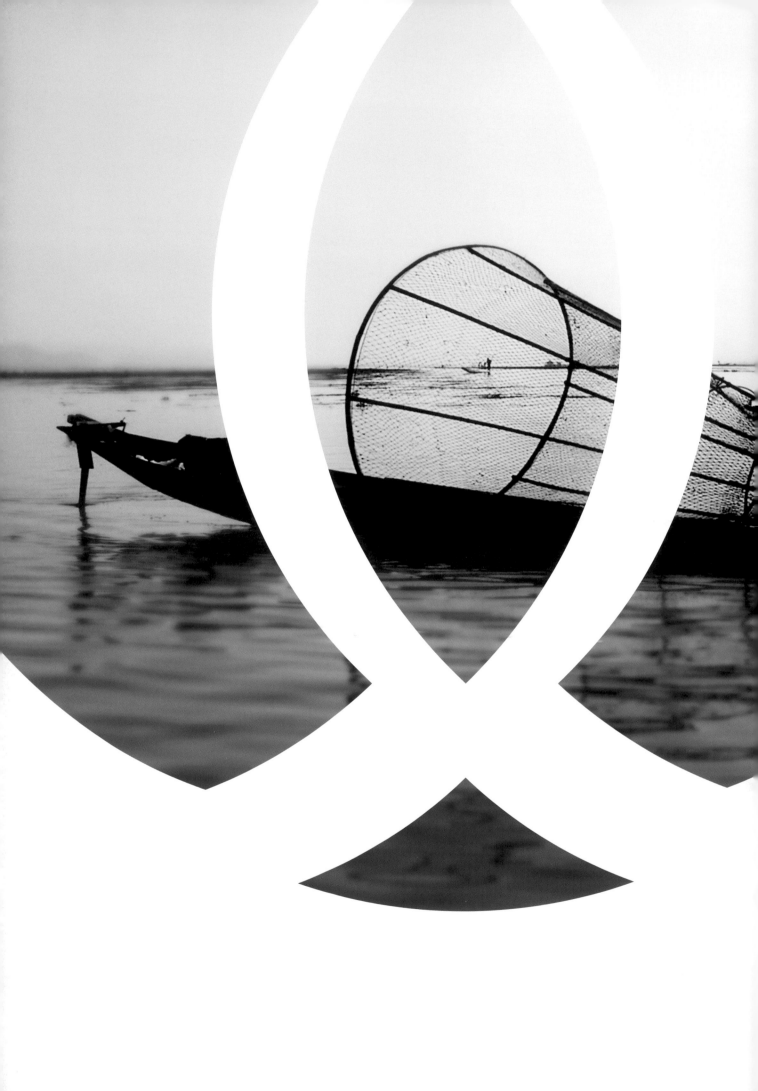

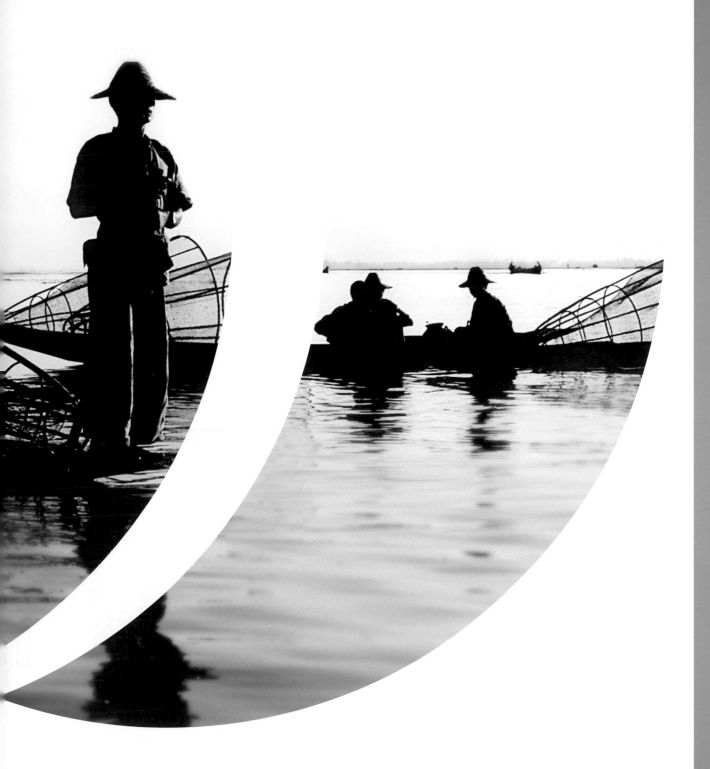

OVERARCHING RECOMMENDATION No. 1
Improve Daily Living Conditions

Improve the well-being of girls and women and the circumstances in which their children are born, put major emphasis on early child development and education for girls and boys, improve living and working conditions and create social protection policy supportive of all, and create conditions for a flourishing older life. Policies to achieve these goals will involve civil society, governments, and global institutions.

Chapter 5: Equity from the Start

Action Area 1: Commit to and implement a comprehensive approach to early life, building on existing child survival programmes and extending interventions in early life to include social/emotional and language/cognitive development.

The Commission recommends that:

5.1. WHO and UNICEF set up an interagency mechanism to ensure policy coherence for early child development such that, across agencies, a comprehensive approach to early child development is acted on (see Rec 15.2; 16.8).

5.2. Governments build universal coverage of a comprehensive package of quality early child development programmes and services for children, mothers, and other caregivers, regardless of ability to pay (see Rec 9.1; 11.6; 16.1).

Action Area 2: Expand the provision and scope of education to include the principles of early child development (physical, social/emotional, and language/cognitive development).

The Commission recommends that:

5.3. Governments provide quality education that pays attention to children's physical, social/emotional, and language/cognitive development, starting in pre-primary school.

5.4. Governments provide quality compulsory primary and secondary education for all boys and girls, regardless of ability to pay, identify and address the barriers to girls and boys enrolling and staying in school, and abolish user fees for primary school (see Rec 6.4; 13.4).

Chapter 6: Healthy Places Healthy People

Action Area 1: Place health and health equity at the heart of urban governance and planning.

The Commission recommends that:

6.1. Local government and civil society, backed by national government, establish local participatory governance mechanisms that enable communities and local government to partner in building healthier and safer cities (see Rec 14.3).

6.2. National and local government, in collaboration with civil society, manage urban development to ensure greater availability of affordable quality housing. With support from UN-HABITAT where necessary, invest in urban slum upgrading including, as a priority, provision of water and sanitation, electricity, and paved streets for all households regardless of ability to pay (see Rec 15.2).

6.3. Local government and civil society plan and design urban areas to promote physical activity through investment in active transport; encourage healthy eating through retail planning to manage the availability of and access to food; and reduce violence and crime through good environmental design and regulatory controls, including control of the number of alcohol outlets (see Rec 12.3).

Action Area 2: Promote health equity between rural and urban areas through sustained investment in rural development, addressing the exclusionary policies and processes that lead to rural poverty, landlessness, and displacement of people from their homes.

The Commission recommends that:

6.4. National and local government develop and implement policies and programmes that focus on: issues of rural land tenure and rights; year-round rural job opportunities; agricultural development and fairness in international trade arrangements; rural infrastructure including health, education, roads, and services; and policies that protect the health of rural-to-urban migrants (see Rec 5.4; 9.3).

Action Area 3: Ensure that economic and social policy responses to climate change and other environmental degradation take into account health equity.

The Commission recommends that:

6.5. International agencies and national governments, building on the Intergovernmental Panel on Climate Change recommendations, consider the health equity impact of agriculture, transport, fuel, buildings, industry, and waste strategies concerned with adaptation to and mitigation of climate change.

Chapter 7: Fair Employment and Decent Work

Action Area 1: Make full and fair employment and decent work a central goal of national and international social and economic policy-making.

The Commission recommends that:

7.1. Full and fair employment and decent work be made a shared objective of international institutions and a central part of national policy agendas and development strategies, with strengthened representation of workers in the creation of policy, legislation, and programmes relating to employment and work (see Rec 10.2; 14.3; 15.2).

Action Area 2: Achieving health equity requires safe, secure, and fairly paid work, year-round work opportunities, and healthy work–life balance for all.

The Commission recommends that:

7.2. National governments develop and implement economic and social policies that provide secure work and a living wage that takes into account the real and current cost of living for health (see Rec 8.1; 13.5).

7.3. Public capacity be strengthened to implement regulatory mechanisms to promote and enforce fair employment and decent work standards for all workers (see Rec 12.3).

7.4. Governments reduce insecurity among people in precarious work arrangements including informal work, temporary work, and part-time work through policy and legislation to ensure that wages are based on the real cost of living, social security, and support for parents (see Rec 8.3).

Action Area 3: Improve working conditions for all workers to reduce exposure to material hazards, work-related stress, and health-damaging behaviours.

The Commission recommends that:

7.5. OHS policy and programmes be applied to all workers – formal and informal – and that the range be expanded to include work-related stressors and behaviours as well as exposure to material hazards (see Rec 9.1).

Chapter 8: Social Protection Across the Lifecourse

Action Area 1: Establish and strengthen universal comprehensive social protection policies that support a level of income sufficient for healthy living for all.

The Commission recommends that:

8.1. Governments, where necessary with help from donors and civil society organizations, and where appropriate in collaboration with employers, build universal social protection systems and increase their generosity towards a level that is sufficient for healthy living (see Rec 7.2; 11.1).

8.2. Governments, where necessary with help from donors and civil society organizations, and where appropriate in collaboration with employers, use targeting only as back up for those who slip through the net of universal systems.

Action Area 2: Extend social protection systems to those normally excluded.

The Commission recommends that:

8.3. Governments, where necessary with help from donors and civil society organizations, and where appropriate in collaboration with employers, ensure that social protection systems extend to include those who are in precarious work, including informal work and household or care work (see Rec 7.4; 11.1; 13.3).

Chapter 9: Universal Health Care

Action Area 1: Build health-care systems based on principles of equity, disease prevention, and health promotion.

The Commission recommends that:

9.1 National governments, with civil society and donors, build health-care services on the principle of universal coverage of quality services, focusing on Primary Health Care (see Rec 5.2; 7.5; 8.1; 10.4; 13.6; 14.3; 15.2; 16.8).

Action Area 2: Ensure that health-care system financing is equitable.

The Commission recommends that:

9.2. National governments ensure public sector leadership in health-care systems financing, focusing on tax-/insurance-based funding, ensuring universal coverage of health care regardless of ability to pay, and minimizing out-of-pocket health spending (see Rec 10.4; 11.1; 11.2).

Action Area 3: Build and strengthen the health workforce, and expand capabilities to act on the social determinants of health.

The Commission recommends that:

9.3. National governments and donors increase investment in medical and health personnel, balancing health-worker density in rural and urban areas (see Rec 6.4; 16.5).

9.4. International agencies, donors and national governments address the health human resources brain drain, focusing on investment in increased health human resources and training, and bilateral agreements to regulate gains and losses.

OVERARCHING RECOMMENDATION No. 2

Tackle the Inequitable Distribution of Power, Money, and Resources

In order to address health inequities, and inequitable conditions of daily living, it is necessary to address inequities – such as those between men and women – in the way society is organized. This requires a strong public sector that is committed, capable, and adequately financed. To achieve that requires more than strengthened government – it requires strengthened governance: legitimacy, space and support for civil society, for an accountable private sector, and for people across society to agree public interests and reinvest in the value of collective action. In a globalized world, the need for governance dedicated to equity applies equally from the community level to global institutions.

Chapter 10: Health Equity in All Policies, Systems, and Programmes

Action Area 1: Place responsibility for action on health and health equity at the highest level of government, and ensure its coherent consideration across all policies.

The Commission recommends that:

10.1. Parliament and equivalent oversight bodies adopt a goal of improving health equity through action on the social determinants of health as a measure of government performance (see Rec 13.2; 15.1).

10.2. National government establish a whole-of-government mechanism that is accountable to parliament, chaired at the highest political level possible (see Rec 11.1; 11.2; 11.5; 12.2; 13.2; 16.6).

10.3. The monitoring of social determinants and health equity indicators be institutionalized and health equity impact assessment of all government policies, including finance, be used (see Rec 12.1; 15.1; 16.2; 16.7).

Action Area 2: Get the health sector right – adopt a social determinants framework across the policy and programmatic functions of the ministry of health and strengthen its stewardship role in supporting a social determinants approach across government.

The Commission recommends that:

10.4. The health sector expands its policy and programmes in health promotion, disease prevention, and health care to include a social determinants of health approach, with leadership from the minister of health (see Rec 9.1).

10.5. WHO support the development of knowledge and capabilities of national ministries of health to work within a social determinants of health framework, and to provide a stewardship role in supporting a social determinants approach across government (see Rec 15.3; 16.8).

Chapter 11: Fair Financing

Action Area 1: Strengthen public finance for action on the social determinants of health.

The Commission recommends that:

11.1. Donors, multilateral agencies and Member States build and strengthen national capacity for progressive taxation (see Rec 8.1; 8.3; 9.2; 10.2).

11.2. New national and global public finance mechanisms be developed, including special health taxes and global tax options (see Rec 9.2; 10.2).

Action Area 2: Increase international finance for health equity, and coordinate increased finance through a social determinants of health action framework.

The Commission recommends that:

11.3. Donor countries honour existing commitments by increasing aid to 0.7% of GDP; expand the Multilateral Debt Relief Initiative; and coordinate aid use through a social determinants of health framework (see Rec 13.6; 15.2).

11.4. International finance institutions ensure transparent terms and conditions for international borrowing and lending, to help avoid future unsustainable debt.

Action Area 3: Fairly allocate government resources for action on the social determinants of health.

The Commission recommends that:

11.5. National and local governments and civil society establish a cross-government mechanism to allocate budget to action on social determinants of health (see Rec 10.2).

11.6. Public resources be equitably allocated and monitored between regions and social groups, for example, using an equity gauge (see Rec 5.2; 14.3; 16.2).

Chapter 12: Market Responsibility

Action Area 1: Institutionalize consideration of health and health equity impact in national and international economic agreements and policy-making.

The Commission recommends that:

12.1. WHO, in collaboration with other relevant multilateral agencies, supporting Member States, institutionalize health equity impact assessment, globally and nationally, of major global, regional and bilateral economic agreements (see Rec 10.3; 16.7).

12.2. Government policy-setting bodies, with support from WHO, ensure and strengthen representation of public health in domestic and international economic policy negotiations (see Rec 10.2).

Action Area 2: Reinforce the primary role of the state in the provision of basic services essential to health (such as water/ sanitation) and the regulation of goods and services with a major impact on health (such as tobacco, alcohol, and food).

The Commission recommends that:

12.3. National governments, in collaboration with relevant multilateral agencies, strengthen public sector leadership in the provision of essential health-related goods/services and control of health-damaging commodities (see Rec 6.3; 7.3).

Chapter 13: Gender Equity

Action Area 1: Address gender biases in the structures of society – in laws and their enforcement, in the way organizations are run and interventions designed, and the way in which a country's economic performance is measured.

The Commission recommends that:

13.1. Governments create and enforce legislation that promotes gender equity and makes discrimination on the basis of sex illegal (see Rec 14.1).

13.2. Governments and international institutions set up within the central administration and provide adequate and long-term funding for a gender equity unit that is mandated to analyse and to act on the gender equity implications of policies, programmes, and institutional arrangements (see Rec 10.2; 15.2).

13.3. Governments include the economic contribution of household work, care work, and voluntary work in national accounts and strengthen the inclusion of informal work (see Rec 8.3).

Action Area 2: Develop and finance policies and programmes that close gaps in education and skills, and that support female economic participation.

The Commission recommends that:

13.4. Governments and donors invest in expanding girls' and women's capabilities through investment in formal and vocational education and training (see Rec 5.4).

13.5 Governments and employers support women in their economic roles by guaranteeing pay-equity by law, ensuring equal opportunity for employment at all levels, and by setting up family-friendly policies that ensure that women and men can take on care responsibilities in an equal manner (see Rec 7.2).

Action Area 3: Reaffirm commitment to addressing sexual and reproductive health and rights universally.

The Commission recommends that:

13.6. Governments, donors, international organizations, and civil society increase their political commitment to and investment in sexual and reproductive health services and programmes, building to universal coverage (see Rec 9.1; 11.3).

Chapter 14: Political Empowerment – Inclusion and Voice

Action Area 1: Empower all groups in society through fair representation in decision-making about how society operates, particularly in relation to its effect on health equity, and create and maintain a socially inclusive framework for policy-making.

The Commission recommends that:

14.1. National government strengthens the political and legal systems to ensure they promote the equal inclusion of all (see Rec 13.1; 16.1).

14.2. National government acknowledges, legitimizes, and supports marginalized groups, in particular Indigenous Peoples, in policy, legislation, and programmes that empower people to represent their needs, claims, and rights.

14.3. National- and local-level government ensure the fair representation of all groups and communities in decision-making that affects health, and in subsequent programme and service delivery and evaluation (see Rec 6.1; 7.1; 9.1; 11.6).

Action Area 2: Enable civil society to organize and act in a manner that promotes and realizes the political and social rights affecting health equity.

The Commission recommends that:

14.4. Empowerment for action on health equity through bottom-up, grassroots approaches requires support for civil society to develop, strengthen, and implement health equity-oriented initiatives.

Chapter 15: Good Global Governance

Action Area 1: Make health equity a global development goal, and adopt a social determinants of health framework to strengthen multilateral action on development.

The Commission recommends that:

15.1. By 2010, the Economic and Social Council, supported by WHO, should prepare for consideration by the UN the adoption of health equity as a core global development goal, with appropriate indicators to monitor progress both within and between countries (see Rec 10.1; 10.3; 16.3).

15.2. By 2010, the Economic and Social Council, supported by WHO, prepare for consideration by the UN the establishment of thematic social determinants of health working groups – initially on early child development, gender equity, employment and working conditions, health-care systems, and participatory governance – including all relevant multilateral agencies and civil society stakeholders, reporting back regularly (see Rec 5.1; 6.2; 9.1; 13.2).

Action Area 2: Strengthen WHO leadership in global action on the social determinants of health, institutionalizing social determinants of health as a guiding principle across WHO departments and country programmes.

The Commission recommends that:

15.3. WHO institutionalizes a social determinants of health approach across all working sectors, from headquarters to country level (see Rec 10.5; 16.8).

OVERARCHING RECOMMENDATION No. 3
Measure and Understand the Problem and Assess the Impact of Action

Acknowledging that there is a problem, and ensuring that health inequity is measured – within countries and globally – is a vital platform for action. National governments and international organizations, supported by WHO, should set up national and global health equity surveillance systems for routine monitoring of health inequity and the social determinants of health and should evaluate the health equity impact of policy and action. Creating the organizational space and capacity to act effectively on health inequity requires investment in training of policy-makers and health practitioners and public understanding of social determinants of health. It also requires a stronger focus on social determinants in public health research.

Chapter 16: Social Determinants of Health: Monitoring, Training, and Research

Action Area 1: Ensure that routine monitoring systems for health equity and the social determinants of health are in place, locally, nationally, and internationally.

The Commission recommends that:

16.1. Governments ensure that all children are registered at birth without financial cost to the household. This should be part of improvement of civil registration for births and deaths (see Rec 5.2; 14.1).

16.2. National governments establish a national health equity surveillance system, with routine collection of data on social determinants of health and health inequity (see Rec 10.3).

16.3. WHO stewards the creation of a global health equity surveillance system as part of a wider global governance structure (see Rec 15.1).

Action area 2: Invest in generating and sharing new evidence on the ways in which social determinants influence population health and health equity and on the effectiveness of measures to reduce health inequities through action on social determinants.

The Commission recommends that:

16.4. Research funding bodies create a dedicated budget for generation and global sharing of evidence on social determinants of health and health equity, including health equity intervention research.

Action area 3: Provide training on the social determinants of health to policy actors, stakeholders, and practitioners and invest in raising public awareness.

The Commission recommends that:

16.5. Educational institutions and relevant ministries make the social determinants of health a standard and compulsory part of training of medical and health professionals (see Rec 9.3).

16.6. Educational institutions and relevant ministries act to increase understanding of the social determinants of health among non-medical professionals and the general public (see Rec 10.2).

16.7. Governments build capacity for health equity impact assessment among policy-makers and planners across government departments (see Rec 10.3; 12.1).

16.8. WHO strengthens its capacity to provide technical support for action on the social determinants of health globally, nationally, and locally (see Rec 5.1; 9.1; 10.5; 15.3).

Commissioner Biographies

Michael Marmot is Chair of the Commission on Social Determinants of Health. He is Director of the International Institute for Society and Health and Head of the Department of Epidemiology and Public Health at University College London. In 2000, he was knighted for services to epidemiology and understanding health inequalities.

Frances Baum is Head of Department and Professor of Public Health at Flinders University and Foundation Director of the South Australian Community Health Research Unit. She is Co-Chair of the Global Coordinating Council of the People's Health Movement.

Monique Bégin is Professor at the School of Management, University of Ottawa, Canada, and twice-appointed Minister of National Health and Welfare. She was the first woman from Quebec elected to the House of Commons.

Giovanni Berlinguer is a Member of the European Parliament. He has recently been a member of the International Bioethics Committee of UNESCO (2001–2007) and rapporteur of the project Universal Declaration on Bioethics.

Mirai Chatterjee is the Coordinator of Social Security for India's Self-Employed Women's Association, a trade union of over 900 000 self-employed women. She was recently appointed to the National Advisory Council and the National Commission for the Unorganised Sector.

William H. Foege is Emeritus Presidential Distinguished Professor of International Health, Emory University. He was Director of the United States Centers for Disease Control and Prevention (CDC), Chief of the CDC Smallpox Eradication Program, and Executive Director of The Carter Center. He also served as Senior Medical Advisor for the Bill and Melinda Gates Foundation.

Yan Guo is a Professor of Public Health and Vice-President of the Peking University Health Science Centre. She is Vice-Chairman of the Chinese Rural Health Association and Vice-Director of the China Academy of Health Policy.

Kiyoshi Kurokawa is Professor at the National Graduate Institute for Policy Studies, Tokyo. He also serves as a Member of the Science and Technology Policy Committee of the Cabinet Office. Previously he was President of the Science Council of Japan and the Pacific Science Association.

Ricardo Lagos Escobar is the former President of Chile, and former Education Minister and Minister of Public Works. An economist and lawyer by qualification, he also worked as an economist for the United Nations.

Alireza Marandi is Professor of Pediatrics at Shaheed Beheshti University, Islamic Republic of Iran. He is former two-term Minister of Health (and Medical Education). In addition, he served as Deputy Minister and Advisor to the Minister. He was recently elected to be a member of the Iranian Parliament.

Pascoal Mocumbi is the High Representative of the European and Developing Countries Clinical Trials Partnership and former Prime Minister of the Republic of Mozambique. Prior to that, he headed the Ministry of Foreign Affairs and the Ministry of Health.

Ndioro Ndiaye is the Deputy Director-General of the International Organization for Migration and was formerly Minister for Social Development and Minister for Women's, Children's and Family Affairs in Senegal.

Charity Kaluki Ngilu is Minister of Health of Kenya. Before taking office, she was a member of the National Assembly of Kenya representing the Democratic Party. Since 1989, she has been the leader of the Macnbeleo ya Wanawake organization, the national women's movement.

Hoda Rashad is Director and Research Professor of the Social Research Center of the American University in Cairo. She is a member of the Senate, one of the two parliamentary bodies in Egypt. She serves on the National Council for Women, which reports to the President of Egypt.

Amartya Sen is Lamont University Professor and Professor of Economics and Philosophy at Harvard University. In 1998, he was awarded the Nobel Prize in Economics.

David Satcher is Director of the Center of Excellence on Health Disparities and the Satcher Health Leadership Institute Initiative. He served as United States Surgeon General and Assistant Secretary for Health. He also served as Director of the Centers for Disease Control and Prevention.

Anna Tibaijuka is Executive Director of UN-HABITAT. She is also the founding Chairperson of the independent Tanzanian National Women's Council.

Denny Vågerö is Professor of Medical Sociology and Director of CHESS (Centre for Health Equity Studies) in Sweden. He is a member of the Royal Swedish Academy of Sciences, and of its Standing Committee on Health.

Gail Wilensky is a senior fellow at Project HOPE, an international health education foundation. Previously she directed the Medicare and Medicaid programmes in the United States and also chaired two commissions that advise the United States Congress on Medicare.

References

Aboriginal and Torres Islander Social Justice Commissioner (2005). *Social justice report*. Sydney, Human Rights & Equal Opportunity Commission. (**http://www.hreoc. gov.au/social_justice/sj_report/sjreport05/pdf/ SocialJustice2005.pdf**, accessed 20 February 2008).

Abramson JH (1988). Community-oriented primary care – strategy, approaches and practice: a review. *Public Health Review*, 16:35-98.

Acosta M (2006). *Identity rights, civil registration and asset accumulation*. Brookings/Ford Workshop Asset-based Approaches. Washington, DC, Brookings Institution (**http:// www.brookings.edu/**, accessed March 2008).

Action for Healthy Kids (2007). Action for Healthy Kids 2005-2006 Annual Report. Skokie, IL, Action for Healthy Kids. (**http://www.actionforhealthykids.org/pdf/AFHK_ report_FINAL_5_7_07.pdf**, accessed 13 May 2008)

Adlung R (2006). Public Services and the GATS. *Journal of International Economic Law*, 9:455-485.

Agency for Healthcare Research and Quality (2003). *National Healthcare Disparities Report: inequality in quality exists*. Rockville, MD, Agency for Healthcare Research and Quality. (**http://www.ahrq.gov/QUAL/nhdr03/nhdrsum03. htm#Inequality**, accessed 7 March 2008).

Aiyer A (2007). The allure of the transnational: notes on some aspects of the political economy of water in India. *Cultural Anthropology*, 22:640-658.

Akin JS et al. (2005). Changes in access to health care in China, 1989-1997. *Health Policy and Planning*, 20:80-89.

Akin JS, Dow WH & Lance PM (2004). Did the distribution of health insurance in China continue to grow less equitable in the nineties? Results from a longitudinal survey. *Social Science and Medicine*, 58:293-304.

Alam KR (2006). Ganokendras: an innovative model for poverty reduction in Bangladesh. *International Review of Education*, 52:343-352.

Alliance for Healthy Cities (nd). *Alliance for Healthy Cities website*. Tokyo: Alliance for Healthy Cities (**http://www. alliance-healthycities.com**, accessed 10 April 2008).

Ambrose S (2006). Preserving disorder: IMF policies and Kenya's health care crisis. *Pambazuka News*. (**http://www. pambazuka.org/en/category/features/34800**, accessed 27 May 2008).

Arslanalp S & Henry PB (2006). Policy watch: debt relief. *Journal of Economic Perspectives*, 20:207-220.

Artazcoz L et al. (2005). Social inequalities in the impact of flexible employment on different domains of psychosocial health. *Journal of Epidemiology and Community Health*, 59:761-767.

Baez C & Barron P (2006). *Community voice and role in district health care systems in east and southern Africa: a literature review.*

Harare, EQUINET. (**http://www.equinetafrica.org/ bibl/docs/DIS39GOVbaez.pdf**, accessed 27 May 2008) (Discussion paper 39).

Bajpai N, Sachs JD & Volavka N (2005). *India's challenge to meet the Millennium Development Goals*. New York, The Earth Institute at Columbia University. (**http://www. earthinstitute.columbia.edu/cgsd/documents/bajpai_ indiamdgchallenge.pdf**, accessed 13 May 2008) (CGSD Working Paper No. 24).

Balabanova D (2007). *Health sector reform and equity in transition*. Prepared for the Health Care Systems Knowledge Network of the Commission on Social Determinants of Health. Geneva, World Health Organization.

Barriento S, Kabeer N & Hossain N (2004). *The gender dimensions of the globalization of production*. Geneva, Policy Integration Department, World Commission on the Social Dimension of Globalization, International Labour Office.

Barrientos A & Lloyd-Sherlock P (2000). Reforming health insurance in Argentina and Chile. *Health Policy and Planning*, 15:417-423.

Barrientos A & Lloyd-Sherlock P (2003). Health insurance reforms in Latin America – cream skimming, equity and cost containment. In: Haagh L & Helgo CT, eds. *Social policy reform and market governance in Latin America*. London, MacMillan, pp. 183-199

Barrientos S & Smith S (2007). Do workers benefit from ethical trade? Assessing codes of labour practice in global production systems. *Third World Quarterly*, 28:713-729.

Barrios S, Bertinelli L & Strobl E (2006). Climatic change and rural-urban migration: the case of sub-Saharan Africa. *Journal of Urban Economics*, 60:357-371.

Bartley M (2005). Job insecurity and its effect on health. *Journal of Epidemiology and Community Health*, 59:718-719.

Barton A et al. (2007). The Watcombe Housing Study: the short term health of residents. *Journal of Epidemiology and Community Health*, 61:771-777.

Bates I et al. (2004). Vulnerability to malaria, tuberculosis, and HIV/AIDS infection and disease. Part II: Determinants operating at environmental and institutional level. *Lancet Infectious Diseases*, 4:368-375.

Bauer PT (1981). *Equality, the third world, and economic delusion*. Cambridge, Harvard University Press.

Baum F (1995). Researching public health: behind the qualitative-quantitative methodological debate. *Social Science and Medicine*, 40:459-468.

Baum F, ed. (1995). *Health for all: the South Australian experience*. Adelaide, Wakefield Press.

Baum F (2007). Cracking the nut of health equity: top down and bottom up pressure for action on the social determinants of health, *Promotion and Education*, 14:90-95.

Baum F (2008). *The new public health*. New York, Oxford University Press.

Baum F, Fry D & Lennie I, eds. (1992). *Community health in Australia: practice and policy*. Sydney, Pluto Press.

Baunsgaard T & Keen M (2005). *Tax revenue and (or?) trade liberalization*. Report No. WP/05/112. Washington, DC, International Monetary Fund.

Bégin M (1998). Gender issues in health care. Presentation at the Symposium on Women Health in Women's Hands, Brandon, Manitoba, Canada, 2 May 1998.

Benach J & Muntaner C (2007). Precarious employment and health: developing a research agenda. *Journal of Epidemiology and Community Health*, 61:276-277.

Bennett S & Gilson L (2001). *Health financing: designing and implementing pro-poor policy*. London, Health Systems Resource Centre.

Bettcher D, Yach D & Emmanuel Guindon G (2000). Global trade and health: key linkages and future challenges. *Bulletin of the World Health Organization*, 78:521-534.

Bhorat H (2003). A universal income grant scheme for South Africa: an empirical assessment. In: Standing G & Samson M, eds. *A basic income grant for South Africa*. Cape Town, UCT Press, pp. 77-101.

Bidani B & Ravaillon M (1997). Decomposing social indicators using distributional data. *Journal of Econometrics*, 77:125-139.

Bird G & Milne A (2003). Debt relief for low income countries: is it effective and efficient? *The World Economy*, 26:43-59.

Birdsall N (2006). *The world is not flat: inequality and injustice in our global economy*. WIDER Annual Lecture 2005. Helsinki, World Institute for Development Economics Research.

Black RE, Morris SS & Bryce J (2003). Where and why are 10 million children dying every year? *Lancet*, 361:2226-2234.

Black RE et al. (2008). Maternal and child undernutrition: global and regional exposures and health consequences. *Lancet*, 371:243-260.

Bloom DE (2007). *Education, health, and development*. Cambridge, MA, American Academy of Arts and Sciences. (**http://www.amacad.org/publications/ubase_edu_health_dev.pdf**, accessed 4 September 2007).

Blouin C (2007). Trade policy and health: from conflicting interests to policy coherence. *Bulletin of the World Health Organization* 85:169-172.

Blouin C et al. (2007). *Trade liberalisation*. Globalisation Knowledge Network synthesis paper 4. Background document of the Globalisation Knowledge Network of the Commission on Social Determinants of Health. Geneva, World Health Organization.

Blumenthal D & Hsiao W (2005). Privatization and its discontents – the evolving Chinese health care system. *New England Journal of Medicine*, 353:1165-1170.

Bokhari F, Gottret P & Gai Y (2005). *Government health expenditures, donor funding and health outcomes*. Washington, DC, World Bank.

Bond P & Dor G (2003). *A critique of uneven health outcomes and neoliberalism in Africa*. Johannesburg, EQUINET. (**http://www.equinetafrica.org/bibl/docs/DIS2trade.pdf**, accessed 26 March 2007) (Discussion Paper 2).

Boone P (1996). Politics and the effectiveness of foreign aid. *European Economic Review*, 40:289-328.

Bourguignon F (2006). *The case for equity*. Francois Bourguignon was Senior Vice-President and Chief Economist of the World Bank between 2003 and 2007. Washington, DC, World Bank (**http://go.worldbank.org/XY6WQUQOZ0**, accessed 9 May 2008).

Braveman P (1998). *Monitoring equity in health: a policy-oriented approach in low- and middle-income countries*. Geneva: World Health Organization (WHO/CHS/HSS/98.1).

Budds J & McGranahan G (2003). Are the debates on water privatization missing the point? Experiences from Africa, Asia and Latin America. *Environment and Urbanization*, 15:87-114.

Burnham G et al. (2006). Mortality after the 2003 invasion of Iraq: a cross-sectional cluster sample survey. *Lancet*, 368:1421-1428.

Buss P & Carvalho A (2007). Health promotion in Brazil. *Promotion and Education*, 14:209-213.

Caffery M & Frelick G (2006). *Attracting and retaining nurse tutors in Malawi*. Health workforce "Innovative Approaches and Promising Practices" study: the Capacity Project. (**http://www.interchurch.org/resources/uploads/files/242Malawi_Prompractices_Report_First_Official_Draft.doc**, accessed 8 February 2007).

Caldwell JC (1986). Routes to low mortality in poor countries. *Population and Development Review*, 12:171-220.

Campbell T & Campbell A (2007). Emerging disease burdens and the poor in cities of the developing world. *Journal of Urban Health*, 84:i54-i64.

Campbell-Lendrum D & Corvalan C (2007). Climate change and developing-country cities: implications for environmental health and equity. *Journal of Urban Health*, 84:i109-i117.

Canadian Health Services Research Foundation (2007). *Incorporate lay health workers to promote health and prevent disease*. Ottawa, Canadian Health Services Research Foundation. (**http://www.chsrf.ca/mythbusters/html/boost11_e.php**, accessed 24 January 2008).

Carrin G, Waelkens MP & Criel B (2005). Community-based health insurance in developing countries: a study of its contribution to the performance of health financing systems. *Tropical Medicine and International Health*, 10:799-811.

CASEL (nd). *How evidence-based SEL programs work to produce greater student success in school and life*. Chicago, Collaborative for Academic, Social and Emotional Learning. (**http://www.casel.org/downloads/academicbrief.pdf**, accessed 1 February 2008).

Catford J (2005). The Bangkok Conference: steering countries to build national capacity for health promotion. *Health Promotion International*, 20:1-6.

Chan M (2007). Speech to the Eleventh Global Forum for Health Research, Beijing, China, 29 October 2007. Geneva, World Health Organization. (**http://www.who.int/dg/speeches/2007/20071029_beijing/en/index.html**, accessed 10 April 2008).

Chan (2008). Speech to the International Federation of Red Cross and Red Crescent Societies Global Health and Care Forum 2008: primary health care starts with people, Geneva, 14 May 2008. (http://www.who.int/dg/speeches/2008/20080514/en/index.html, accessed 29 May 2008).

Chandler MJ & Lalonde CE (1998). Cultural continuity as a hedge against suicide in Canada's First Nations. *Horizons*, 10:68-72.

Chen S & Ravallion M (2004). How have the world's poorest fared since the early 1980s? *The World Bank Research Observer*, 19:141-169.

Chinyama V (2006). *Kenya's abolition of school fees offers lessons for the whole of Africa*. New York, UNICEF. (http://www.unicef.org/infobycountry/kenya_33391.html, accessed 5 February 2008).

Choi S-H (2002). *Integrating early childhood into education: the case of Sweden*. UNESCO Policy Brief on Early Childhood. Paris, UNESCO. (http://portal.unesco.org/education/en/ev.php-URL_ID=43971&URL_DO=DO_TOPIC&URL_SECTION=201.html, accessed 3 April 2008).

Chu KY, Davoodi H & Gupta S (2004). Income distribution and tax and government spending policies in developing countries. In: Cornia GA, ed. *Inequality, growth and poverty in an era of liberalisation and structural adjustment*. Oxford, Oxford University Press.

Cleland JG & Van Ginneken JK (1988). Maternal education and child survival in developing countries: the search for pathways of influence. *Social Science and Medicine*, 27:1357-1368.

Clemens M, Radelet S & Bhavnani R (2004). *Counting chickens when they hatch: the short-term effect of aid on growth*. Washington DC, Center for Global Development (Working Paper 44).

CMH (2001). *Macroeconomics and health: investing in health for economic development*. Report of the Commission on Macroeconomics and Health. Geneva, World Health Organization.

COAG (2007). *Communique of the Working Group on Indigenous reform*. Canberra, Council of Australian Governments (http://www.coag.gov.au/meetings/201207/index.htm#ind, accessed 2 May 2008).

Cobham A (2005). *Taxation policy and development*. Oxford, The Oxford Council on Good Governance (OCGG Economy Analysis no. 2).

Cohen PN (2007). *Closing the gap: equal pay for women workers*. Statement prepared for the Health, Education, Labor, and Pensions Committee of the US Senate, 12 April 2007. (http://help.senate.gov/Hearings/2007_04_12/Cohen.pdf, accessed 5 May 2008).

Collier P & Dollar D (2000). *Aid allocation and poverty reduction*. Washington, DC, World Bank (Policy Research Working Paper 2041).

Collier P (2006). *Rethinking assistance for Africa*. Oxford, Institute of Economic Affairs.

Connect International (nd). Connect International website. Leiden, Connect International (http://www.connectinternational.nl, accessed 9 May 2008).

Côté R (2002/3). Pay equity at last in Quebec? *Labour Education*, 128:57-60 (http://www.oit.org/public/english/dialogue/actrav/publ/ledpubl.htm, accessed 5 May 2008).

Countdown Group (2008). Countdown to 2015 for maternal, newborn, and survival: the 2008 report on tracking coverage and interventions. *Lancet*, 371:1247-1258.

Cruz-Saco MA (2002). *Global insurance companies and the privatisation of pensions and health care in Latin America – the case of Peru*. Presented at the Globalism and Social Policy Programme (GASPP) Seminar, Dubrovnik, Croatia.

CS (2007). *Civil society report*. Final report of the Civil Society work stream of the Commission on Social Determinants of Health. Geneva, World Health Organization.

Curriculum Corporation (nd). Mind Matters website. Melbourne, MindMatters (http://cms.curriculum.edu.au/mindmatters, accessed 13 May 2008.)

Cutler D & Lleras-Muney A (2006). *Education and health: evaluating theories and evidence*. Ann Arbor, National Poverty Center (National Poverty Center Working Paper Series: # 06-19) (http://www.npc.umich.edu/publications/workingpaper06/paper19/working-paper06-19.pdf, accessed 25 September 2007).

CW (2007). *Translating the social determinants evidence into a health equity agenda at the country level*. Report of the Country work stream of the Commission on Social Determinants of Health. Geneva, World Health Organization.

Dambisya Y, Modipa S & Legodi M (2005). *The distribution of pharmacists trained at the University of the North, South Africa*. Harare: EQUINET (http://www.equinetafrica.org/bibl/docs/Dis31HRdambisya.pdf, accessed 27 June 2007) (Discussion Paper 31).

Das Gupta M et al. (2005). *Improving child nutrition outcomes in India: can the Integrated Child Development Services programme be more effective?* Washington, DC, World Bank (World Bank Policy Research Working Paper 3647).

DAC (2005). Creditor Reporting System, Aid database. Paris, Organisation for Economic Cooperation and Development (http://www.oecd.org/department/0,2688,en_2649_34447_1_1_1_1_1,00.html, accessed 16 May 2008).

Davies JB et al. (2006). *The world distribution of household wealth*. Research of the United Nations University (UNU-WIDER). Helsinki, World Institute for Development Economics.

Davis KK, Scott Collins K & Hall AG (1999). *Community health centres in a changing US health care system*. New York, The Commonwealth Fund.

de Ferranti D et al. (2004). *Inequality in Latin America & the Caribbean: breaking with history?* Washington, DC, World Bank.

De Maeseneer J et al. (2007). *Primary health care as a strategy for achieving equitable care*. Paper prepared for the Health Care Systems Knowledge Network of the Commission on Social Determinants of Health. Geneva, World Health Organization.

Deacon B et al. (2003). *Global social governance: themes and prospects*. Helsinki, Ministry of Foreign Affairs for Finland.

Deaton A (2003). Health, inequality, and economic development. *Journal of Economic Literature*, 41:113-158.

Deaton A (2004). Health in an age of globalization. *Brookings Trade Forum*, 83-130.

Deaton A (2006a). Global patterns of income and health. WIDER Annual Lecture. WIDER Angle Newsletter, 2:1-3. (http://www.wider.unu.edu/publications/newsletter/en_GB/angle-introduction/_files/78200687251423272/default/angle2006-2.pdf, accessed 20 March 2008).

Deaton A (2006b). *Global patterns of income and health: facts, interpretations, and policies.* Helsinki, WIDER Annual Lecture.

Debbane AM (2007). The dry plight of freedom: commodifying water in the Western Cape, South Africa. *Antipode*, 39:222-226.

Deere CD & Leon M (2003). The gender asset gap: land in Latin America. *World Development*, 31:925-947.

Delhi Group on Informal Sector Statistics (nd). Delhi Group on Informal Sector Statistics website. New York, UN. (http://unstats.un.org/unsd/methods/citygroup/delhi.htm, accessed 28 May 2008).

Department for Communities and Local Government (2006). *Government action plan: implementing the Women and Work Commission recommendations.* London, Government Equalities Office (http://www.womenandequalityunit.gov.uk/publications/wwc_govtactionplan_sept06.pdf, accessed 5 May 2008).

Department of Health (2005). *Tackling health inequalities: status report on the Programme for Action.* London, Department of Health.

Department of Health (2007). *Review of the health inequalities infant mortality PSA target.* London, Department of Health.

Dervis K (2005). *The challenge of globalization: reinventing good global governance.* Keynote address. Washington, DC, George Washington Center for the Study of Globalization.

Dervis K & Birdsall N (2006). A stability and social investment facility for high-debt countries. Washington, DC, Center for Global Development (CGD Working Paper No. 27).

Devernam R (2007). On solid ground: preserving the quality of place. *Environmental Practice*, 9:3-5.

DFID (2008). *Helping Bolivia's poor to access their rights.* London, Department for International Development (http://www.dfid.gov.uk/news/files/south-america/bolivia-identity.asp, accessed March 6 2008).

DHS (nd). *Demographic and Health Surveys.* Calverton, MD, MEASURE DHS. (http://www.measuredhs.com, accessed 15 February 2008).

Dixon J et al. (2007). The health equity dimension of urban food systems. *Journal of Urban Health*, 84:i118-i129.

Doherty J & Govender R (2004). *The cost-effectiveness of primary care services in developing countries: a review of the international literature.* A background paper commissioned by the Disease Control Priorities Project. Washington, DC, World Bank.

Dorling D, Shaw M & Davey Smith G (2006). Global inequality of life expectancy due to AIDS. *BMJ*, 332;662-664.

Douglas M & Scott-Samuel A (2001). Addressing health inequalities in health impact assessment. *Journal of Epidemiology and Community Health*, 55:450-451.

Dreze J (2003). Food security and the right to food. In: Mahendra Dev S, Kannan K, Ramachandran N, eds. *Towards a food secure India: issues and policies.* New Delhi and Hyderabad, Institute for Human Development and Centre for Economic and Social Studies.

Dummer TJB & Cook IG (2007). Exploring China's rural health crisis: processes and policy implications. *Health Policy*, 83:1-16.

Easterly W (2006). *Planners vs. searchers in foreign aid.* ADB Distinguished Speakers Program, Asian Development Bank, 18 January 2006.

Eastwood R & Lipton M (2000). *Rural-urban dimensions of inequality change.* Helsinki, World Institute for Development.

ECDKN (2007a). *Early child development: a powerful equalizer.* Final report of the Early Child Development Knowledge Network of the Commission on Social Determinants of Health. Geneva, World Health Organization.

ECDKN (2007b). *Total environment assessment model for early child development.* Evidence report. Background document of the Early Child Development Knowledge Network of the Commission on Social Determinants of Health. Geneva, World Health Organization.

ECOSOC (1997). Agreed Conclusions 1997/2, 18 July 1997.

ECOSOC (nd). *Background information on the United Nations Economic and Social Council.* New York, United Nations (http://www.un.org/ecosoc/about, accessed 28 May 2008).

Edward P (2006). The ethical poverty line: a moral quantification of absolute poverty. *Third World Quarterly*, 27:377-393.

EFILWC (2007). *Industrial relations developments in Europe in 2006.* Dublin, European Foundation for the Improvement of Living and Working Conditions.

Eichler M, Reisman AL & Borins EM (1992). Gender bias in medical research. *Women and Therapy: a Feminist Quarterly*, 12:61-70.

Elinder LS (2005). Obesity, hunger, and agriculture: the damaging role of subsidies. *BMJ*, 331:1333-1336.

EMCONET (2007). *Employment conditions and health inequalities.* Final report of the Employment Conditions Knowledge Network of the Commission on Social Determinants of Health. Geneva, World Health Organization.

Engle PL et al. (2007). Strategies to avoid the loss of developmental potential in more than 200 million children in the developing world. *Lancet*, 369:229-242.

Epping-Jordan JE et al. (2005). Preventing chronic diseases: taking stepwise action. *Lancet*, 366:1667-1671.

EU (1997). Decision No. 1400/97/EC of the European Parliament and of the Council of 30 June 1997 adopting a programme of Community action on health monitoring within the framework for action in the field of public health (1997 to 2001). *Official Journal of the European Communities*, 40:1-10.

European Commission (1996). *A code of practice on the implementation of equal pay for work of equal value for women and men.* Brussels, European Commission (http://aei.pitt.edu/3963/, accessed 5 May 2008) (COM (96) 336 final, 17.07.1996).

EUROTHINE (2007). *Tackling health inequalities in Europe: an integrated approach.* EUROTHINE final report. Rotterdam, Department of Public Health, ErasmusMC University Medical Centre Rotterdam.

Farley M (2006). 14 nations will adopt airline tax to pay for AIDS drugs. *Los Angeles Times*, 3 June.

Farmer P (1999). Pathologies of power: rethinking health and human rights. *American Journal of Public Health*, 89:486-1496.

Fathalla MF et al. (2006). Sexual and reproductive health for all: a call for action. *Lancet*, 368:2095-100.

Felstead A et al. (2002). Opportunities to work at home in the context of work-life balance. *Human Resource Management Journal*, 12:54-76.

Fernald LC, Gertler PJ & Neufeld LM (2008). Role of cash in conditional cash transfer programmes for child health, growth, and development: an analysis of Mexico's Oportunidades. *Lancet*, 371:828-37.

Ferrie JE et al. (2002). Effects of chronic job insecurity and change of job security on self-reported health, minor psychiatry morbidity, psychological measures, and health related behaviours in British civil servants: the Whitehall II study. *Journal of Epidemiology and Community Health*, 56:450-454.

Forman L (2007). Right and wrongs: what utility for the right to health in reforming trade rules on medicines. Briefings volume four: comparative program on health and society and Lupina Foundation Working Paper Series. Toronto, Munk Centre for International Studies.

French HW (2006). Wealth grows, but health care withers in China. *New York Times*, January 14.

Friedman M (1958). Foreign economic aid: means and objectives. *The Yale Review*, 47.

Friel S, Chopra M & Satcher D (2007). Unequal weight: equity oriented policy responses to the global obesity epidemic. *BMJ*, 335:1241-1243.

Fröbel F, Heinrichs J & Kreye O (1980). *The new international division of labour*. Cambridge, Cambridge University Press.

Frumkin H, Frank L & Jackson R, eds. (2004). *Urban sprawl and public health: designing, planning and building for healthy communities*. Washington, DC, Island Press.

Galea S & Vlahov D (2005). *Handbook of urban health*. New York, Springer.

Galiani S, Gertler P & Schargrodsky E (2005). Water for life: the impact of the privatization of water services on child mortality. *Journal of Political Economy*, 113:83-120.

Ganesh-Kumar A, Mishra S & Panda M (2004). Employment guarantee for rural India. *Economic and Political Weekly*, 39:5359-5361.

Garau P, Sclar ED & Carolini GY (2005). *A home in the city*. UN Millennium Project: Taskforce on Improving the Lives of Slum Dwellers. London, Earthscan.

GEGA (nd). The equity gauge: concepts, principles, and guidelines. Durban, Global Equity Gauge Alliance & Health Systems Trust (**http://www.gega.org.za/download/gega_gauge.pdf**, accessed 5 May 2008).

Geiger H (1984). Community health centres. In: Sidel V, Sidel R, eds. *Reforming medicine: lessons of the last quarter century*. New York: Pantheon Books, pp. 11-31.

Geiger H (2002). Community-oriented primary care: a path to community development. *American Journal of Public Health*, 92:1713-1716.

Gender Promotion Programme ILO (2001). Promoting gender equality – a resource kit for trade unions. Geneva, International Labour Organization. (**http://www.ilo.org/public/english/employment/gems/eeo/tu/tu_toc.htm**, accessed 5 May 2008).

GKN (2007). *Towards health-equitable globalisation: rights, regulation and redistribution*. Final report of the Globalisation Knowledge Network of the Commission on Social Determinants of Health. Geneva, World Health Organization.

Glasier A et al. (2006). Sexual and reproductive health: a matter of life and death. *Lancet*, 368:1595-607.

Glenday G (2006). *Toward fiscally feasible and efficient trade liberalization*. Durham, NC, Duke Center for Internal Development, Duke University.

Glewwe P, Zhao M & Binder M (2006). *Achieving universal basic and secondary education: how much will it cost?* Cambridge, MA, American Academy of Arts and Sciences. (*http://www.amacad.org/publications/Glwwe.pdf*, accessed 4 September 2007).

Global Forum for Health Research (2006). *Monitoring financial flows for health research: the changing landscape of health research for development*. Geneva, Global Forum for Health Research. (**http://www.globalforumhealth.org/filesupld/monitoring_financial_flows_06/Financial%20Flows%202006.pdf**, accessed 9 May 2008).

Goetz A & Gaventa J (2001). *Bringing citizen voice and client focus into service delivery*. Brighton, UK, Institute of Development Studies. (**http://www.ids.ac.uk/ids/bookshop/wp/wp138.pdf**, accessed 27 June 2007) (Institute of Development Studies Working Papers – 138).

Gordon R & Lei W (2005). *Tax structures in developing countries: many puzzles and a possible explanation, 2005*. University of California San Diego and University of Virginia (**http://econ.ucsd.edu/~rogordon/puzzles16.pdf**, accessed February 2008).

Gostin L (2007). The 'Tobacco Wars' – global litigation strategies. *JAMA*, 298:2537-2539.

Gostin LO, Boufford JI & Martinez RM (2004). The future of the public's health: vision, values, and strategies. *Health Affairs*, 23:96-107.

Gottret P & Schieber G (2006). *Health financing revisited: a practitioner's guide*. Washington, DC, World Bank.

Govender V & Penn-Kekana L (2007). *Gender biases and discrimination: a review of health care interpersonal interactions*. Background document of the Women and Gender Equity Knowledge Network of the Commission on Social Determinants of Health. Geneva, World Health Organization.

Government of Canada (2007). *Tripartite First Nations Health Plan*. Vancouver, The First Nations Leadership Council, Government of Canada and Government of British Columbia.

Graham H (1987). Women's smoking and family health. *Social Science and Medicine*, 25:47-56.

Graham H & Kelly MP (2004). *Health inequalities: concepts, frameworks and policy*. London, Health Development Agency. (**http://www.nice.org.uk/page.aspx?o=502453**, accessed 5 May 2008).

Graham WJ et al. (2004). The familial technique for linking maternal death with poverty. *Lancet*, 363:23-27.

Grantham-McGregor SM et al. (1991). Nutritional supplementation, psychosocial stimulation, and mental development of stunted children: the Jamaican Study. *Lancet*, 338:1-5.

Grantham-McGregor SM et al. (2007). Developmental potential in the first 5 years for children in developing countries. *Lancet*, 369:60-70.

Grimsrud B (2002). *The next steps. Experiences and analysis of how to eradicate child labour*. Oslo, Fafo.

Grown C, Gupta GR & Pande R. (2005). Taking action to improve women's health through gender equality and women's empowerment. *Lancet*, 365:541-543.

Gupta S, Verhoeven M & Tiongson ER (2003). Public spending on health care and the poor. *Health Economics*, 12:685-696.

Gwatkin D & Deveshwar-Bahl (2001). *Immunization coverage inequalities: an overview of socio-economic and gender differentials in developing countries*. New York, World Bank.

Gwatkin D, Bhuiya A & Victoria C (2004). Making health care systems more equitable. *Lancet*, 364:1272-1280.

Gwatkin D, Wagstaff A & Yazbeck A, eds. (2005). *Reaching the poor with health, nutrition, and population services: what works, what doesn't, and why*. Washington DC, World Bank.

Gwatkin DR et al. (2007). *Socio-economic differences in health, nutrition, and population within developing countries: an overview*. Washington, DC, World Bank.

Halstead S, Walsh J & Warren K (1985). *Good health at low cost*. New York, Rockefeller Foundation.

Hamdad M (2003). *Valuing households' unpaid work in Canada, 1992 and 1998: trends and sources of change*. Ottawa: Statistics Canada.

Hanlon P, Walsh D & Whyte B (2006). *Let Glasgow flourish*. Glasgow, Glasgow Centre for Population Health.

Hargreaves S (2000). Call for increased commitment to promote reproductive health of refugees. *Lancet*, 356:1910.

Harris E (2007). *NSW Health HIA Capacity Building Program: mid-term review*. Sydney, Centre for Primary Health Care and Equity, University of New South Wales.

Harris E, Harris P & Kemp L (2006). *Rapid equity focused health impact assessment of the Australia Better Health Initiative: assessing the NSW components of priorities 1 and 3*. Sydney, UNSW Research Centre for Primary Health Care and Equity.

Hartmann H, Allen K & Owens C (1999). *Equal pay for working families; national and state data on the pay gap and its costs*. Washington, Institute for Women's Policy Research. (http://www.aflcio.org/issues/jobseconomy/women/equalpay/EqualPayForWorkingFamilies.cfm, accessed 28 May 2008).

Hawkes C (2002). Marketing activities of global soft drink and fast food companies in emerging markets: a review. In: *Globalization, diets and non-communicable diseases*. Geneva, World Health Organization.

Hawkes C et al. (2007). Globalisation, food and nutrition transitions. Background paper of the Globalisation Knowledge Network, Commission on Social Determinants of Health. Geneva, World Health Organization.

Hayward D (2007). Tackling health inequalities in England – policy development and progress. Case study prepared by Department of Health UK for the Commission on Social Determinants of Health. London, Department of Health.

Health Disparities Task Group (2004). Reducing health disparities – role of the health sector. Discussion paper. Ottawa, Public Health Agency Canada. (http://www.phac-aspc.gc.ca/ph-sp/disparities/pdf06/disparities_discussion_paper_e.pdf, accessed 11 April 2008).

Health Inequalities Unit (2008). *Tackling health inequalities: 2007 status report on the Programme for Action*. London: Department of Health.

Health Metrics Network (nd). *Assessing the National Health Information System: an assessment tool*. Geneva, Health Metrics Network (http://www.who.int/healthmetrics/tools/hisassessment/en/index.html, accessed 5 May 2008).

Health Systems Trust (nd). *The South African equity gauge*. Durban, Health Systems Trust (http://www.hst.org.za/generic/28, accessed 9 May 2008).

Healy J (2004). *Housing, fuel poverty and health. a pan-European analysis*. Aldershot, Ashgate Publishing Ltd.

HelpAge International (2006a). *Why social pensions are needed now*. London, HelpAge International (www.helpage.org/Resources/Briefings/main_content/LVqT/Pensionbriefing_web.pdf, accessed 5 May 2008).

HelpAge International (2006b). *Social pensions in Bolivia*. London, HelpAge International (http://www.helpage.org/Researchandpolicy/Socialprotection/PensionWatch/Bolivia, accessed 5 May 2008).

HelpAge International (2007). *Jakarta forum highlights importance of social protection*. London, HelpAge International (http://www.helpage.org/News/Latestnews/KQKY, accessed 5 May 2008).

HelpAge International (nd). *Social pensions in low and middle income countries*. London, HelpAge International. (http://www.helpage.org/Researchandpolicy/PensionWatch/Feasibility, accessed 5 May 2008).

Heymann J (2006). *Forgotten families: ending the growing crisis confronting children and working parents in the global economy*. Oxford, Oxford University Press.

HIFX (2007). Global foreign exchange turnover. Windsor: HIFX Foreign Exchange. (http://www.hifx.co.uk/marketwatch/market_news/headlines/uk_Daily_Global_Foreign_Exchange_turnover_rises_to_USD_3,-d-,2%20trillion.aspx, accessed 20 March 2008).

Hillman D, Kapoor S & Spratt S (2006). *Taking the next step: implementing a currency transaction development levy*. Oslo, Norwegian Ministry of Foreign Affaris.

Homedes N & Ugalde A (2005). Why neoliberal health reforms have failed in Latin America. *Health Policy*, 71:83-96.

Houweling TAJ et al. (2007). Huge poor-rich inequalities in maternity care: an international comparative study of maternity and child care in developing countries. *Bulletin of the World Health Organization*, 85:745-754.

Houweling TAJ (2007). *Socio-economic inequalities in childhood mortality in low and middle income countries* [thesis]. Rotterdam, Erasmus MC University Medical Center Rotterdam (http://hdl.handle.net/1765/11023, accessed 5 May 2008).

Houweling TAJ et al. (2005). Determinants of under-5 mortality among the poor and the rich. A cross-national analysis of 43 developing countries. *International Journal of Epidemiology*, 43:1257-1265.

Houweling TAJ et al. (2007). Huge poor-rich inequalities in maternity care: an HSKN (2007). *Final report of the Health Systems Knowledge Network of the Commission on Social Determinants of Health*. Geneva, World Health Organization.

Huisman M, Kunst AE & Mackenbach JP (2003). Socioeconomic inequalities in morbidity among the elderly; a European overview. *Social Science and Medicine*, 57:861-873.

Hunt P (2003). *Panel discussion on the rights to sexual and reproductive health*. Ottawa: Action Canada pour la Population et le Développement. (**http://www.acpd.ca/acpd.cfm/en/section/csih/articleid/223**, accessed 17 April 2008).

Hunt P (2006). *Economic, social and cultural rights: report of the Special Rapporteur on the right of everyone to the enjoyment of the highest attainable standard of physical and mental health, Paul Hunt. Addendum: mission to Uganda.* UN Economic and Social Council, New York, United Nations (**http://www2.essex.ac.uk/human_rights_centre/rth/docs/Uganda.pdf**, accessed March 08).

Hunt P (2007). Right to the highest attainable standard of health. *Lancet*, 370:369-371.

Hutchison B, Abelson J & Lavis JN (2001). Primary care in Canada: so much innovation, so little change. *Health Affairs*, 20:116-131.

Hutton G (2004). *Charting the path to the World Bank's "No blanket policy on user fees": A look over the past 25 years at the shifting support for user fees in health and education, and reflections on the future.* London, DFID Health Systems Resource Centre.

Huxley VH (2007). Sex and the cardiovascular system: the intriguing tale of how women and men regulate cardiovascular function differently. *Advances in Physiology Education*, 31:17-22.

IDMC (2007). *Internal displacement: global overview of trends and developments in 2006*. Geneva, Internal Displacement Monitoring Centre.

ILO (2002). *Women and men in the informal economy: a statistical picture*. Geneva, International Labour Organization.

ILO (2003). *ILO launches global campaign on social security for all*. Geneva, International Labour Organization (**http://www.ilo.org/global/About_the_ILO/Media_and_public_information/Press_releases/lang--en/WCMS_005285/index.htm**, accessed 8 May 2008).

ILO (2004a). Resolution concerning the promotion of gender equality, pay equity and maternity protection. 92nd Session of the International Labour Conference. Geneva, International Labour Organization.

ILO (2004b). *Breaking through the glass ceiling: women in management. Update 2004*. Geneva, International Labour Organization.

ILO (2005). *Decent work – safe work*. Introductory report to the XVIIth World Congress on Safety and Health at Work, 2005. Geneva, International Labour Organization (**www.ilo.org/public/english/protection/safework/wdcongrs17/intrep.pdf**, accessed 3 March 2008).

ILO (2006a). *The end of child labour: within reach*. Global report under the follow-up to the ILO declaration on fundamental principles and rights at work 2006. Geneva, International Labour Organization.

ILO (2006b). Facts on labour migration. Geneva, International Labour Organization.

ILO (2007a). *The end of child labour: millions of voices, one common hope. World of work, No. 61*. Geneva, International Labour Organization.

ILO (2007b). *The decent work agenda in africa: 2007-2015*. Report of the Director-General to the Eleventh African Regional Meeting, Addis Ababa, April 2007. Geneva: International Labour Organization (**http://www.ilo.org/wcmsp5/groups/public/---dgreports/---dcomm/---webdev/documents/publication/wcms_082282.pdf**, accessed 5 May 2008).

ILO (2008). *Global employment trends*. Geneva, International Labour Organization.

ILO (nd). *In Africa*. Web page of the Social Security Department. Geneva, International Labour Organization. (**http://www.ilo.org/public/english/protection/secsoc/projects/africa.htm**, accessed 21 February 2008).

ILOLEX (2007). International Labour Standards [online database]. Geneva, International Labour Organization (**http://www.ilo.org/ilolex/english/**, accessed December 2007).

Indian Government (1992). The Constitution (Seventy-Second Amendment) Act, 1992. (**http://indiacode.nic.in/coiweb/fullact1.asp?tfnm=73**, accessed March 08).

Indigenous Health Group (2007). Social determinants and indigenous health: the international experience and its policy implications. Presented at the Adelaide Symposium of the Commission on Social Determinants of Health.

Ingleby D et al. (2005). The role of health in integration. In: Fonseca L & Malheiros J, eds. *Social integration and mobility: education, housing and health.* IMISCOE Cluster B5 state of the art report. Lisbon, Centro de Estudos Geográficos.

IOM (2006). *Migration health annual report 2006*. Geneva, International Office of Migration.

IPCC (2007). *Climate change 2007: the physical science basis*. New York, Cambridge University Press.

Irwin A & Scali E (2005). *Action on the social determinants of health: learning from previous experiences*. Background document for the Commission on Social Determinants of Health. Geneva, World Health Organization.

IUHPE (2007). Shaping the future for health promotion: priority actions. *Promotion and Education*, 14:199-202.

IUHPE/CEU (1999). *The evidence of health promotion effectiveness: shaping public health in a new Europe. Part 2 Evidence book.* Vanves: International Union for Health Promotion and Education.

Iyer A, Sen G & Östlin P (2007). *The intersections of gender and class in health status and health care*. Background document of the Women and Gender Equity Knowledge Network of the Commission on Social Determinants of Health. Geneva, World Health Organization.

Jacobs G, Aeron-Thomas A & Astrop A (2000). *Estimating global road fatalities*. Wokingham: Transport Research Laboratory (TRL Report 445).

Jaglin S (2002). The right to water versus cost recovery: participation, urban water supply and the poor in sub-Saharan Africa. *Environment and Urbanization*, 14:231-245.

Jolly R (1991). Adjustment with a human face: a UNICEF record and perspective on the 1980s. *World Development*, 19:1807-1821.

Jubilee Debt Campaign (2007). *Debt and education*. London, Jubilee Debt Campaign (**http://www. jubileedebtcampaign.org.uk/Debt%20and%20Educatio n+3198.twl**, accessed 29 May 2008).

JUNJI (nd). JUNJI website [in Spanish]. Santiago, Junta Nacional de Jardines Infantiles (**http://www.junji.cl**, accessed 14 May 2008).

Kark SL & Kark E (1983). An alternative strategy in community health care: community-oriented primary health care. *Israel Journal of Medical Science*, 19:707-713.

Kelly MP et al. (2006). *Guide for the Knowledge Networks for the presentation of reports and evidence about the social determinants of health*. Background document of the Commission on Social Determinants of Health. Geneva, World Health Organization.

Kemp M (2001). *Corporate social responsibility in Indonesia: quixotic dream or confident expectation?* Geneva, UNRISD (Technology, Business and Society Programme Paper Number 6).

Kickbusch I (2003). The contribution of the World Health Organization to a new public health and health promotion. *American Journal of Public Health*, 93:383-388.

Kickbusch I (2007). Health promotion: not a tree but a rhizome. In: O'Neill M et al., eds. *Health promotion in Canada: critical perspectives*, 2nd ed. Toronto, Canadian Scholars Press Inc.

Kickbusch I & Payne L (2004). *Constructing global public health in the 21st century*. Presented to the Meeting on Global Health Governance and Accountability, 2-3 June 2004, Harvard University, Cambridge, MA. (**http://www.ilonakickbusch. com/en/global-health-governance/GlobalHealth.pdf**, accessed 28 May 2008).

Kickbusch I, Wait S & Maag D (2006). *Navigating health: the role of health literacy*. London, Alliance for Health and the Future, International Longevity Centre-UK. (**http://www.ilcuk.org. uk/files/pdf_pdf_3.pdf**, accessed 5 May 2008).

Kida T & Mackintosh M (2005). Public expenditure allocation and incidence under health care market liberalization: a Tanzanian case study. In: Mackintosh M & Koivusalo M, eds. *Commercialisation of health care: global and local dynamics and policy responses*. Basingstoke: Palgrave Macmillan, Chapter 17.

Kim IH et al. (2006). The relationship between nonstandard working and mental health in a representative sample of the South Korean population. *Social Science and Medicine*, 63:566-74.

Kivimäki M et al. (2003). Temporary employment and risk of overall and cause-specific mortality. *American Journal of Epidemiology*, 158:663-668.

Kivimäki M et al. (2006). Work stress in the aetiology of coronary heart disease – a meta-analysis. *Scandinavian Journal of Work and Environmental Health*, 32:431-442.

KNUS (2007). *Our cities, our health, our future: acting on social determinants for health equity in urban settings*. Final Report of the Urban Settings Knowledge Network of the Commission on Social Determinants of Health. Geneva, World Health Organization.

Koçak AA (2004). *Evaluation report of the Father Support Program*. Istanbul: Mother Child Education Foundation.

Koivusalo M & Mackintosh M (2005). Health systems and commercialisation: in search of good sense. In: Mackintosh M & Koivusalo M, eds. *Commercialization of health care: global and local dynamics and policy responses*. Basingstoke, UK: Palgrave Macmillan, pp. 3-21.

Korpi W (2001). Contentious institutions: an augmented rational-action analysis of the origins and path dependency of welfare state institutions in Western countries. *Rationality and Society*, 13:235-283.

Korpi W & Palme J (1998). The paradox of redistribution and strategies of equality: welfare state institutions, inequality, and poverty in Western countries. *American Sociological Review*, 63:661-687.

Kunst AE & Mackenbach JP (1994). *Measuring socio-economic inequalities in health*. Copenhagen, WHO Regional Office for Europe.

Kurowski C, Wyss K & Abdulla S (2007). Scaling up priority health interventions in Tanzania – the human resources challenge. *Health Policy and Planning*. 22:113-127.

Lagarde M & Palmer P (2006). *Health financing. Evidence from systematic reviews to inform decision making regarding financing mechanisms that improve access for poor people*. Presented to the meeting of the Alliance for Health Policy and Systems Research, Khon Kaen, Thailand. (**http://www.who.int/ rpc/meetings/HealthFinancingBrief.pdf**, accessed 4 May 2007).

Landers C (2003). *Early learning and the transition to school: implications for girls' education*. New York, UNICEF.

Landon Pearson Resource Centre for the Study of Childhood and Children's Rights (2007). *Shaking the movers: speaking truth to power: civil and political rights of children*. Ottawa, Landon Pearson Resource Centre for the Study of Childhood and Children's Rights.

Lang T, Rayner G & Kaelin E (2006). *The food industry, diet, physical activity and health: a review of reported commitments and practice of 25 of the world's largest food companies*. London, Centre for Food Policy, City University.

Langer A (2006). Cairo after 12 years: successes, setbacks, and challenges. *Lancet*, 368:1552-1554.

Leon DA et al. (1997). Huge variation in Russian mortality rates 1984-94: artefact, alcohol, or what? *Lancet*, 350:383-388.

Levine R (2004). *What's worked? Accounting for success in global health*. Washington, DC, Centre for Global Development.

Levine R et al. (2008). *Girls count: a global investment and action agenda*. Washington, DC, Center for Global Development.

LHC (2000). *The London Health Strategy 2000*. London: London Health Commission.

Lister J (2007). *Globalisation and health care systems change*. Background document of the Health Care Systems Knowledge Network of the World Health Organization's Commission on Social Determinants of Health.

Locke K (2004). Opportunities for inter-sector health improvement in new Member States. In: McKee M et al., eds. *Health policy and European Union enlargement*. Maidenhead, Open University Press.

Locke K (2006). *Health impact assessment of foreign and security policy*. Background paper: the role of health impact assessment. London, Nuffield Foundation.

Loewenson R (2003). *Civil society – state interactions in national health care systems*. Annotated bibliography on civil society and health. Harare: WHO/Training and Research Support Center (TARSC). (**http://www.tarsc.org/WHOCSI/**, accessed 26 June 2007).

Loftus AJ & McDonald DA (2001). Of liquid dreams: a political ecology of water privatization in Buenos Aires. *Environment and Urbanization*, 13:179-200.

Logie DE (2006). An affordable and sustainable health service for Africa in the 21st century. Ottawa, International Development Research Center (**http://www.crdi.ca/es/ev-99716-201-1-DO_TOPIC.html**, accessed 28 May 2008).

Lokshin M et al. (2005). Improving child nutrition? The Integrated Child Development Services in India. *Development and Change*, 36:613-640.

Lopez A et al., eds. (2006). *Global burden of disease and risk factors*. Oxford: Oxford University Press and World Bank.

Luciano D, Esim S & Duvvury N (2005). How to make the law work? Budgetary implications of domestic violence Laws in Latin America, Central America and the Caribbean. *Journal of Women, Politics & Policy*, 27:123-133.

Lundberg O et al. (2007). *The Nordic experience: welfare states and public health (NEWS)*. Report for the Commission on Social Determinants of Health. Stockholm, Centre for Health Equity Studies (CHESS).

Lynch RG (2004). *Exceptional returns: economic, fiscal, and social benefits of investment in early childhood development*. Washington, DC, Economic Policy Institute.

McCoy D et al. (2004). Pushing the international health research agenda towards equity and effectiveness. *Lancet*, 364:1630-1631.

McDonald D & Smith L (2004). Privatising Cape Town: from apartheid to neo-liberalism in the mother city. *Urban Studies*, 41:1461-1484.

McGillivray M et al. (2005). *It works; it doesn't; it can, but that depends...: 50 years of controversy over the macroeconomic impact of development aid*. Helsinki, World Institute for Development Economics Research (Research Paper No. 2005/54).

Macinko J et al. (2006). Evaluation of the impact of the Family Health Program on infant mortality in Brazil, 1990-2002. *Journal of Epidemiology and Community Health*, 60:13-19.

Mackenbach JP (2005). *Health inequalities: Europe in profile*. An independent, expert report commissioned by the UK Presidency of the EU. Rotterdam: ErasmusMC University Medical Center Rotterdam.

Mackenbach JP & Bakker MJ (2003); for the European Network on Interventions and Policies to Reduce Inequalities in Health. Tackling socioeconomic inequalities in health: an analysis of recent European experiences. *Lancet*, 362:1409-1414.

Mackenbach JP & Kunst AE (1997). Measuring the magnitude of socio-economic inequalities in health: an overview of available measures illustrated with two examples from Europe. *Social Science and Medicine*, 44:757-771.

Mackenbach JP, Meerding WJ & Kunst AE (2007). *Economic implications of socio-economic inequalities in health in the European Union*. Luxembourg: European Commission.

McKinnon R (2007). Tax-financed old-age pensions in lower-income countries. In: *International Social Security Association. Developments and trends: supporting dynamic social security*. World Social Security Forum, 29th ISSA General Assembly. Geneva, International Social Security Association, pp. 31-37 (**http://www.issa.int/pdf/publ/2DT07.pdf**, accessed 5 May 2008).

McMichael AJ et al. (2007). Food, livestock production, energy, climate change and health. *Lancet*, 370:55-65.

McMichael AJ et al. (2008). Global environmental change and health: impacts, inequalities, and the health sector. *BMJ*, 336:191-194.

Macpherson AK et al. (2002). Impact of mandatory helmet legislation on bicycle-related head injuries in children: a population-based study. *Pediatrics*, 110:e60-e65.

Madsen PR (2006). Contribution to the EEO Autumn Review 2006 'Flexicurity'. Denmark: European Employment Observatory.

Magnussen L, Ehiri J & Jolly P (2004). Comprehensive versus selective primary health care: lessons for global health policy. *Health Affairs*, 23:167-176.

Mahapatra P et al. (2007). Civil registration systems and vital statistics: successes and missed opportunities. *Lancet*, 370:1653-1663.

Mandel S (2006). *Debt relief as if people mattered: a rights-based approach to debt sustainability*. London, New Economics Foundation.

Marmot M (2004). *The status syndrome: how your social standing affects your health and life expectancy*. London, Bloomsbury.

Marmot M (2007). Achieving health equity: from root causes to fair outcomes. *Lancet*, 370:1153-1163.

Marmot M & Wilkinson RG, eds. (2006). *Social determinants of health*. Oxford, Oxford University Press.

Marshall TH (1950). *Citizenship and social class and other essays*. Cambridge: Cambridge University Press.

Martens J (2007). Strengthening domestic public finance for poverty eradication. *Development*, 50:56-62.

Mathers CD & Loncar D (2005). *Updated projections of global mortality and burden of disease, 2002-2030: data sources, methods and results*. Evidence and information for Policy Working Paper. Geneva, World Health Organization.

MDG Report (2007). The Millennium Development Goals report 2007. New York, United Nations (**http://www.un.org/millenniumgoals/pdf/mdg2007.pdf**, accessed 13 May 2008).

Mehta L & Madsen BL (2005). Is the WTO after your water? The General Agreement on Trade in Services (GATS) and poor people's right to water. *Natural Resources Forum*, 29:154-164.

MEKN (2007a). *The social determinants of health: developing an evidence base for political action*. Final report of the Measurement and Evidence Knowledge Network of the Commission on Social Determinants of Health. Geneva, World Health Organization.

MEKN (2007b). *Constructing the evidence base on the social determinants of health: a guide*. Background document of the Measurement and Evidence Knowledge Network of the Commission on Social Determinants of Health. Geneva, World Health Organization.

Meng Q (2007). *Developing and implementing equity-promoting health care policies in China.* Background paper for the Health Systems Knowledge Network of the Commission on Social Determinants of Health. Geneva, World Health Organization.

Mercado S et al. (2007). Urban poverty: an urgent public health issue. *Journal of Urban Health*, 84:i7–i15.

Micheletti M & Stolle D (2007). Mobilizing consumers to take responsibility for global social justice. *Annals of the American Academy of Political and Social Science*, 611:157-175.

Millennium Villages Project (nd). Millennium Promise website. New York, Millennium Promise (**http://www. millenniumpromise.org**, accessed 8 February 2008)

Mills A (2007). *Strategies to achieve universal coverage.* Paper prepared for the Health Care Systems Knowledge Network of the Commission on Social Determinants of Health. Geneva, World Health Organization.

Ministries of the Economy (2006). *Solidarity and globalisation.* Paris Conference on Innovative Development Financing Mechanisms, 28 February-1 March 2006. Paris, Government of France.

Mishra P & Newhouse D (2007). *Health aid and infant mortality.* Washington, DC, IMF (Working Paper 07/100).

Mitlin D (2007). Finance for low-income housing and community development. *Environment and Urbanization*, 19:331.

Mizunoya S et al. (2006). *Costing of basic social protection benefits for selected Asian countries: first results of a modelling exercise.* Issues in Social Protection, Geneva, Social Security Department, International Labour Organization (*http://www.ilo.org/public/ english/protection/secsoc/downloads/publ/1527sp1.pdf*, accessed 5 May 2008) (Discussion paper 17).

Mongella G (1995). Address by the Secretary-General of the 4th World Conference on Women at the formal opening of the Plenary Session 4th September 1995 (**http://www.un.org/ esa/gopher-data/conf/fwcw/conf/una/950904201423. txt**, accessed 5 May 2008).

Montgomery MR et al., eds. (2004). *Cities transformed: demographic change and its implications in the developing world.* London, Earthscan.

Morris JN & Deeming C (2004). Minimum incomes for healthy living (MIHL): next thrust in UK social policy? *Policy & Politics*, 32:441-454.

Morris JN et al. (2000). A minimum income for healthy living. *Journal of Epidemiology and Community Health*, 54:885-889.

Morris JN et al. (2007). Defining a minimum income for healthy living (MIHL): older age, England. *International Journal of Epidemiology*, 36:1300-7.

Moser K, Shkolnikov V & Leon DA (2005). World mortality 1950-2000: divergence replaces convergence from the late 1980s. *Bulletin of the World Health Organization*, 83:202-209.

Muntaner C et al. (1995). Psychosocial dimensions of work and the risk of drug dependence among adults. *American Journal of Epidemiology*, 142:183-190.

Murphy M et al. (2006). The widening gap in mortality by educational level in the Russian Federation, 1980-2001. *American Journal of Public Health*, 96:1293-1299.

Murray CJL et al. (2006). Eight Americas: investigating mortality disparities across races, counties, and race-counties in the United States. *PLoS Medicine*, 3:1513-1525.

Murray CJ et al. (2007). Validation of the symptom pattern method for analyzing verbal autopsy data. *PLoS Medicine*, 4: e327.

Murthy R (2007). *Accountability to citizens on gender and health.* Paper commissioned by the Women and Gender Equity Knowledge Network of the Commission on the Social Determinants of Health. Geneva, World Health Organization.

Musgrove P (2006). *Disability in late middle age and after in low and middle-income countries: a summary of some findings from the Disease Control Priorities Project (DCPP).* Paper prepared for the Behavioral and Social Research Program. Washington, DC, National Institute on Aging.

Mustard JF (2007). Experience-based brain development: scientific underpinnings of the importance of early child development in a global world. In: Young ME, Richardson LM, eds. *Early child development: from measurement to action.* Washington, DC, World Bank, pp. 43-71.

Musuka G & Chingombe I (2007). *Building equitable, people-centred national health systems: the role of Parliament and parliamentary committees on health in East and Southern Africa.* A literature review commissioned by the Health Systems Knowledge Network of the Commission on Social Determinants of Health. Geneva: World Health Organization.

NAS Panel on Aging (2006). Panel on Aging of the National Academies Committee on Population, convened for the Commission on Social Determinants of Health, August 2006. Washington, DC, National Institute on Aging.

National Coalition on Health Care (2008). *Health insurance cost.* Washington, DC, National Coalition on Health Care (**http:// www.nchc.org/facts/cost.shtml**, accessed 7 March 2008).

Newman L et al. (2007). *A rapid appraisal case study of South Australia's Social Inclusion Initiative.* Paper for the Social Exclusion Knowledge Network of the Commission on the Social Determinants of Health. Geneva, World Health Organization.

NHF (2007). *Building health. Creating and enhancing places for healthy, active lives: blueprint for action.* London, UK National Heart Forum.

NHS (2000). *The London Health Strategy.* London, NHS Executive London Regional Office.

Nicholson A et al. (2005). Socio-economic influences on self-rated health in Russian men and women--a life course approach. *Social Science and Medicine*, 61:2345-54.

Nissanke M (2003). Revenue potential of the Tobin Tax for Development Finance: a critical appraisal. In: Atkinson A, ed. *New sources of development finance.* Oxford, Oxford University Press for UNU-WIDER.

NNC (2001). *Smart growth for neighborhoods: affordable housing and regional vision.* USA, National Neighborhood Coalition.

O'Donnell O et al. (2005). *Who benefits from public spending on health care in Asia?* Rotterdam and Colombo: Erasmus University and IPS. (**http://www.equitap.org/ publications/wps/EquitapWP3.pdf**, accessed 12 October 2006) (EQUITAP Project Working Paper #3).

O'Donnell O et al. (2007). The incidence of public spending on healthcare: comparative evidence from Asia. *World Bank Economic Review*, 21:93-123.

ODI (1999). *Global governance – an agenda for the renewal of the United Nations.* London, Overseas Development Institute.

OECD (2001). *Starting strong: early childhood education and care*. Paris, Organisation for Economic Cooperation and Development.

OECD (2005). *From employment to work*. Paris, Organisation for Economic Cooperation and Development.

Office of the Mayor (2007). Mayor Bloomberg and major philanthropic foundations unveil size, scope, and schedule of Opportunity NYC, the nation's first-ever conditional cash transfer program. Press release, 29 March. New York: Office of the Mayor. (**http://www.nyc.gov**, accessed 5 May 2008).

Ogawa S, Hasegawa T & Carrin G (2003). Scaling up community health insurance: Japan's experience with the 19th century Jyorei scheme. *Health Policy and Planning*, 18:270-278.

Oldfield S & Stokke K (2004). *Building unity in diversity: social movement activism in the Western Cape Anti-Eviction Campaign*. A case study for Globalisation, Marginalisation and New Social Movements in post-Apartheid South Africa. Durban, University of KwaZulu-Natal. (**http://www.ukzn.ac.za/ccs/files/Oldfield%20&%20Stokke%20WCAEC%20Research%20Report.pdf**, accessed March 2008)

Ooi GL & Phua KH (2007). Urbanization and slum formation. *Journal of Urban Health*, 84;i27-i34.

Ooms G & Schrecker T (2005). Viewpoint: expenditure ceilings, multilateral financial institutions, and the health of poor populations. *Lancet*, 365:1821-1823.

Oxfam (2002). *Milking the CAP: how Europe's dairy regime is devastating livelihoods in the developing world*. London, Oxfam. (Briefing Paper 34).

Oxfam Great Britain (2000). *Tax havens: releasing the hidden billions for poverty eradication*. Oxford, Oxfam.

Paes de Barros R et al. (2002). *Meeting the Millennium Poverty Reduction Targets in Latin America and the Caribbean*. Santiago: United Nations Economic Commission for Latin America and the Caribbean.

PAHO (2001). *Investment in health*. Washington, DC, Pan-American Health Organization (Social and Economic Returns Scientific and Technical Publication No.582).

PAHO (2005). PAHO Healthy Municipalities, Cities and Communities. *Bulletin of the Healthy Settings Units*, 1 (**http://www.paho.org/English/ad/sde/municipios.htm**, accessed 10 May 2008).

PAHO (2006). *Mission Barrio Adentro: the right to health and social inclusion in Venezuela*. Caracas, Pan-American Health Organization.

PAHO (2007). *Renewing primary health care in the Americas*. A position paper of the Pan American Health Organization. Washington, DC, Pan-American Health Organization (**http://www.paho.org/English/AD/THS/primaryHealthCare.pdf**, accessed 27 June 2007).

Pal K et al. (2005). *Can low income countries afford basic social protection? First results of a modelling exercise*. Geneva, International Labour Organization (**http://www.ilo.org/public/english/protection/secsoc/downloads/policy/1023sp1.pdf**, accessed 5 May 2008) (Issues in Social Protection, discussion paper 13).

Palmer N et al. (2004). Health financing to promote access in low income settings – how much do we know? *Lancet*, 364:1365-1370.

Parent-Thirion A et al. (2007). *Fourth European Working Conditions Survey*. Dublin, European Foundation for the Improvement of Living and Working Conditions.

Partnership for Child Development (nd). A FRESH start to improving the quality and equity of education. London, Partnership for Child Development. (**www.freshschools.org**, accessed 13 May 2008).

Pasha O et al. (2003). The effect of providing fansidar (sulfadoxine-pyrimethane) in schools on mortality on school-age children in Malawi. *Lancet*, 361:577-578.

Patel V et al. (2004). Effect of maternal mental health on infant growth in low income countries: new evidence from South Asia. *BMJ*, 328:820-823.

Paul J & Nahory C (2005). *Theses towards a democratic reform of the UN Security Council*. New York, Global Policy Forum.

Paxson C & Schady N (2007). *Does money matter? The effects of cash transfers on child health and development in rural Ecuador*. Washington, DC, World Bank (**http://www-wds.worldbank.org/external/default/WDSContentServer/IW3P/IB/2007/05/03/000016406_20070503092958/Rendered/PDF/wps4226.pdf**, accessed 5 May 2008) (Impact Evaluation Series No. 15. World Bank Policy Research Working Paper 4226).

Petchesky RP & Laurie M (2007). *Gender, health and human rights in sites of political exclusion*. Background document of the Women and Gender Equity Knowledge Network of the Commission on Social Determinants of Health. Geneva, World Health Organization.

PHAC (2007). *Crossing sectors – experiences in intersectoral action, public policy and health*. Ottawa, Public Health Agency of Canada.

PHAC & WHO (2008). *Enhancing health and improving health equity through cross-sectoral action: an analysis of national case studies*. Ottawa, Public Health Agency of Canada.

PHM (2000). *People's charter for health*. Cairo: People's Health Movement.

PHM, Medact & GEGA (2005). *Global Health Watch, 2005-2006: an alternative world health report*. London, Zed Books.

Picciotto R (2004). *Institutional approaches to policy coherence for development*. OECD Policy Workshop May 2004. Paris, Organisation for Economic Cooperation and Development.

Pierson P (2000). Increasing returns, path dependence, and the study of politics. *American Political Science Review*, 94:251-267.

Pierson P (2001). Investigating the welfare state at century's end. In: Pierson P, ed. *The new politics of the welfare state*. Oxford, Oxford University Press, pp. 1-14.

Pogge T (2008). Growth and inequality: understanding recent trends and political choices. *Dissent Magazine* [online], (**http://dissentmagazine.org/article/?article=990**, accessed 10 April 2008).

PPHCKN (2007a). *Inequities in the health and nutrition of children*. Report of the Priority Public Health Conditions Knowledge Network of the Commission on Social Determinants of Health. Geneva, World Health Organization.

PPHCKN (2007b). *Alcohol and social determinants of health*. Report from the alcohol node to the Priority Public Health Conditions Knowledge Network of the Commission on Social Determinants of Health. Geneva, World Health Organization.

PPHCKN (2007c). Interim report of the Priority Public Health Conditions Knowledge Network of the Commission on Social Determinants of Health. Geneva, World Health Organization.

PPHCKN (2007d). *Social determinants of mental disorders.* Report from the mental health node to the Priority Public Health Conditions Knowledge Network of the Commission on Social Determinants of Health. Geneva, World Health Organization.

Prince M et al. (2007). No health without mental health. *Lancet*, 370:859-877.

Prüss-Üstün A & Corvalán C (2006). *Preventing disease through healthy environments. Towards an estimate of the environmental burden of disease.* Geneva, World Health Organization.

Public Health Agency of Canada (nd). *Canada's response to WHO Commission on Social Determinants of Health.* Ottawa, Public Health Agency of Canada (**http://www.phac-aspc.gc.ca/sdh-dss/crg-grc-eng.php**, accessed 14 May 2008).

Quan J (1997). *The important of land tenure to poverty eradication and sustainable development in Africa. Summary of findings.* Chatham, UK, National Resources Institute (**http://www.oxfam.org.uk/resources/learning/landrights/downloads/quanpov.rtf**, accessed 30April 2008).

Quartey P (2005). *Innovative ways of making aid effective in Ghana: tied aid versus direct budgetary support.* Helsinki, UNU-WIDER (WIDER Research Paper No. 2005/58).

Rajan R & Subramanian A (2005). *Aid and growth: what does the cross-country evidence really show?* Washington, DC, IMF (IMF Working Paper 05/127).

Randel J, German A & Ewing D, eds. (2004). *The reality of aid 2004: an independent review of poverty reduction and development assistance, the Reality of Aid Project.* London, IBON Books Manila/Zed Books.

Ranson M, Hanson K & Oliveira Cruz V (2003). Constraints to expanding access to health interventions: an empirical analysis and country typology. *Journal of International Development*, 15:15-39.

Ravindran T & de Pinho H, eds. (2005). *The right reforms? Health sector reforms and sexual and reproductive health.* Johannesburg: The Initiative for Sexual and Reproductive Rights and Health Reforms (**www.wits.ac.za/whp/rightsandreforms/globalvolume.htm**, accessed 27 March 2007).

Ravindran TKS & Kelkar-Khambete A (2007). *Women's health policies and programmes and gender-mainstreaming in health policies, programmes and within health sector institutions.* Background document of the Women and Gender Equity Knowledge Network of the Commission on Social Determinants of Health. Geneva, World Health Organization.

Rifkin S & Walt G (1986). Why health improves: defining the issues concerning "comprehensive primary health care" and "selective primary health care. *Social Science and Medicine*, 23:559-566.

Rihani MA (2006). *Keeping the promise: 5 benefits of girls' secondary education.* Washington, DC, AED Global Learning Group (**http://siteresources.worldbank.org/EDUCATION/Resources/Summary_Book_Girls_Education_MayRIHANI.pdf**, accessed 24 September 2007).

Ritakallio V-M & Fritzell J (2004). *Societal shifts and changed patterns of poverty.* New York: Luxembourg & Syracuse (LIS Working Paper Series, no. 393).

Roberts H & Meddings DR (2007). *What can be done about the social determinants of violence and unintentional injury.* Background paper of the Priority Public Health Conditions Knowledge Network of the Commission on Social Determinants of Health. Geneva, World Health Organization.

Rodrik D (2001). *The global governance of trade as if development really mattered.* New York, United Nations Development Programme.

Romeri E, Baker A & Griffiths C (2006). Mortality by deprivation and cause of death in England and Wales, 1999-2003. *Health Statistics Quarterly*, 32:19-34.

Rootman I & Gordon-El-Bihbety D (2008). *A vision for a health literate Canada: report of the expert panel on health literacy.* Ottawa: Canadian Public Health Association.

Rose G (1985). Sick individuals and sick populations. *International Journal of Epidemiology*, 14:32-38.

Ross CE & Wu C-L (1995). The links between education and health. *American Sociological Review*, 60:719-745.

Ruger JP & Kim HJ (2006). Global health inequalities: an international comparison. *Journal of Epidemiology and Community Health*, 60:928-936.

RWJF Commission (2008). *Perceived health challenges in the United States.* National survey results of a public opinion poll commissioned by the Robert Wood Johnson Foundation. Princeton: Robert Wood Johnson Foundation.

Sachs J (2004). Health in the developing world: achieving the Millennium Development Goals (MDGs). *Bulletin of the World Health Organization*, 82:947-952.

Sachs J (2007). Beware false tradeoffs. *Foreign Affairs* [online], (**http://www.foreignaffairs.org/special/global_health/sachs**, accessed 14 March 2008).

Sachs J (2005). *The end of poverty: how we can make it happen in our lifetime?* London, Penguin Books.

Saltman R, Busse R & Figueras J, eds. (2004). *Social health insurance systems in western Europe.* European Observatory on Health Systems and Policies Series. Maidenhead, UK, Open University Press.

Sanders D (1985). *The struggle for health: medicine and the politics of underdevelopment.* London, Macmillan.

Sanders D et al. (2004). Making research matter: a civil society perspective on health research. *Bulletin of the World Health Organization*, 82:757-763.

Save the Children UK, HelpAge International & Institute of Development Studies (2005). *Making cash count: lessons from cash transfer schemes in east and southern Africa for supporting the most vulnerable children and households.* London: Save the Children UK, HelpAge International and Institute of Development Studies.

Schirnding YE (2002). Health and sustainable development: can we rise to the challenge? *Lancet*, 360:632-637.

Schneider A (2005). Aid and governance: doing good and doing better. *IDS Bulletin*, 36(3).

Schubert B (2005). *The pilot social cash transfer scheme, Kalomo District – Zambia.* Manchester, Insitute for Development Policy and Management/Chronic Poverty Research Centre (Chronic Poverty Research Centre Working Paper 52).

Schurmann A (2007). *Microcredit, inclusion and exclusion in Bangladesh.* Background paper for the Social Exclusion Knowledge Network of the Commission on Social Determinants of Health. Geneva, World Health Organization.

Schweinhart L (2004). *The High/Scope Perry preschool study through age 40: summary, conclusions, and frequently asked questions.* Ypsilanti, High/Scope Educational Research Foundation.

Schweinhart LJ, Barnes HV & Weikart DP (1993). *Significant benefits: the High/Scope Perry preschool study through age 27.* Ypsilanti, High/Scope Press.

Scott-McDonald K (2002). Elements of quality in home visiting programmes: three Jamaican models. In: Young ME, ed. *From early child development to human development: investing in our children's future.* Washington, DC, World Bank, pp. 233-253.

SEKN (2007). *Understanding and tackling social exclusion.* Final Report of the Social Exclusion Knowledge Network of the Commission on Social Determinants of Health. Geneva, World Health Organization.

Sen A (1999). *Development as freedom.* New York, Alfred A Knopf Inc.

Setel PW et al. (2007). A scandal of invisibility: making everyone count by counting everyone. *Lancet,* 370:1569-77.

SEWA Bank (nd). SEWA Bank web page. Ahmedabad, Self-employed Women's Association (**http://www.sewa.org/ services/bank.asp**, accessed 7 April 2008).

SEWA Social Security (nd). Childcare section of the SEWA Social Security web page. Ahmedabad, Self Employed Women's Association (**http://www.sewainsurance.org/childcare. htm#Childcare**, accessed 5 May 2008).

Shaw M (2004). Housing and public health. *Annual Review of Public Health,* 25:397-418.

Sheuya S, Howden-Chapman P & Patel S (2007). The design of housing and shelter programs: the social and environmental determinants of inequalities. *Journal of Urban Health,* 84:i98-i108.

Sibal B (2006). People's power in people's hands: the lesson we need to learn. *Journal of Epidemiology and Community Health,* 60:521.

Siegel P, Alwang J & Canagarajah S (2001). *Viewing microinsurance as a social risk management instrument.* Washington, DC, World Bank (Social Protection Discussion Paper Series, no. 0116).

SIGN (2006). Newsletter of the Schoolfeeding Initiative Ghana-Netherlands, issue 1. Amsterdam, Schoolfeeding Initiative Ghana-Netherlands (**http://www.sign-schoolfeeding.org/_dynamic/downloads/Augustus_ 2006.doc**, accessed 30 April 2008).

Simmons R & Shiffman J (2006). Scaling up health service innovations: a framework for action. Chapter 2. In: Simmons R, Fajans P & Ghiron L, eds. Scaling up health services delivery: from pilot innovations to policies and programmes. Geneva, World Health Organization (**http://www.expandnet.net/ volume.htm**, accessed 26 June 2007).

Smith L & Haddad L (2000). *Explaining child malnutrition in developing countries: a cross-country analysis.* Washington, DC, International Food Policy Research Institute (Research Report No.111).

Solar O & Irwin A (2007). *A conceptual framework for action on the social determinants of health.* Discussion paper for the Commission on Social Determinants of Health. Geneva, World Health Organization.

Son M et al. (2002). Relation of occupational class and education with mortality in Korea. *Journal of Epidemiology and Community Health,* 56:798-799.

Ståhl T et al., eds. (2006). *Health in All Policies: prospects and potentials.* Helsinki, Ministry of Social Affairs and Health and the European Observatory on Health Systems and Policies.

Standing Committee on Nutrition (nd,a). United Nations System Standing Committee on Nutrition website. Geneva, Standing Committee on Nutrition (**http://www.unsystem. org/SCN/Default**, accessed 4 May 2008)

Standing Committee on Nutrition (nd,b). *Strategic framework.* Geneva: Standing Committee on Nutrition Secretariat (**http://www.unsystem.org/SCN/Publications/SCN%2 0Strategic%20Framework%20130407.pdf**, accessed 8 May 2008)

Stansfeld S & Candy B (2006). Psychosocial work environment and mental health – a meta-analytic review. *Scandinavian Journal of Work and Environmental Health,* 32:443-462.

Starfield B (2006). State of the art research on equity in health. *Journal of Health Politics Policy Law,* 31:11–32.

Starfield B, Shi L & Macinko J (2005). Contribution of primary care to health systems and health. *Milbank Quarterly,* 83:457-502.

Stern N (2006). *Stern review: the economics of climate change.* London, HM Treasury.

Stern N, Dethier J-J & Rogers H (2004). *Growth and empowerment: making development happen.* Cambridge, MA, MIT Press.

Stiglitz JE (2002). *Globalization and its discontents.* London, Penguin Books.

Stiglitz JE (2006). *Making globalization work.* New York, WW Norton.

Strazdins L, Shipley M & Broom DH (2007). What does family-friendly really mean? Well-being, time, and the quality of parents' jobs. *Australian Bulletin of Labour,* 33:202-225.

Svensson J (2000). Foreign aid and rent-seeking. *Journal of International Economics,* 51:437-461.

Swaminathan M (2006). *2006-7 Year of Agricultural Renewal.* 93rd Indian Science Congress, Hyderabad.

Szreter S (1988). The importance of social intervention in Britain's mortality decline c. 1850-1914: a re-interpretation of the role of public health. *Social History of Medicine,* 1:1-37.

Szreter S (2002). Rethinking McKeown: the relationship between public health and social change. *American Journal of Public Health,* 92:722-725.

Szreter S (2004). Health, economy, state and society in modern Britain: the long-run perspective. *Hygiea Internationalis,* 4:205-228 (special issue).

Szreter S (2007). The right of registration: development, identity registration, and social security-a historical perspective. *World Development,* 35:67-86.

Tajer D (2003). Latin American social medicine: roots, development during the 1990s, and current challenges. *American Journal of Public Health*, 93:2023-2027.

Tanahashi T (1978). Health service coverage and its evaluation. *Bulletin of the World Health Organization*, 56:295-303.

Tanzi V (2001). Globalization and the work of fiscal termites. *Finance and Development*, 38.

Tanzi V (2002). Globalization and the future of social protection. *Scottish Journal of Political Economy*, 49:116-127.

Tanzi V (2004). Globalization and the need for fiscal reform in developing countries. *Journal of Policy Modeling*, 26:525-542.

Tanzi V (2005). Social protection in a globalizing world. *Rivista di Politica Economica*, 25-45.

Tax Justice Network (2005). *Briefing paper – the price of offshore*. Tax Justice Network, UK [online] (**http://www.taxjustice. net/cms/upload/pdf/Price_of_Offshore.pdf**, accessed 27 February 2008).

The Age (2008). *Text of PM Rudd's 'sorry' address*. Melbourne, The Age (**http://www.theage.com. au/news/national/bfull-textb-pms-sorry-address/2008/02/12/1202760291188.html**, accessed 28 May 2008).

The Hindu (2008). *Lifeline for the rural poor*. Chennai, The Hindu (**http://www.hindu.com/2008/01/25/ stories/2008012555601000.htm**, accessed 30 January 2008).

Thorson A, Long NH & Larsson LO (2007). Chest X-ray findings in relation to gender and symptoms: a study of patients with smear positive tuberculosis in Vietnam. *Scandinavian Journal of Infectious Diseases*, 39:33-37.

Tolstoy L (1877). *Anna Karenina*. London, Allen Lane/Penguin, 2000.

Townsend P (2007). *The right to social security and national development: lessons from OECD experience for low-income countries*. Geneva, International Labour Organization (**http://www. ilo.int/public/english/protection/secsoc/downloads/ publ/1595sp1.pdf**, accessed 5 May 2008) (Issues in Social Protection, Discussion Paper 18).

Tudor Hart J (1971). The inverse care law. *Lancet*, 1:405-12.

UIS (2008). *75 million children out of school, according to new UIS data*. Paris, United Nations Educational, Scientific, and Cultural Organization (**http://www.uis.unesco.org/ev_ en.php?ID=7194_201&ID2=DO_TOPIC**, accessed 20 May 2008).

UN (1948). *Universal Declaration of Human Rights*. Adopted and proclaimed by General Assembly resolution 217 A (III) of 10 December 1948 (**http://www.un.org/Overview/rights. html**, accessed 28 May 2008).

UN (2000a). *General Comment No. 14 (2000). The right to the highest attainable standard of health (article 12 of the International Covenant on Economic, Social and Cultural Rights)*. Geneva, United Nations Economic and Social Council (**http://www. unhchr.ch/tbs/doc.nsf/(symbol)/E.C.12.2000.4.En**, accessed 1 March 2008).

UN (2000b). *Millennium Development Goals*. New York, United Nations.

UN (2001). Africa's capacity to deliver is huge. *Africa Recovery* 15:12 (**http://www.un.org/ecosocdev/geninfo/afrec/ vol15no1/151aids3.htm**, accessed 16 May 2008).

UN (2005). Resolution 60/1 adopted at the World Summit 2005 (60th Session of the General Assembly of the UN). New York, United Nations.

UN (2006a). *General comment no. 7: implementing child rights in early childhood*. Geneva, United Nations Committee on the Rights of the Child (**http://www2.ohchr. org/english/bodies/crc/docs/AdvanceVersions/ GeneralComment7Rev1.pdf**, accessed 8 May 2008).

UN (2006b). The Status of Women in the United Nations System. United Nations Office of the Special Adviser on Gender Issues and Advancement of Women (**http://www. un.org/womenwatch/osagi/pdf/Fact%20sheet%2028% 20september.pdf**, accessed 21 February 2008).

UN Millennium Project (2005). *Investing in development: a practical plan to achieve the Millennium Development Goals*. London, Earthscan.

UNCTAD (2004). *Economic development in Africa – debt sustainability: oasis or mirage*. New York and Geneva, United Nations.

UNCTAD (2006). *Trade and Development Report 2006: global partnership and national policies for development*. Geneva, United Nations Conference on Trade and Development.

UNDESA (2006). *World economic situation and prospects, 2006*. New York, United Nations Department of Economic and Social Affairs.

UNDESA, *Population Division (2006)*. Population ageing 2006. New York, United Nations Department of Economic and Social Affairs, Population Division (**http://www.un.org/ esa/population/publications/ageing/ageing2006.htm**, accessed 5 May 2008).

UNDP (1998). *Human development report. Consumption for human development*. New York, United Nations Development Programme.

UNDP (1999). *Human development report. Gobalization with a human face*. New York, United Nations Development Programme.

UNDP (2007). *Fighting climate change: human solidarity in a divided world*. New York, United Nations Development Programme.

UNDP & Ministry of Planning and Development Cooperation (2005). *Iraq Living Conditions Survey 2004*. Volume I: tabulation report. Baghdad, Central Organisation for Statistics and Information Technology, Ministry of Planning and Development Cooperation.

UNESCO (2001). *Handbook on effective implementation of continuing education at the grassroots*. Bangkok, United Nations Educational, Scientific and Cultural Organization Principal Regional Office for Asia and the Pacific.

UNESCO (2006a). *Water: a shared responsibility*. The United Nations World Water Development Report 2. Paris, United Nations Educational, Scientific and Cultural Organization.

UNESCO (2006b). *Strong foundations: early childhood care and education*. EFA Global Monitoring Report 2007. Paris: United Nations Educational, Scientific and Cultural Organization (**http://unesdoc.unesco.org/images/0014/001477/ 147794E.pdf**, accessed 5 May 2008).

UNESCO (2007a). *Education for All by 2015: will we make it?* EFA Global Monitoring Report 2008. Paris, United Nations Educational, Scientific and Cultural Organization.

UNESCO (2007b). Literacy Initiative for Empowerment LIFE 2006-2015. Vision and strategy paper. Hamburg, United Nations Educational, Scientific and Cultural Organization Institute for Lifelong Learning.

UN-HABITAT (2006). *State of the worlds' cities 2006/7. The millennium development goals and urban sustainability*. Nairobi, UN-HABITAT.

UN-HABITAT (2007a). UN-HABITAT website. Nairobi, UN-HABITAT (**http://www.unhabitat.org/**, accessed 10 Dec 2007).

UN-HABITAT (2007b). *The emerging global order: the city as a catalyst for stability and sustainability*. Address by Executive Director Anna Tibaijuka. Nairobi, UN-HABITAT (**http://www.unhabitat.org/content.asp?cid=5389&catid=14&typeid=8&subMenuId=0**, accessed April 30, 2008).

UNHCR (2005). *Measuring protection by numbers*. Geneva, Office of the United Nations High Commissioner for Refugees.

UNHCR (2007). The United Nations Refugee Agency website. Geneva, Office of the United Nations High Commissioner for Refugees (**http://www.unhcr.org**, accessed December 2007).

UNICEF (1997). *The role of men in the lives of children*. New York, United Nations Children's Fund.

UNICEF (2000). *The state of the world's children 2001*. New York, United Nations Children's Fund.

UNICEF (2001). *We the children: meeting the promises of the World Summit for Children*. New York, United Nations Children's Fund.

UNICEF (2004). *The state of the world's children 2005: childhood under threat*. New York, United Nations Children's Fund.

UNICEF (2005). *The 'rights' start to life 2005: a statistical analysis of birth registration*. New York, United Nations Children's Fund.

UNICEF (2006). *The state of the world's children 2007. Women and children: the double dividend of gender equality*. New York, United Nations Children's Fund.

UNICEF (2007a). *Progress for children: a world fit for children*. New York, United Nations Children's Fund (Statistical Review, Number 7).

UNICEF (2007b). *Can the Kenyan State put the 300,000 most vulnerable children in the country on a cash transfer programme by the end of 2010?* New York, United Nations Children's Fund.

UNICEF (2007c). *The state of the world's children 2008: child survival*. New York, United Nations Children's Fund.

UNICEF (nd,a). *Child protection information sheets*. New York, UNICEF.

UNICEF (nd,b). Life skills website. New York, UNICEF (**http://www.unicef.org/lifeskills**, accessed 1 May 2008).

UNICEF (nd,c) *Life skills: a special case for HIV/AIDS preventions*. New York, UNICEF (**http://www.unicef.org/lifeskills/index_7323.html**, accessed 1 May 2008).

UNICEF (nd,d). *Child friendly schools*. New York, UNICEF. (**http://www.unicef.org/lifeskills/index_7260.html**, accessed 20 March 2008) and *Fact Sheet: The CRC@ 18: its impact on a generation of children*. New York, UNICEF. (**http://www.unicef.org/media/files/Fact_Sheet.doc**, accessed 20 March 2008).

US Social Security Administration (2004). Social security is important to women. Fact Sheet. Baltimore, MD, Press Office of the Social Security Administration (**http://ssa.gov/pressoffice/factsheets/women.htm**, accessed 5 May 2008).

Vågerö D (1995). Health inequalities as policy issues – reflections on ethics, policy and public health. *Sociology of Health & Illness*, 17:1-19.

Van Ginneken W (2003). *Extending social security: Policies for developing countries*. Geneva, International Labour Organization (ESS Paper No. 13).

Vega J & Irwin A (2004). Tackling health inequalities: new approaches in public policy. *Bulletin of the World Health Organization*, 82:482-483.

Vega-Romero R & Torres-Tovar M (2007). *The role of civil society in building an equitable health system*. Paper prepared for the Health Care Systems Knowledge Network of the Commission on Social Determinants of Health. Geneva, World Health Organization.

Victora CG et al. (2000). Explaining trends in inequities: evidence from Brazilian child health studies. *Lancet*, 356:1093-1098.

Victora CG et al. (2008). Maternal and child undernutrition: consequences for adult health and human capital. *Lancet*, 371:340-357.

Villaveces A et al. (2000). Effect of a ban on carrying firearms on homicide rates in 2 Colombian cities. *JAMA*, 283:1205-1209.

Vincent I (1999). Collaboration and integrated services in the NSW public sector. *Australian Journal of Public Administration*, 58:50-54.

Vlahov D et al. (2007). Urban as a determinant of health. *Journal of Urban Health*, 84;i16-i26.

Voas RB et al. (2006). A partial ban on sales to reduce high-risk drinking south of the border: seven years later. *Journal of Studies of Alcohol*, 67:746-753.

Wagstaff A (2003). Child health on a dollar a day: some tentative cross-country comparisons. *Social Science and Medicine*, 57:1529-1538.

Wagstaff A (2007). Social health insurance reexamined. Washington, DC, World Bank (World Bank Policy Research Working Paper 4111).

Wagstaff A et al., (1999). Redistributive effect, progressivity and differential tax treatment: personal income taxes in twelve OECD countries. *Journal of Public Economics* 72:25.

Waring M (1988). *If women counted: a new feminist economics*. San Fransisco, HarperCollins.

Waring M (1999). *Counting for nothing: what men value and what women are worth*. Toronto: University of Toronto Press.

Waring M (2003). Counting for something! Recognizing women's contribution to the global economy through alternative accounting systems. *Gender and Development*, 11:35-43.

Watts S et al. (2007). *Social determinants of health in countries in conflict and crises: the eastern Mediterranean perspective*. Background paper for the Commission on Social Determinants of Health. Geneva, World Health Organization.

WGEKN (2007). *Unequal, unfair, ineffective and inefficient – gender inequity in health: why it exists and how we can change it.* Final report of the Women and Gender Equity Knowledge Network of the Commission on Social Determinants of Health. Geneva, World Health Organization.

WHO (1986). Ottawa Charter for Health Promotion. Geneva, World Health Organization.

WHO (2002a). *World report on violence and health.* Geneva, World Health Organization.

WHO (2002b). *World health report 2002: reducing risks, promoting healthy life.* Geneva, World Health Organization.

WHO (2005a). *WHO multi-country study on women's health and domestic violence – initial results on prevalence, health outcomes and women's responses.* Geneva, World Health Organization.

WHO (2005b). *World health report 2005: make every mother and child count.* Geneva, World Health Organization.

WHO (2005c). *Preventing chronic diseases: a vital investment.* Geneva, World Health Organization.

WHO (2005d). *Bangkok Charter for Health Promotion.* Geneva, World Health Organization.

WHO (2005e). *The Health and Environment Linkages Initiative.* Geneva, World Health Organization (**http://www.who.int/ heli/risks/risksmaps/en/index5.html**, accessed May 2008).

WHO (2006). *The world health report 2006: working together for health.* Geneva, World Health Organization.

WHO (2007a). *Medium-term Strategic Plan 2008-2013.* Geneva, World Health Organization (**http://www.who.int/gb/e/ e_amtsp.html**, accessed 14 February 2008).

WHO (2007b). *Women's health and human rights: monitoring the implementation of CEDAW.* Geneva: World Health Organization.

WHO (2007c). *World health statistics.* Geneva, World Health Organization. (**http://www.who.int/whosis/whostat2007. pdf**, accessed 28 March 2008).

WHO (2007d). *Global age-friendly cities: a guide.* Geneva, World Health Organization.

WHO (2007e). *Preventing injuries and violence: a guide for ministries of health.* Geneva, World Health Organization.

WHO (2008a). Monitoring of health-related Millennium Development Goals. EB 122/33. Executive Board, 122nd session, 22 January 2008. Agenda Item 4.14,.

WHO (2008b). *Eliminating female genital mutilation: an interagency statement.* Geneva, World Health Organization.

WHO (2008c). *Preventing violence and reducing its impact: how development agencies and governments can help.* Geneva, World Health Organization.

WHO (nd,a). *Cardiovascular diseases: what are cardiovascular diseases?* Geneva, World Health Organization. (**http://www. who.int/mediacentre/factsheets/fs317/en/index.html**, accessed 17 March 2008) (Factsheet No 317).

WHO (nd,b). *Management of substance abuse: alcohol.* Geneva, World Health Organization (**http://www.who.int/ substance_abuse/facts/alcohol/en/index.html**, accessed 15 March 2008).

WHO (nd,c). *Quick diabetes facts.* Geneva, World Health Organization (**http://www.who.int/diabetes/en/**, accessed 17 March 2008).

WHO (nd,d). *Child and adolescent health and development.* Geneva, World Health Organization (**http://www.who.int/ child-adolescent-health/integr.htm**, accessed 4 May 2008).

WHO & PHAC (2007). Improving health equity through intersectoral action. Geneva, World Health Organization and Public Health Agency of Canada Collaborative Project.

WHO & UNICEF (1978). *Declaration of Alma-Ata.* Geneva, World Health Organization. (**http://www.who.int/hpr/ NPH/docs/declaration_almaata.pdf**, accessed 28 May 2008).

WHO et al. (2007). *Maternal mortality in 2005: estimates developed by WHO, UNICEF, UNFPA and the World Bank.* Geneva, World Health Organization. (**http://www.who/ reproductive-health/publications/maternal mortality 2005/mme 2005.pdf**, accessed 16 July 2008).

WHO Healthy Cities (nd). Healthy Cities website. Copenhagen, World Health Organization (**http://www.euro. who.int/healthycities**, accessed April 10, 2008).

Wilkinson RG (1996). *Unhealthy societies: the affliction of inequality.* London, Routledge.

Williams K & Borins EF (1993). Gender bias in a peer-reviewed medical journal. *Journal of the American Medical Women's Association,* 48:160-162.

Wilthagen T, Tros F & van Lieshot H (2003). *Towards 'flexicurity': balancing flexicurity and security in EU member states.* Invited paper for the 113th World Congress of the International Industrial Relations Association, Berlin.

Wirth M et al. (2006). *Monitoring health equity in the MDGs: a practical guide.* New York; CIESIN and UNICEF.

Wismar M et al. (2007). *The effectiveness of health impact assessment: scope and limitations of supporting decision-making in Europe.* Copenhagen, European Observatory on Health Systems and Policies.

Women and Work Commission (2006). *Shaping a fairer future.* London, Government Equalities Office (**http://www. equalities.gov.uk/publications/wwc_shaping_fairer_ future06.pdf**, accessed 30 April 2008).

Wood A (2006). *IMF macroeconomic policies and health sector budgets.* Amsterdam: Wemos Foundation.

Woodward D (2005). The GATS and trade in health services: implications for health care in developing countries. *Review of International Political Economy,* 12:511-534.

Woodward D & Simms A (2006a). *Growth isn't working: the unbalanced distribution of benefits and costs from economic growth.* London, New Economics Foundation (**http:// www.neweconomics.org/NEF070625/NEF_ Registration070625add.aspx?returnurl=/gen/uploads/ hrfu5w555mzd3f55m2vqwty502022006112929.pdf**, accessed 5 May 2008).

Woodward D & Simms A (2006b). *Growth is failing the poor: the unbalanced distribution of the benefits and costs of global economic growth.* New York, United Nations (ST/ESA/2006/DWP/20), based on Woodward D & Simms A (2006a).

Woolf SH et al. (2004). The health impact of resolving racial disparities: an analysis of US mortality data. *American Journal of Public Health*, 94:2078-2081.

Woolf SH et al. (2007). Giving everyone the health of the educated: an examination of whether social change would save more lives than medical advances. *American Journal of Public Health*, 97:679-683.

World Bank (1997). Designing effective safety net programmes. *Poverty Lines*, 7:1-2. (**http://www.worldbank.org/html/ prdph/lsms/research/povline/pl_n07.pdf**, accessed 5 May 2008).

World Bank (1999). *Global development finance*. Washington, DC, World Bank.

World Bank (2006a). *Global monitoring report 2006*. Washington, DC, World Bank.

World Bank (2006b). *World development indicators, 2006*. Washington, DC, World Bank.

World Bank (2007). *Global economic prospects 2007*: managing the next wave of globalization. Washington, DC, World Bank.

World Bank (2008). *The world development report 2008 – agriculture for development*. Washington, DC, World Bank.

World Bank Independent Evaluation Group (2006). *Debt relief for the poorest: an evaluation update of the HIPC Initiative*. Washington, DC, World Bank.

World Commission on the Social Dimension of Globalization (2004). *A fair globalization: creating opportunities for all*. Geneva, International Labour Organization.

WorldWatch Institute (2007). *State of the world 2007: our urban future*. Washington DC, The WorldWatch Institute.

Xu K et al. (2007). Protecting households from catastrophic health spending. *Health Affairs*, 26:972-983.

YouGov Poll (2007). Commissioned by the Fabian Society. London, YOUGOV (**http://www.yougov.com/uk/ archives/pdf/fabian%20toplines.pdf**, accessed 20 March 2008).

Young ME (2002). Ensuring a fair start for all children: the case of Brazil. In: Young ME ed. *From early child development to human development: investing in our children's future*. Washington, DC, World Bank, pp. 123-142.

Yusuf S et al. (2001). Global burden of cardiovascular diseases. Part I: General considerations, the epidemiologic transition, risk factors, and impact of urbanization. *Circulation*, 104:2746-2753.

Zedillo E et al. (2001). *Recommendations of the High-level Panel on Financing for Development*. New York, United Nations (A/55/1000).

Ziersch A & Baum F (2004). Involvement in civil society groups: is it good for your health? *Journal of Epidemiology and Community Health*, 58:493-500.

Acronyms

ADB	Asian Development Bank
AFRO	African Regional Office (WHO)
CEDAW	Convention on the Elimination of All forms of Discrimination Against Women
CIDA	Canadian International Development Agency
CMH	Commission on Macroeconomics and Health
DAC	Development Assistance Committee
DAH	Development assistance for health
DALY	Disability-adjusted life year
DFID	Department for International Development
DHS	Demographic and Health Surveys
ECD	Early child development
ECDKN	Early Childhood Development Knowledge Network of the Commission on Social Determinants of Health
ECOSOC	Economic and Social Council
EMCONET	Employment Conditions Knowledge Network of the Commission on Social Determinants of Health
EMRO	Eastern Mediterranean Regional Office (WHO)
ESCAP	Economic and Social Commission for Asia and the Pacific
EU	European Union
EURO	European Regional Office (WHO)
FAO	Food and Agriculture Organization of the United Nations
FCTC	Framework Convention on Tobacco Control
FDI	Foreign direct investment
FGM	Female genital mutilation
G7/8	Group of Seven/Eight
GATS	General Agreement on Trade in Services
GATT	General Agreement on Tariffs and Trade
GBS	General budget support
GDP	Gross domestic product
GEGA	Global Equity Gauge Alliance
GHI	Global Health Initiative
GKN	Globalization Knowledge Network of the Commission on Social Determinants of Health
GNI	Gross national income
GNP	Gross national product
HALE	Health-adjusted life expectancy
HDI	Human Development Index
HEIA	Health Equity Impact Assessment
HIA	Health Impact Assessment
HIV/AIDS	Human immunodeficiency virus/auto-immune deficiency syndrome
HIPC	Highly Indebted Poor Country
HSKN	Health Systems Knowledge Network of the Commission on Social Determinants of Health
ISA	Intersectoral action
ILO	International Labour Organization
IMCI	Integrated Management of Childhood Illness
IMF	International Monetary Fund
IOM	International Organization for Migration
IPCC	Intergovernmental Panel on Climate Change
KN	Knowledge Network
KNUS	Knowledge Network on Urban Settings of the Commission on Social Determinants of Health
LEB	Life expectancy at birth
MEKN	Measurement and Evidence Knowledge Network of the Commission on Social Determinants of Health
MDGs	Millennium Development Goals
MTEF	Medium-Term Expenditure Framework
NGO	Nongovernmental organization
ODA	Official development assistance
OECD	Organisation for Economic Cooperation and Development
OHS	Occupational Health and Safety
PAHO	Pan-American Health Organization
PEPFAR	President's Emergency Plan for AIDS Relief
PHC	Primary Health Care
PPHCKN	Priority Public Health Conditions Knowledge Network of the Commission on Social Determinants of Health
PRSP	Poverty Reduction Strategy Paper

SCN	UN System Standing Committee on Nutrition
SAP	Structural Adjustment Programme
SDH	Social determinants of health
SEARO	South-East Asian Regional Office (WHO)
SEKN	Social Exclusion Knowledge Network of the Commission on Social Determinants of Health
SEWA	Self-Employed Women's Association
STI	Sexually transmitted infection
TRIPS	Trade-related Intellectual Property Rights
UN	United Nations
UNAIDS	Joint United Nations Programme on HIV/AIDS
UNCTAD	United Nations Conference on Trade and Development
UNDP	United Nations Development Programme
UNESCO	United Nations Educational, Scientific and Cultural Organization
UNFPA	United Nations Population Fund
UN-HABITAT	United Nations Human Settlements Programme
UNHCR	Office of the United Nations High Commissioner for Refugees
UNICEF	United Nations Children's Fund
UNSNA	UN System of National Accounts
UNRISD	United Nations Research Institute for Social Development
WFP	World Food Programme
WGEKN	Women and Gender Equity Knowledge Network of the Commission on Social Determinants of Health
WHO	World Health Organization
WPRO	Western Pacific Regional Office (WHO)
WTO	World Trade Organization

LIST OF BOXES, FIGURES, AND TABLES

Figures

Tables

Index

women's contribution in national accounts 150

gradient, social see social gradient in health

Greece 32

greenhouse gas emissions 60–62, 63, 66, 71

Guo, Yan 207

H

health
    returns from investing in 39
    right to 158, 165, 173, 174
    urban populations 62–63
    WHO definition 33

health and safety, occupational see occupational health and
         safety

Health and Safety Executive (HSE), UK 83

health care 94–106
    financing 8, 100–103, 104
    gender equity 97, 145, 146
    inequitable distribution 94
    private sector regulation 133–134
    public accountability 97
    regulation to ensure equity 139
    social determinants of health approach 116
    Tanahashi model 99
    targeted 99
    universal see universal health care

health-care systems 95
    civil registration and 179
    early child development role 50, 56
    role 27, 35

health equity 110–119
    coherent approach 10–11, 111–118
    as global goal 170, 171
    goals and targets 196–198
    mainstreaming 195
    as marker of societal progress 111–112
    milestones 198
    sectors and actors involved 110–111

health equity impact assessment 114–115
    building capacity 190–191
    economic agreements 135–136
    recommendations 206

health equity surveillance systems 180–185
    comprehensive 181–183
    global 184–185
    minimum 180–181
    national 180–183

    recommendations 206
    role of communities 183
    using data for policy-making 185

health expenditure 36

"Health for All" approach 33, 34

health gap, closing see closing the health gap in a generation

health impact assessment (HIA) 115, 136

health inequities 1, 26, 29–34
    causes and solutions 35–39
    between and within countries 29, 167–168
    feasibility of change 32–33
    global 167–168
    in health conditions 30
    measuring and understanding 20–21, 44, 206
    poorest of the poor 31–32
    social gradient 31
    structural drivers see structural drivers

health insurance 100–103, 116
    evaluation 186
    private, regulation 139
    social 102, 103

health literacy 189

Health Metrics Network 180, 181

health promotion 97, 116

health sector 117
    action within 116
    recommendations 204
    reform 95, 185
    representation in trade agreements 137–138
    stewardship role 111–112

health services, rural 70–71

health systems knowledge network (HSKN) 42

health workers 103–105
    aid for 105
    brain drain 35, 105, 106
    rural–urban distribution 103–104
    training 188

Healthy Cities movement 63, 111, 186, 196

healthy eating, promoting 66, 67–68

Healthy Settings approach 63

heart disease 35

Helsinki Process on Globalisation and Democracy 169

high-income countries
    development assistance 120
    domestic revenues 121
    inequity in health conditions 30